AMBULATORY CARE MANAGEMENT AND PRACTICE

Edited by

Albert E. Barnett, MD

Chief Executive Officer
Friendly Hills HealthCare Network
La Habra, California

Gloria Gilbert Mayer, RN, EdD, FAAN

Friendly Hills HealthCare Network
La Habra, California

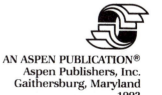

AN ASPEN PUBLICATION®
Aspen Publishers, Inc.
Gaithersburg, Maryland
1992

Library of Congress Cataloging-in-Publication Data

Barnett, Albert E.
Ambulatory care management and practice/Albert E. Barnett,
Gloria Gilbert Mayer.
p.   cm.
Includes bibliographical references and index.
ISBN: 0-8342-0313-8
1. Ambulatory medical care—Management.   I. Mayer, Gloria G.
II. Title.
[DNLM: 1. Ambulatory Care—organization & administration. WX 205
B261a]
RA974.B27   1992
610'.65—dc20
DNLM/DLC
for Library of Congress
91-47124
CIP

Aspen Publishers, Inc., grants permission for photocopying for limited personal or
internal use. This consent does not extend to other kinds of copying, such as copying
for general distribution, for advertising or promotional purposes, for creating new
collective works, or for resale. For information, address Aspen Publishers, Inc.,
Permissions Department, 200 Orchard Ridge Drive, Suite 200,
Gaithersburg, Maryland 20878.

Editorial Services: Ruth Bloom

Library of Congress Catalog Card Number: 91-47124
ISBN: 0-8342-0313-8

Printed in the United States of America

1 2 3 4 5

No matter how dramatically you think health care has changed in the last decade, now is the time before the revolution, year by year, the existing system is coming unstuck.

Paul Starr, professor of sociology at
Princeton University and author of
The Social Transformation of American Medicine

* * * *

There is a tide in the affairs of men, which, taken at the flood, leads on to fortune; Omitted, all the voyage of their life is bound in shallows and in miseries. On such a full sea are we now afloat, and, we must take the current when it serves, or lose our ventures.

Shakespeare

This book is dedicated to all those workers who strive to improve the quality and effectiveness of the nation's health care. Those studying health care will find excitement and gratification in their chosen field, which after thousands of years is still in its infancy.

Table of Contents

Contributors

Brad L. Armstrong, BS, MBA
Manager
The Warner Group
Woodland Hills, California

Albert E. Barnett, MD
CEO
Friendly Hills HealthCare Network
La Habra, California

Amy Bernard, RN, BSN, MS
Clinical Educator
Department of Education and Development
Patient Advisory Nurse
Carle Clinic Association
Champaign, Illinois

Helga Bonfils, BS, RN
Administrator
Home Health Resource Center, Inc.
La Habra, California

Nancy Parliman Brown, RN
Director of Education
Friendly Hills HealthCare Network
La Habra, California

Judith M. Bulau, MSN, PHN
Health Care Consultant
Minneapolis, Minnesota

Ann Casstevens, BS
Staff Development Coordinator
Department of Education and Development
Carle Clinic Association
Champaign, Illinois

Susan Cejka, CPA
President
Cejka & Company
St. Louis, Missouri

Loretta Crowell, RN, BS
Staff Development Coordinator
Department of Education and Development
Carle Clinic Association
Champaign, Illinois

Linda D'Angelo, RNC, MSN, MBA
Director of Patient Care
Carle Clinic Association
Adjunct Faculty
University of Illinois College of Medicine
University of Illinois College of Nursing
Champaign, Illinois

Steve Daily
Daily Planet Marketing & Corporate Communications
Santa Monica, California

Martin D. Goldberg, MS
Vice President
Organization Development
Imperial Bank
Inglewood, California

Sharon Guller, RN, PHN, MSN
Assistant Director of Professional Services
Home Health Resource Center, Inc.
La Habra, California

Nicolet A. Handy, RRA
Manager
Medical Records
Friendly Hills HealthCare Network
La Habra, California

Robert Hanna
Executive Director
Patient Services and Facilities
Friendly Hills HealthCare Network
La Habra, California

Shannon Hodges, MBA
Marketing Director
Nurse On Call
Mohomet, Illinois

Linda K. Jackson, BSN, MS
Director of Nursing
Friendly Hills HealthCare Network
La Habra, California

Judith Moore Johnson, BA, RN
Senior Consultant
Health Management Systems Associates
and
Nurse Specialist
Hennepin Faculty Associates
Minneapolis, Minnesota

Rebekah Jones, RN, BS, MEd
Conference Manager/Education Specialist
Department of Education and Development
Carle Clinic Association
Champaign, Illinois

Ellen Kaufman, MS
Consultant
William M. Mercer, Incorporated
San Francisco, California

Allan Korn, MD
Principal
William M. Mercer, Incorporated
Chicago, Illinois

Roger A. Krissman
Executive Director of Finance
Friendly Hills HealthCare Network
La Habra, California

Michael E. Kurtz, MS, AAHC
Organizational Psychologist
Herndon, Virginia

Edward Lipson, MD, MS
Principal
Ernst and Young
San Francisco, California

Mary Jo Littlefield
Director of Business Development
Friendly Hills HealthCare Network
La Habra, California

Meryl D. Luallin
Partner
Sullivan/Luallin
San Diego, California

Judy M. Marsh
Director of Human Resources
Friendly Hills HealthCare Network
La Habra, California

Sandra C. Matherly, RNC, FNP, MA
President
Nurse On Call
Mohomet, Illinois

Gloria Gilbert Mayer, RN, EdD, FAAN
Executive Director of Patient Care
    Management
Friendly Hills HealthCare Network
La Habra, California

Thomas Mayer, MD, MBA
Principal
William M. Mercer, Incorporated
Huntington Beach, California

Thomas P. McCabe, JD, MBA
Executive Counsel
Assistant to the CEO
Friendly Hills HealthCare Network
La Habra, California

Arnold Milstein, MD, MPH
Managing Director
William M. Mercer, Incorporated
Huntington Beach, California

David R. Morgan, BS, MA
Health Services Administrator
Friendly Hills HealthCare Network
La Habra, California

Robert A. Nelson, FACMGA
Executive Director
Harriman Jones Medical Group
Long Beach, California

Marjory A. O'Connor, RN, BS, CIC
Infection Control
Friendly Hills HealthCare Network
La Habra, California

Judy Pierson, MSN
President
The Pierson Company
Los Angeles, California

Susan Andrea Ritchie, LVN
Manager of Neighborhood Office
Friendly Hills HealthCare Network
La Habra, California

Noah D. Rosenberg, MSSW, JD
Rosenberg and Kaplan
Beverly Hills, California

Elan Rubinstein, Pharm D., MPH
E/B Rubinstein Associates
Canoga Park, California

Denise E. Stanton, BS
Supervisor for Nursing and Therapy Services
Home Health Resource Center, Inc.
La Habra, California

Annie Stoeckmann, RN, JD
Division Manager
HealthCare Professional Liability Division
Farmers Insurance Group of Companies
Los Angeles, California

Kevin W. Sullivan
Partner
Sullivan/Luallin
San Diego, California

Paul E. Terry, PhD
Vice President of Education
Park Nicollett Medical Foundation
Minneapolis, Minnesota

Todd A. Walike, MBA
The Warner Group
Woodland Hills, California

Michael L. Wiley
Director
Management Information Systems
Friendly Hills HealthCare Network
La Habra, California

Jeffrey V. Winston, MD
Department Chairman, Vision Services
Friendly Hills HealthCare Network
La Habra, California
and
Assistant Clinical Professor
Jules Stein Eye Institute
UCLA Medical Center
Los Angeles, California

Julie Yen, BA
Vice President
Commercial Loan Office
Imperial Bank
Inglewood, CA 90301

Introduction

The health care industry is currently changing as rapidly and comprehensively as any major industry in the United States. Whereas most people associate health care with hospitals and high technology, the vast majority of care is actually provided in ambulatory settings and involves routine, nonemergency health care services such as routine physical examinations, management of chronic diseases, and outpatient surgery. Therefore, patients generally access the health system via ambulatory care, and for many it is their only point of contact with that system.

In order to write a book dealing with a subject as dynamic as health care, a series of premises had to be made regarding the future of the ambulatory component. It was necessary to consider not only how ambulatory medicine is practiced today but also what ambulatory care encompasses and what it might encompass in the future. It was widely believed in the 1980s that medical care consisted of three major components: (1) outpatient providers, (2) the hospital industry, and (3) third-party payers (the insurance industry and government programs). But as the hospital industry fragments and as methods of payment become similarly decentralized, ambulatory care providers are increasingly playing a more dominant role in the provision of care.

A brief history of the American health care industry may be useful in trying to understand the course the industry is likely to take in the future. Although we may take current health practices largely for granted, many of the components of health care today are of very recent origin. Much has been written of the many forces impacting American health care at the present time, including the hospital industry, insurance plans, and government programs. But until recently, many of these forces either did not exist or were ineffective. The doctor-patient relationship, the traditional foundation of medical care, had remained relatively unaltered over two millennia. The generic term *provider* was unnecessary, because the physician was the generally accepted healer. Furthermore, the patient was essentially the only customer. Until recently, then, American medicine could easily trace its roots back to the time of Aesculapius.

Within this historical perspective, the hospital merits particular attention. Prior to the middle of the nineteenth century, there were not even any "ancillary services," much less hospitals as we know them. There were few trained nurses, prescription pharmacists, and technologists. Physicians generally filled all the necessary roles. If patients were not ambulatory, they were treated at home. American rural physicians often had back rooms where a seriously ill patient could be treated or observed. Medicine was not, of course, unique in this regard. In the early nineteenth century, almost all goods and services were provided or manufactured within a 20-mile radius of even the smallest population center.

However, wars act as catalysts for change, and the Civil War, no exception to the rule, spurred significant developments in health care. The need to standardize everything from uniforms to gun barrels to railroad gauges affected medicine as well. The appalling weaknesses of the medical establishment became apparent. Unable to cope with injury or disease on a large scale, medicine was propelled from its former lethargy into an increasingly dynamic mode, resulting in change and experimentation. It was in the decade after the war ended, when Sir William Osler began to tend the disabilities of veterans under the awnings at Blockley in Philadelphia, that the modern hospital was born.

At first, in the mid-nineteenth century, hospitals were closely affiliated with training programs and universities. They served the dual purpose of patient care and education of physicians and nurses. They usually started as charitable institutions such as almshouses, insane asylums, or places to segregate victims of contagious diseases.

The transformation of inpatient health care into a large-scale industry is very recent. Huge injections of capital during the early cost-plus years of Medicare accelerated the establishment of the hospital as a defined and profitable economic entity. Single hospitals merged into large profit-making chains. But soon the hand that had given began to take away. DRGs and other reductions in government and third-party payer reimbursements impaired hospital financial performance. Physicians and other entrepreneurs created profit-making entities such as imaging centers and surgicenters, using elements from the hospital's traditional spectrum of services. Many institutions, unable to adapt to this competitive environment, languished, struggled, and finally began to founder.

In short, the modern hospital does not enjoy a very long history as an institution. Its star burst within our lifetime, and we are now witnessing its waning. It seems unlikely to regain its luster.

The hospitals of the future may well service only a small segment of the population. They will be used mostly for severe illness or injury and for short periods of time. Like our ancestors, many of us will go through life without ever being an inpatient. Already, in many of the more progressive health care systems, those who are under age 65 are hospitalized at a rate of less than 200 days per thousand population. Given an average length of stay of 4 days, simple arithmetic affords proof that, on average, a person can expect to be hospitalized only once in 20 years. If normal childbirth is excluded as an inpatient "illness," the incidence of hospitalization is even lower. In comparison, the average individual seeks ambulatory health care four or five times a year. With the decline in inpatient utilization, the ambulatory arena can be expected to continue to grow in importance, both in terms of provision of health care and consumption of health care dollars. Although the hospital industry will always have a role to play, it can be expected to further fragment into tertiary care and teaching centers or to be dominated and controlled by the more powerful ambulatory care entities.

The payer sector has similarly experienced a very recent emergence and a mercurial rise. The decline of this sector as an independent entity is not yet so evident, but signs of ill health are emerging. In contrast to the hospital industry, government programs and private insurance companies are strongly buoyed by unlimited borrowing power on the one hand and tremendous resources on the other, yet they seem to focus more on cutting losses than on achieving substantial economic benefits from health care investments.

A brief look at what insurance companies and particularly the HMOs are paid for provides an interesting insight. The main function of any insurance company is to transfer risk from an individual to a strong organization with a broad membership base. Secondary functions include maintaining reserves, paying claims, marketing, and performing certain administrative duties. Therefore, if the insurance company does not shoulder risk, it becomes merely an administrator or sales agent. In the early years of the HMO movement, HMOs did fulfill this risk-taking function and were rightfully compensated. This is still the case with small groups and IPAs. But, again, as the better organized provider groups have achieved financial strength, they have become increasingly willing and able to take on the necessary risk themselves. This leaves HMOs with only marketing and administrative functions, which certainly do not justify huge rewards. In fact, many large provider medical groups, especially those with predominantly prepaid managed care practices, have preempted many of the claims-paying and marketing functions as well. Industrial leaders have already recognized this and are increasingly looking for ways to contract directly with provider groups, bypassing both the insurance industry and the hospital industry in the process.

We have thus, in a sense, come almost full circle. Over the centuries, individual physicians had been the dominant providers of medical care. Both the hospital and the insurance industry then arose to challenge that dominance. Finally, in the 1990s, physicians, especially in group practices, are reasserting their importance. These physicians, however, are quite different from their predecessors, since they have had to meet many new challenges and accommodate new types of customers.

There are many scenarios for the form that outpatient care might take in the future, but each reasonable scenario must include the concept of "managed care." We are committed to that as a basic assumption. And we have further assumed that the major payment methods of the future will be more akin to the prepayment methods used by HMOs than to any form of traditional fee-for-service payment. We have anticipated that the emerging provider entities will be dominated by medium to large medical groups, the strongest of which will be multispecialty in nature. These large multispecialty groups will differ vastly from current configurations. They will have sophisticated organizational structures and professional management. They will integrate all levels of care, including home health, inpatient, and preventive medicine.

The newer payment methods, with incentives for controlling costs, will also dictate massive changes in practice patterns. This will translate into new definitions for the various health care providers. The high cost of physician labor will limit the use of physicians to those areas requiring their unique skills and training. Nurses will achieve more prominence in the provision of care, and other nonphysician providers will assume increased responsibility and control. This may eventually limit the need for large numbers of new physicians, allowing a true team approach to health care to develop.

The editors and most of the authors of this book live and work in California, where these developments are no longer theoretical. However, we feel that in all parts of the country, no matter how seemingly distant in time from similar developments, events will move with increasing rapidity in the direction indicated above. In order to help smooth the change, we have attempted, in this book, to describe the dynamics of multispecialty groups comprising physicians, allied health professionals, nurses, technicians, and professional administrative staff, to analyze the characteristics that will contribute most to their success, and to predict those areas that are most likely to ensure their future prosperity.

Finally, we assume it is obvious to any reader that a work of this magnitude could not be accomplished without the help and support of many individuals. In particular, we wish to acknowledge Donna Espenhain and Joyce Hall for their time and effort and the partners of Friendly Hills Medical Group, who contributed their resources and moral support to this endeavor.

Albert E. Barnett, MD
Gloria Gilbert Mayer, RN, EdD, FAAN

Part I

Organization and Leadership

1

The Medical Organization

Albert E. Barnett

INTRODUCTION

In no human endeavor is the concept of teamwork more central than in the practice of health care. Teamwork is evident, for example, in the operating room, where the players not only are referred to as the "OR team" but even wear scrubsuits of the same style and color. Similarly, we talk of "team nursing" or the "cardiac resuscitation team" and cannot help but recognize the prevalence of collaborative effort. Indeed, the merging of highly specialized skills and individual egos into a functioning group is absolutely necessary for complex patient care to occur.

In discussing outpatient medical organizations, it is therefore essential to keep in mind the importance of teamwork. Although perhaps not as dramatic as teamwork in the OR, the management of the enormous number of patients treated in outpatient settings is the most significant element in maintaining and restoring health to the nation's population. Combining all the involved skills and technologies in a smooth, effective, and continuing effort is not an easy task. In a large multispecialty medical group, for example, employees may fall into as many as 200 different job categories. There is a physician hierarchy as well as an administrative hierarchy. And since 80 percent of the employees in any group practice are trained workers with at least some kind of credential, certification, or license, these employees will often have strong opinions regarding their value and function within the organizational matrix. Because of this, the major function of management is to organize these individuals into a cohesive unit. A health care organization requires an appropriate and workable matrix in order for this to happen.

There is no single or correct way to organize all the human and physical resources that come together in a health care enterprise. Probably no two medical practices are organized in precisely the same manner, and frequently there are significant differences in the nomenclature, duties, and responsibilities of the various positions. This is especially true in the case of large health care organizations.

Generally, in the past, the vast majority of medical organizations seemed to work, some better than others. But in the present intensely competitive environment, success is not as easily assured. Putting into place an effective and efficient organizational structure has therefore become essential for survival and continued growth.

This chapter addresses many of the organizational issues involved in outpatient medical practice and presents one of many workable systems.

ORGANIZATIONAL GOALS

The best type of structure for an organization is one based on the organization's goals. What are the goals of a medical organization? In many ways they are no different than the goals of most business enterprises. Furthermore, very small medical partnerships up to the largest multispecialty, vertically integrated medical practices share most of the same goals. In outpatient medicine, the organizational format should help the entity to accomplish the following goals, at the very least:

- successful pursuit of its chosen mission
- financial survival
- political survival
- provision of a matrix that enhances quality and productivity
- provision of a "playing field" that nurtures teamwork
- provision of a "playing field" that nurtures creativity and innovation

Pursuing the Organizational Mission

An established, well-considered mission and a strategy for pursuing it are necessary for the judicious allocation of any company's human and financial resources. They can also challenge and motivate the entire staff. Likewise, the mission that the company has committed itself to will be carefully scrutinized by potential lenders and joint venture partners. These players are vital to success and must be given careful consideration in the organizational plan. The mission of a company is generally manifested in three elements: the mission statement, the strategic plan, and the business plan.

The Mission Statement

In order for any organization to create its own identity, distinguish itself from similar enterprises, and motivate its staff effectively, it must first establish a sense of its own mission. The formal expanded mission statement or vision statement thus becomes the organization's constitution, or at least a constitutional preamble. The mission statement need not be lengthy, perhaps little more than a page or two, but it should clearly state in general terms what the organization perceives itself to be and what it intends to accomplish.

To create a meaningful mission statement, many issues must be thought through. For example, what is the product? Who are the customers? As mentioned previously, customers are usually no longer restricted to individual patients but include employers, health plans, the government, and the community in which the organization is located. Many good mission statements devote specific paragraphs to certain major areas such as finance, human resources, quality of care, and marketing.

The mission statement is designed for internal use. It is not a single statement or slogan of the type that might be used for outside marketing such as "We Light up the World" or "Better Living through Chemistry." An effective mission statement should have a certain permanence, but it is also dynamic. The external or internal environment will change, so from time to time the mission statement should be critically reviewed. However, the mission statement must always express the fundamental goals of the company—goals that are often lofty, not always achieved, but always pursued.

An effective mission statement should be collaborative, since it requires the efforts of all members of the organization. Both physician representatives and upper levels of management should participate in its creation under the direction of the chief executive officer (CEO) or physician leader. The completed statement should be distributed to all physicians and managers at all levels at the very least.

The Strategic Plan

Using the principles of the mission statement, the organization should develop and adopt a strategic plan. If the mission statement describes what the company wants to be and where it wants to go, the strategic plan outlines how to get there. It is a much more comprehensive document, far more researched and detailed. Some strategic plans are created by outside consultants, and others are created internally by those who have the necessary skills and the necessary time. (See Chapter 2 for a description of the strategic planning process.)

The Business Plan

The business plan converts the contents of the strategic plan into a specific blueprint for action. It indicates time frames, establishes annual budgets for operations and capital expenditures, and refines the more general forecasts of the strategic plan into specific needs. For example, the strategic plan might forecast a shortage of laboratory technologists and the corresponding need to increase recruitment efforts. The business plan would then present the numbers needed, the expected costs for salary and for recruitment and retention, and possible sources for the money.

In developing a meaningful business plan, a small or medium-sized organization that does not employ an experienced chief financial officer might find it helpful to follow a template suggested by the organization's accountant or by a prospective lender. Each lender usually desires a format that fits well with the needs of its loan committee.

Thus, the business plan, while very valuable internally as a resource management tool, is also an important link to the outside financial community. In addition, it completes and gives substance to the organizational goals.

Ensuring Financial Survival

Evident as it might seem, financial survival should nevertheless be forthrightly stated as the most important goal of any business enterprise. Obviously no mission or plan can proceed after the bankruptcy or death of the company. Following are some of the issues that must be considered in attempting to achieve financial viability:

- structure (corporation vs. partnership)
- retained earnings
- financing for growth
- credibility

Structure

There is no one ideal business structure for an outpatient medical practice. Besides the various needs and backgrounds of the individuals involved, state laws differ greatly regarding the corporate practice of medicine and other matters. Appropriate legal counsel is a necessity in dealing with these issues. However, there are some generalizations that can be made.

Incorporation is generally desirable inasmuch as it provides an accepted format. Corporate accounting is a template easily recognized by lenders, potential joint venture candidates, and vendors. A partnership, on the other hand, is generally the most effective vehicle for reducing individual tax liability, since it allows direct write-off of certain expenses and eliminates risk of double taxation. Furthermore, most physicians today are already organized financially as individuals, since many of the previously available advantages of professional corporations have been systematically eliminated. Converting from a corporation to a partnership mode can have severe financial consequences for an individual and should be done only after professional advice has been sought. Additionally, some partnerships have become so corporatelike that they risk being treated as corporations by the federal government, with potential adverse consequences. Is there an ideal format? Many factors must be considered, many of which should already have been addressed in the preceding section. There are very large legal and accounting firms that are partnerships and others that have incorporated and the same is true in the case of medical practices.

Retained Earnings

It may seem strange to single out retained earnings as an organizational financial goal, but its importance cannot be overemphasized. Individual physician practices and small partnerships almost universally withdraw all earnings on an ongoing basis. No one wants to be taxed on cash left undistributed in the bank account, and even as the organization grows larger, the partners rationalize their needs so as to justify withdrawing all cash available for distribution. It has been suggested that part of the physician psyche is to seek immediate gratification, just as surgeons like to see immediately the results of their interventions. But whatever the reason, few individual practitioners and no large group practices can survive this behavior.

The discipline imposed on medical professionals by their financial partners increasingly dictates how they handle business. Much has been written (including many complaints) in medical circles regarding onerous regulations imposed by various state and federal government agencies as well as those imposed by medicolegal considerations. But the discipline imposed by today's financial marketplace is equally stringent and is neglected at great peril. Virtually every lender has covenants requiring the orderly building of net equity that can only be accomplished by a systematic retention of earnings, and this necessity must be clearly understood by the entire organization and scrupulously budgeted as a first priority. The maturity of an organization and the prognosis for its success as a growth company can be assessed by its accomplishment in retaining earnings. The plan of organization must provide the leadership with sufficient strength to ensure retention of earnings.

The Foundation Model

Although not applicable to the large majority of ambulatory practices, mention should at least be made of the medical foundation model of medical group organization. This complex model, utilized in various formats by the nation's largest group practices (including the Mayo, Ochsner, Cleveland, Scripps, and Palo Alto clinics), solves many of the problems alluded to in this section. In this model, the medical group or professional corporation sells or otherwise transfers its assets (often with the aid of a tax-exempt bond issue) to a foundation. The newly created foundation then becomes the care provider and contracts with the medical group for provision of that care. Political permanence is established through the structure of the foundation's board of trustees. The foundation can access tax-exempt debt, and it can also minimize tax burdens for the physician group, since the foundation cannot be taxed on retained earnings. Selling to the foundation allows a group to escape the problem of unfunded buy-outs of senior partners and it mitigates the problem of expensive buy-ins of prospective new partners.

The medical foundation model exists in many variations, but basically it can be differentiated into the more autonomous, free-standing form and the health system or hospital-affiliated form. In any case, this model should be considered as an option only by the largest group practices, since conversion is intricate and expensive and is heavily controlled by state and federal statutes and regulations. Medical foundations, for example, must demonstrate a genuine community charitable purpose that also includes teaching and research. The foundation model is mentioned here only for the sake of completeness. Although medical foundations are highly visible, most local markets contain no integrated medical groups capable of making the transition.

Financing for Growth

The intense competition in the medical arena leaves little room for an organization merely to exist. The adage "grow or die" has much relevance in the health care industry. The growth of managed care itself has dictated massive growth in provider organizations. In most cases, financing this growth has remained the province of these organizations instead of being provided by the insurance companies. In order to ensure financial survival, medical organizations must organize for and secure financing for this growth.

The importance of securing lenders to aid in needed capital formation has already been touched upon. As noted, a viable business plan and a rigid policy of retaining earnings are requisites. Even so, many lenders are concerned about health care financing. They point to the desperate straits of many hospitals, the red ink and bankruptcies in health plans, and the many individual physicians who have lately proved to be poor financial risks. The large multispecialty group practices, which have generally been blessed with financial success, are to a great extent invisible to lenders, since they are not publicly held corporations with published balance sheets. Furthermore, the successful practices, those with rapid growth characteristics and in need of the greatest financial support, often are involved in providing health care for HMOs and other forms of prepaid managed care. This is unfamiliar territory for the always conservative lender, since it does not involve accounts receivable, the traditional bastion of a lender's security. The evaluation of contracts, the accounting of Incurred but Not Received Obligations (IBNRs), and the inverse relationship of hospital census and number of office visits to the bottom line tend to make most loan committees feel uncomfortable.

Therefore, the medical organization must take into account these financing difficulties and structure itself so as to be as easily scrutinized and evaluated by prospective lenders as possible. Anything complex or arcane, added to the other difficulties lenders have in evaluating medical enterprises, might be viewed as an attempt to mask some piece of unpleasant financial information.

In this discussion of the need to organize so as to present the best face to the financial community, it would be remiss not to mention the necessity for cooperative banking relationships. Besides its ability to offer lines of credit and cash management, a good bank will provide considerable assistance in negotiations with outside lenders and in evaluations of outside opportunities. An organization should select a bank on the basis of its officers' knowledge of and experience in health care. The bank should be large enough to accommodate reasonable forecasts for future growth, yet small enough to regard the health care organization as a valuable customer. The interested banker, as an outside expert, can often be helpful in supporting necessary financial stringency (see Chapter 15).

Financial Credibility

Often overlooked in the internal arena of organizational politics is the value of appearing credible to the financial community. Such credibility is not important just for getting loans but also for obtaining contracts from health plans and buying and leasing equipment. It is surprising how many medical groups and small partnerships allow wrenching political and organizational changes to occur without giving any thought to the possible effects on their financial support framework.

How is credibility established and enhanced by a medical practice? Creating and adhering to financial plans, such as the business plan, is one important means of achieving financial credibility. Therefore, the planning must be done well, growth must be forecast realistically, and the strengths and weaknesses of the organization must be accurately portrayed.

Tied in with financial planning is the need to create and adhere to budgets. Budgeting in small medical organizations has not been universally practiced. It has always been a difficult exercise to do well, and in the old days any budget deficits could easily be corrected by raising fees or working a few extra hours. Today, of course, medical practices are caught between rising costs on the one hand and smaller annual capitation and Medicare increases on the other. For many physicians, working additional hours has ceased to be an option. Operational budgets are now a fact of life for successful medical enterprises, and for growing practices, capital budgets are equally necessary. Budgeting should be looked upon not only as a way of internally controlling the company's finances but as a means of establishing financial credibility.

Any health care organization that has gone into the financial marketplace and secured lending has not solved all its problems. Accompanying a lender's dollars is an abundance of small print setting out the financial covenants. It is important that these covenants, which involve various ratios, net equity gains, and other financial constraints, are carefully adhered to. By neglecting them, the borrower runs the risk of adverse financial statements and a stringent restructuring of the loan. Again, before signing loan documents, the covenants should be scrutinized and negotiated with the help of the organization's accountant and banker. Timely payments on loans are not sufficient to ensure credibility if the associated financial covenants are not met.

Finally, it is necessary to emphasize the value of personal relationships, which must be structured into the organizational framework from the outset. The chosen leadership must be viewed by all outsiders as honest, fair, and stable. It must be seen as flexible and dynamic, yet prudent and disciplined. Because credibility and personal relationships are so important to the success of a practice, good leadership should be structured for the long term. Any change will be viewed negatively by outsiders, especially lenders, and the new leadership will require months and years to prove itself. Of course, mediocrity should not be enshrined, but a good management team should not be replaced simply because partner distributions decline for a year or because someone else would "like a turn."

In the past, most outpatient medical groups have not needed to pay much attention to their financial appearance when creating their organizational framework. Today any group that aspires to be something beyond a "medical boutique" ignores these issues at its peril.

Ensuring Political Survival

Political considerations are as important as financial considerations in a medical organization. They are also always extremely complex. Most medical groups that fail to survive self-destruct over political issues, not because of financial reverses. Listed here are several common political issues, which are discussed in the following pages and later in this chapter:

- medical staff–lay leadership relations
- the need for strong leadership
- the need for consensus
- leadership issues
- organizational issues

Medical Staff–Lay Leadership Relations

Probably unique to outpatient medical groups is the dual hierarchy consisting of a physician staff, often owners, on the one hand and a lay administrative team on the other. This creates the knotty problem of two organizations within one, which often leads to disruption. Furthermore, whereas few lay medical managers aspire to become physicians, it seems many physicians covet the authority associated with administrative positions. Some physicians have the interest, aptitude, training, and experience to be effective executives. Most do not. To ensure success, physicians must suppress their desires to administrate and instead try to understand and be supportive of the lay administrative team.

Since most medical practices are physician owned, the chairperson of the board is a physician (or the executive committee members are physicians, as the case may be), whereas the CEO or administrator usually is not. To be successful then, the physician leader and the lay CEO must have a smooth and collaborative relationship. Unless they are mutually supportive, each will risk demotion or dismissal, since the partners or stockholders will strive to affix blame. As noted above, change in leadership, even if perceived appropriately by the group, is almost always viewed negatively by the outside community. In fact, changes in the top-level nonphysician administration are often viewed far more negatively than changes in the physician leadership. Therefore, it is essential to search carefully and choose wisely when selecting candidates for both positions. Once the selection is accomplished, the best advice is to allow the administration to manage and the physicians to practice medicine (which often is more easily said than done).

Cohesion between the lay administrators and the physicians is partly the responsibility of the medical director. The position requires strength, hard work, intelligence, and fairness, and the ideal candidate is not the benign elderly physician who has befriended everyone in the organization (see Chapter 4). If an appropriate synergistic relationship is able to be achieved between the chairperson of the board, the CEO, and the medical director, this would represent an enormous organizational resource. If two of the positions could be successfully combined, management would be even further enhanced.

A few words might be said about the practice of training physicians for administrative roles. Some large organizations have made a commitment to provide such training. In our experience, the demands of the administrative and managerial roles have become so specialized that few physicians have the time or aptitude to become competent in them. Employee relations, quality assurance, management information systems, finance, and so on, require much formal training or many years of experience before proficiency is attained. People skills, problem-solving skills, and group skills seem better areas for physician training.

Need for Strong Leadership

As mentioned in the preceding section, a medical director should be a strong individual. Similarly, strength and stamina are needed by the two other members of the triumvirate: the chairperson of the board and the CEO. All three individuals must be able to pursue company goals despite the myriad "housekeeping" chores that arise daily, to move the group forward with consistency and ingenuity, to stand firm on agreed principles, and to adhere to unpopular stances if convinced of their correctness.

It is easier to fill these positions if one or more of the physicians are partner-owners, and even easier if they are founders of the organization. Any organization is fortunate if it has a strong owner-founder capable of filling one or more of these vital roles, since that individual would usually be less susceptible to the political stresses and strains.

Need for Consensus

Equally important, and intimately related to the need for strong leadership, is the need for a strong consensus within the ownership. The majority of medical groups appear to lack such a consensus, and they frequently degenerate into squabbling factions that presage organizational demise. A leader who cannot depend on a consensus cannot achieve the flexibility and quickness of response to problems that characterize the successful health care provider group.

The means of building consensus, which are well known, include the following:

- broadening the base of organizational ownership
- sharing and communicating company goals to all members
- expanding leadership responsibilities and empowerments
- broadening the base of physical ownership of real property and equipment
- maintaining a policy of fairness and honesty with respect to all group members
- facilitating free and open communication among the leadership and all group members

Although all of these strategies are obvious and are mentioned in many basic management texts, they are frequently not followed, sometimes because of perceived time constraints, sometimes simply because of greed. Broadening the base of ownership, for example, is much easier said than done. Bringing in new owners or increasing the shares of certain existing owners results in a decrease in the percentage of profits received by some of those already "in the club." Charging prospective members for their shares often makes it too costly for them, and it can also have adverse tax consequences for the existing owners. Nevertheless, groups that have successfully achieved longevity generally have found a way to allow others to achieve the incentive that comes with ownership. Without at least opportunities for ownership, a serious lack of incentive, participation, and motivation will almost certainly occur.

Of course, one way out of the ownership dilemma is to stimulate nonowners to buy emotionally into the goals and successes of the company. This also circumvents a difficulty that exists in many states: the legal barring of certain allied health care professionals (e.g., podiatrists and psychologists) and key nonphysician managers from becoming owners. An emotional or motivational buy-in can be accomplished by sharing such things as problem resolution and rewards and by providing empowerment and job security.

As difficult as it is to broaden ownership in the organizational entity, it is even more challenging to broaden ownership of real property. Many groups have real estate partnerships that become relatively narrow-based as the groups grow in size. The narrowness of such a partnership can be a source of rancor and hostility. For the restricted set of owners to give up a privileged financial position for the benefit of the larger organization is difficult, but this often becomes necessary in order to build the strong consensus needed for overall success. Making real property ownership broadbased and available even to lay administrators is in fact one of the most important building blocks for a strong group practice.

Perceptions of fairness are also important with regard to compensation. The range of compensation in a multispeciality group with a large prepaid component is generally quite compressed compared with the range for individuals in like specialties in the fee-for-service sector. Since all members share in building and marketing the group practice, the generally higher-priced specialists are more dependent on the primary care physicians and on the organization as a whole for their success. The specialist, therefore, cannot generally be compensated at the same level as his solo fee-for-service counterpart, unless the organization as a whole is unusually productive. To establish and maintain a strong consensus for action in the group setting, compensation issues must be addressed from the beginning of the relationship, and unrealistic compensation expectations need to be deflated (see Chapter 6).

Finally, under the heading of consensus, a few words are necessary regarding "productivity." The concept of productivity in medical practice is undergoing rapid redefinition. Some change is inherent in the switch to the Resource Based Relative Value System (RBRVS) payment schedules, with their greater emphasis on cognitive elements than on surgical procedures. But a much more marked and basic redefinition of productivity is entailed by the switch from a fee-for-service to a prepaid form of practice. Productivity in a group with prepaying enrollees must be evaluated on the basis of volume and efficiency, with the denominator being the number of enrollees and the numerator being the group's (or individual physician's) total cost of care. Using this definition, procedures, studies, and time-consuming consults, necessary as they may be, are simply cost factors. Physicians also represent costs, and the primary care physician who can give service to the largest number of patients while maintaining high standards of quality becomes the most valued performer. Therefore, fairness again dictates that specialists decline in value relative to high-volume, patient-moving primary care physicians. Achievement of a consensus demands that these and other concepts be clearly understood and bought into—and not only by the leadership but by all the physicians.

Leadership Issues

Leadership in a medical group must be based on credibility, fairness, and a strong consensus of support. Upon these building blocks are added all the other desirable characteristics of leadership. A complete list would include the following:

- intelligence
- experience
- the ability to attract and retain competent staff members
- the ability to develop and maintain relationships with leaders of outside organizations
- good communication skills
- political awareness
- the ability to build an organization
- the ability to manage effectively
- stamina
- the willingness, in the case of a physician, to give up the active practice of medicine

An additional desirable characteristic for anyone attempting to lead a large number of physicians is, as one medical group administrator once remarked, the ability to "herd cats."

Even a leader who possesses the above characteristics must address the major issues outlined previously in this section early in the organization's evolution so that the leadership can proceed with the confidence that only a strong consensus can provide. Each organization will differ as to how the leadership is established, how the authority and the responsibilities are divided, and whether physicians or nonphysicians are utilized in the various positions.

Terms of Office. Terms of office and compensation are major issues that should be dealt with early in the organization's development. The short "life expectancy" of hospital CEOs is symptomatic of an industry under severe financial duress. Short terms of office in any industry make it more likely that short-term solutions and quick fixes will be relied upon and less likely that an orderly pursuit of long-term goals will occur. It is not ideal to undergo frequent changes in leadership in any organization, but this is especially true in outpatient medicine. The structural complexity of medical organizations, the need for teamwork, the many interactions among staff and other professionals, and the many important outside relationships make leadership change difficult and very costly. For these reasons, short terms of office should not be specified for key leadership positions. Performance evaluations of leadership should consider the time frames needed to address the many and difficult problems faced by any medical group.

One of the ways that some organizations build the necessary length of office terms into their structures is by requiring "supermajorities." If a two-thirds or even three-fourths majority is needed to replace key leaders, upheavals by small majorities at critical times can be prevented. Is this compatible with our concept of democratic process? The answer, of course, is no. But few companies achieve success in an entrepreneurial setting by following a fully democratic format. Good results are achieved by good leaders and managers with the expertise and the time to solve problems.

What then should the term of office be for a CEO or medical director in a medical group? There is so much to learn and the field moves so fast that probably the longer in office, the more effective the leader becomes. Gaining the necessary on-the-job experience, receiving the necessary outside training, and building a competent management team takes years. A term of at least four years, with ample opportunity to continue in office for another term, would appear to be the minimum.

Compensation. Compensation for the leadership positions often brings to light a mindset that most physicians possess. They are trained to regard direct patient care as the most important product of a medical organization and therefore deserving of the highest reward. In the fee-for-service mode especially, they equate financial productivity solely with their own efforts, a view reinforced by the fact that all payments and checks are made out directly to the physicians.

Additionally, physicians and nurses tend to feel that they alone are patient advocates, the controllers of quality, the human link between life and death, sickness and health. Given this bias, conditioned by many years of training and reinforced by innumerable patient encounters, their opinion of administrators is understandable. Instead of seeing administrators as patient advocates as well, but at a more cosmic level, they tend to see administrative management simply as "overhead," as a cost of doing business, like rent or utilities. The situation is compounded if the group practice consists of individuals who have previously practiced independently, since they tend to look back on the success they were able to achieve without having had much knowledge of management or without having devoted much time to it.

For these reasons, no matter how large the medical group nor how successful, it is very difficult for leadership to command salaries commensurate with those in other industries of like size. Despite the knowledge and sophistication now required in order to provide competent professional management, it is the rare group of physicians that willingly give management its just financial reward. And it is for this reason that many potential leaders, both lay and physician, take jobs with insurance companies or seek other related business opportunities.

Among the factors that should be considered by group members in establishing compensation for executive positions is that, in larger groups at least, these are full-time positions. Thus a physician, after serving a term of office as a medical director or CEO, could find it very difficult to return to the practice of clinical medicine and is often precluded from that option entirely. The executive's salary should reflect this fact. Similarly, the time needed to devote to management, if the job is to be done correctly, generally exceeds the time devoted to the practice of medicine by any other individual physician. Finally, as the group grows larger, the management of the group increases in complexity, whereas the practicing physician is largely unaffected by the growth in size. For all these reasons, physicians in management, and lay managers as well, should be regarded as very vital members of the health care team and should be rewarded accordingly.

Today, in larger groups, the physician executive, promoted by organizations such as the College of Physician Executives, is gaining increasingly in status. It is apparent that in the present complex environment good medical management is a very important resource. Similarly, there are an increasing number of programs at university level that are specializing in ambulatory health care rather than traditional hospital administration. It is beginning to be appreciated that, in order to retain competent individuals in leadership roles in outpatient health care, compensation must be brought to the level of the most highly paid medical professionals in a medical organization. There are few industries that are more in need of attracting effective leaders and managers. Hopefully, those preparing for careers in ambulatory care management in the future will benefit from these trends.

Organizational Issues

The Executive Committee. In a small ambulatory care medical group, the leader or administrator generally derives his or her authority from all the physician owners collectively. But as the group grows in size, a point is reached where it is impractical to convene the entire membership on all issues of importance. This problem is usually solved, as in most businesses, by the insertion of an executive committee or board of directors between the partners or shareholders and the CEO or chairperson. Since in most states only physicians can be owners of medical groups, executive committees are almost always composed of physicians, although lay managers usually attend meetings and are allowed various degrees of input. Again, it is not surprising in the light of the usual physician bias against administration that lay managers generally are deprived of any vote.

Careful consideration should be given to the size of the executive committee. As in the case of most committees, the smaller, the better; the ideal size is perhaps five voting members, with a maximum of seven. Since most physicians feel they have the necessary qualifications to be effective committee members and wish to participate in group affairs, it is often difficult to restrict membership to a small number. Yet the larger the number of participants, the longer the meetings become and the fewer the matters that reach conclusion.

The political climate of the group also insinuates itself into the executive committee. The committee generally becomes a microcosm of the entire group— and not surprisingly, since committee members are voted into office by group members and require their support. Once elected, however, committee members should act for the benefit of the whole organization and not as representatives of factions within the organization. If the number of members is kept small, not everyone's interests will be directly represented. In a multispecialty group, not only are there the various specialties, but there are also various levels of ownership, various age cohorts, and various degrees of financial need. Committee members should remember that their duty is to support the mission statement and ensure the continuity of the organization, not to curry favors for their individual coteries.

The question frequently arises as to whether committee members should receive cash compensation for performing their duties. In order to make an effective and intelligent contribution, committee members have the responsibility to be informed on the matters brought before them. This often requires considerable outside reading and research and sometimes attendance at seminars and retreats. Also, in most medical groups, unlike most large publicly held corporations, executive committees do more than just provide direction. Medical group executive committees are often involved with and take responsibility for relatively minor issues of a financial or operational nature. They generally meet at least monthly, and many of them meet weekly. For these reasons it is often held that a financial stipend is appropriate for members of these committees. However, if paid to be on the executive committee, members should not receive additional compensation for serving in other administrative positions such as directorships, in order to avoid appearing self-serving.

In some medical groups the CEO and the medical director are elected by the executive committee, whereas in other groups these officials are elected by the entire set of shareholders or partners. In some groups the medical director is not a voting member of the executive committee. But no matter what the particular format, it is absolutely essential that there exist a close relationship and good communication among these various leadership elements. The consensus necessary for effective management can be easily damaged by any perceived infighting among the principals.

As a group grows larger, especially if it acquires its own health plan or inpatient facilities or becomes involved in other vertically integrated functions, it may find itself transformed into a major health care company. In order to compete at this level, the organization must fill the administrative positions with the most qualified individuals. The role played by trained and effective lay managers increases in this scenario, and in order to retain these managers, they too must be given the opportunity to obtain equity as part of their compensation package and to have a say regarding company policy. They should even be given voting seats on the executive committee. This kind of empowerment is difficult for many physicians to accept, since it threatens their own power in the organization.

Providing a Matrix That Enhances Quality and Productivity

The structure of an ambulatory care organization must enhance productivity and quality of care. For important as financial and political issues are in a group practice, they primarily concern only the physician component. The other 80 percent or 90 percent of employees must also work together smoothly and productively. In short, good solid management of the nonphysician staff is essential as well.

One of the first questions that needs to be answered is how to get quality managers. Should outsiders be hired on the basis of their academic qualifications and experience in outside organizations? Or should there be a well-established career track for people within the organization to move "up through the ranks"? Certainly outsiders with proven credentials and experience can contribute expertise and new ideas. On the other hand, people advanced from within, on the basis of their loyalty to the company as well as their expertise, can provide a very high degree of motivation to their fellow employees.

Most successful organizations take pride in their uniqueness and in their special complexities. Outsiders hired for management positions must cope with a certain degree of prejudice against newcomers and must prove themselves to a skeptical peer group. As already noted, medical groups are very intricate and variable enterprises, with their own singular cultures, politics, and organizational and technical systems. It may take an outsider months, maybe even years, to become an accepted and fully productive member of the management team. No amount of credentials can clear away all of the hurdles.

But before deciding that "up through the ranks" is the better approach, consider a significant fact regarding most medical organizations: The great majority of employees are "knowledge workers," that is, they have a vast amount of technical training in areas such as nursing, various technologies, and data processing. Although these employees are highly intelligent and may excel in their particular field, they are not usually prepared for, or even interested in, a management role. Those who enjoy teaching often make good supervisors, but they frequently fail in middle management positions. Motivation, ambition, and technical skills often mask a serious lack of management ability.

There is, however, a solution to the dilemma: education. No doubt, excellent people from the outside should be hired when available to inject new perspectives, insight, and expertise, especially in the case of upper-level management positions. But most of the middle management positions can be filled by current employees if the proper educational support is provided. Although many medium and large medical groups have management training programs, these programs are generally focused on people skills, problem solving, and communication. These are undoubtedly important areas for the middle manager. But the competition no longer allows the luxury of stopping there. Before an employee moves into management, there should be a testing of the employee's aptitude and a demonstration of a certain level of verbal and mathematical ability. Then there should be ongoing cycles of college-level business courses to provide skills helpful in producing meaningful reports, doing basic accounting, and performing other administrative duties. The management education process can either occur in house or be provided through arrangements with a convenient college or university. With a good selection process and with continuing educational support, most medical groups should be able to meet their middle management needs without having to hire many outsiders.

There are several other general issues that must be considered. Most ambulatory organizations do not have the luxury of sitting down and perfecting a design. They often grow rapidly and increase within a few years from a few doctors and a dozen employees to a staff of hundreds. During these periods of rapid growth, situations arise that require the isolation and establishment of one management function or another. At times, many responsibilities may be held by a single person, then later separated to form the substance of several distinct positions.

Also, during an accelerated growth phase, the organizational chart is frequently redesigned in accordance with the talents of the people on board. For example, the original office manager may serve as controller and purchaser of supplies. The nurse with the longest tenure may become "head nurse" and do most of the hiring and termination of employees. With the maturity of the organization, these roles may eventually be taken over by a chief financial officer, a purchasing officer, a director of nursing, and a director of human resources. As a result, there are probably no two medical groups that are organized exactly the same, even at a similar stage of development.

Nevertheless, there are certain specific areas of management that must be adequately dealt with in order for a medical group to survive and flourish. These key areas include the following, which are not presented in order of importance:

- top-level management
- patient care management
- operations
- finance
- quality assurance
- risk management
- medical and surgical utilization review
- peer review
- medical records
- legal matters and contracting
- management information systems
- marketing
- recruitment and retention of professional staff
- human resources
- prepaid management
- education and training

Top-Level Management

As in any company, the CEO of a medical group must be accountable for the functioning of the entire organization, including the physician component. Because departments often attempt to contain problems within lower levels of management, it is important that there be as few levels of management as possible separating the CEO from the grass roots of the organization. Ideally, the CEO should be visible and accessible to all staff members and physically located so as to facilitate interaction with all top managers, particularly the medical director. In fact, the most vital interaction in the medical group is between the CEO and medical director. They must communicate many times a day on a variety of issues common to both medical and lay staff, and each must be fully informed on all issues of importance. Few groups can survive (and fewer CEOs and medical directors) if this relationship is ever seriously impaired.

Patient Care Management

Although patient care management directly involves physicians and nurses, it would be a mistake to single out these two groups as separate management entities. Ambulatory medicine is a team effort, and patient care should be managed as a whole (with physicians allowed some autonomy under the medical director). The patient care director should have executive status and should possess a strong goal orientation, much experience, good operational skills, and the ability to be flexible and innovative. Although in most groups the patient care manager is a nurse, this is certainly not necessary, and it can even be demoralizing for nonnursing staff members, who may perceive nursing as particularly favored.

Operations

In most medical groups, operations is not assigned as the responsibility of a single person or department. Instead, operational tasks of various kinds are performed by most of the departments. Yet operations is an area where many groups show weakness. Since most groups start with physicians and are directed by physicians, this is not surprising. Physicians are not generally observant of the operational details of their offices. And even within the staffs of large groups, it is rare to find individuals who are oriented to such details. Although virtually all areas benefit from a solid operational approach, it is most important with regard to nursing and nonprofessional staff. Operations also includes such areas as ancillary services and facilities management. Good operations people are not only adept at problem solving, but must also be talented in creating and implementing new programs and systems.

Finance

A chief financial officer is usually responsible for accounting, payroll, billing, and purchasing as well as budgeting and other financial controls. One of the officer's significant duties is to keep the leadership informed about the financial condition of the company on a regular basis and to interact with the outside accountants in the process of providing financial advice and direction. The chief financial officer is, of course, intimately involved with ensuring financial survival, as discussed earlier in this chapter.

Quality Assurance

Ensuring quality in today's marketplace for medical services virtually amounts to ensuring success. The value of quality to health care customers is constantly increasing. Both quality as perceived by patients and quality as defined by the various third-party payers and attested to by accreditation are important. And if a synergy indeed exists between quality and cost containment, ensuring that quality becomes even more vital to the successful enterprise. (For more on quality assurance, see Chapter 21.)

Risk Management

The person in charge of risk management is responsible for medicolegal matters, risk avoidance programs, and credentialing physicians and other professionals. Given the current medicolegal climate, even small groups must have someone who is delegated these duties. (See Chapter 12 for further discussion of risk management.)

Medical and Surgical Utilization Review

Only small fee-for-service practices in certain geographic areas can avoid setting up a management structure for utilization review. In a larger group with a significant prepaid enrollment, the administration of utilization review programs can make or break the company. If the group includes a pharmacy, drug formulary compliance would also be included in utilization review. (See Chapters 18 and 22 for further discussion of utilization review.)

Peer Review

The peer review function is mandated by many payers today, including the federal government. Although generally considered part of the medical director's responsibility, it nevertheless needs administrative support and a formalized process for its implementation.

Medical Records

Medical records management is intimately involved with quality assurance, risk management, peer review, patient care management, and management information systems and other areas of administration (see Chapter 20).

Legal Matters and Contracting

In a group with tens of thousands of managed care patients enrolled, the legal and contracting function will significantly affect the financial health of the company. The person in charge of this function must interact with payers, outside contracted providers, and in-house professionals. This individual would also be involved with joint ventures, leases, and other contractual arrangements. An in-house executive counsel experienced in these matters can be invaluable. Help with these concerns can sometimes also be obtained from associations such as the Unified Medical Group Association. (See Chapters 9 and 10 for further discussion of contracting.)

Management Information Systems

The need for a management information system (MIS) in a medical group increases dramatically as the size of the group increases. The administrative duties usually delegated to an MIS include appointment scheduling, communications, financial and accounting support data, and operational information. Although small groups focus on billing, collections, and accounting, larger groups usually develop an insatiable appetite for operational information and controls. Again, because of the inherent individuality of medical groups, a system developed in house may be better at meeting specific needs, but very useful commercial MIS programs are available from outside software and hardware companies. (See Chapters 13, 14, and 32 for further discussion of the use of financial and scheduling data.)

Marketing

Marketing can be divided into internal marketing and external marketing. The object of internal marketing is to retain the existing patient population, largely by developing an effective patient relations program and by motivating staff (see Chapters 8 and 30). The object of outside marketing is to increase name recognition and make the public aware of the services and unique characteristics of the medical group, which is generally done through advertising (see Chapter 29).

Recruitment and Retention of Professional Staff

Finding physicians, nurses, and allied health care professionals, especially those with personalities and work characteristics suitable for a group practice setting, has become a difficult task. Physician recruitment is discussed in Chapter 5.

Human Resources

The head of human resources (formerly called personnel) directs and oversees employee policies and procedures, hiring, and terminations. The job involves interpreting labor law, collecting wage and salary data, implementing benefit programs, and dealing with other aspects of employee-management relations (see Chapter 31).

Prepaid Management

The individual in charge of prepaid management is responsible for the operation of any prepaid programs. Tracking, validating, and paying outside providers; collecting data on the programs; ensuring that procedures are correct according to contract; and many other functions are under the control of the prepaid management department. In a large group with a heavy prepaid enrollment, many millions of dollars flow through this department (see Chapter 9).

Education and Training

No outpatient ambulatory care enterprise of substance can survive today without providing education and training programs. There is an increasing body of evidence to support the supposition that patient education may reduce the incidence of illness and thus enhance the viability of groups involved in prepaid medicine. Furthermore, there is little doubt that an organized program for developing and training staff is extremely valuable. Providing career ladders for employees has been found to be motivating and useful for retaining skilled personnel in areas such as nursing, and the required in-service education can be done efficiently in house. For these reasons, a director of education would seem a desirable acquisition for a large and well-integrated ambulatory health care company. (See Chapters 16 and 17 for further discussion of staff and patient education.)

Providing a Playing Field That Nurtures Teamwork

The positions, the players' desirable skills, and many of the significant financial and political issues involved in organizing an outpatient medical practice have been discussed above. It is time to try to bring it all together into a workable model.

The model outlined in this section is that employed by Friendly Hills HealthCare Network, based in La Habra, California. This group, although owning its own inpatient facility, primarily is a large ambulatory care provider that records over 600,000 outpatient visits each year. It consists of over 130 physicians and 1,200 full-time employee equivalents and is 90 percent prepaid, with almost 100,000 patients under contract. The ambulatory and inpatient services are highly integrated.

Those who desire a rigid chart of little boxes connected by solid lines will not be disappointed (see Figure 1-1). However, although this kind of model may suffice in an industrial mode, or even for an individual or small group practice, it is not really descriptive of a medium- or large-size medical group. Part of the reason is the duality of the physician-owner hierarchy on the one hand and the lay administrative and employee staff hierarchy on the other. The fact that the physician owners are also workers compounds the difficulties.

Although not most desirable, the existence of two reporting mechanisms must be accepted for practical reasons. However, they should be aligned at every possible juncture by free and open communication and cooperation. To draw fixed boxes and lines graphically seems to separate the two segments, whereas in reality, in many areas, they are merged.

Because of the existence of the two reporting structures—the physician and support staff hierarchies—lateral interactions are necessary. To keep the overall organization as simple as possible, therefore, vertical levels of management are kept to a minimum. There are four levels of management that exist in the organization on the staff side, and three levels on the physician side. Those on the physician side consist of the CEO, the medical director, and the department chairpersons. On the staff side, the levels consist of (1) the CEO, (2) the executive and nonexecutive directors, (3) the managers, and (4) the working supervisors.

The CEO and the Medical Director

Let us begin at the top of the organizational plan (Figure 1-1). The close interplay necessary between the CEO and the medical director (executive director of medical affairs) has already been described. However, it is also true that only one individual can have final authority. That individual should be the CEO for two reasons. First, giving the physicians ultimate dominance, despite the fact that they are also owners, might send the wrong message to the other 90 percent of employees, and it also might serve to preserve a system of physician dominance that may be archaic in today's competitive business climate. The second reason is simply that the CEO is ultimately accountable for the financial performance of the company, upon which, in a business sense, all else is judged.

Executive and Nonexecutive Directors

Directors are similar to vice presidents in the corporate model. The only difference between executive directors and nonexecutive directors in this model

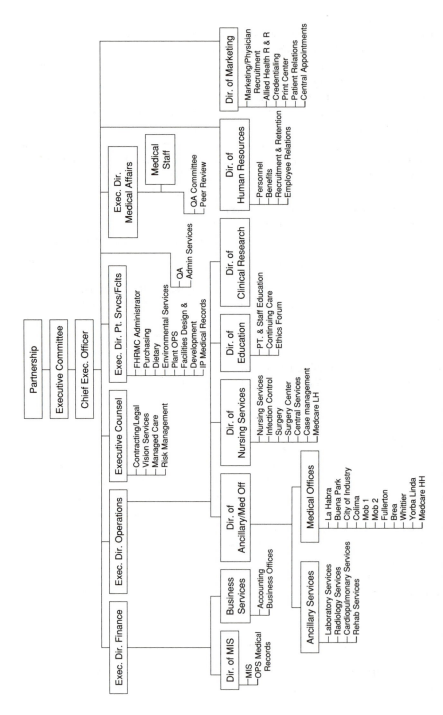

Figure 1-1 Organizational Chart for Friendly Hills HealthCare Network

is the degree of autonomy necessary for doing their jobs. The ambulatory sector executive director positions at Friendly Hills also include the executive counsel in charge of contracting and the administration of prepaid programs, the executive director of finance (CFO), and the executive director of operations. The medical director in this model is also at this level of management. The nonexecutive director positions are in all the other areas of accountability noted in this chapter. Of course, even in a group the size of Friendly Hills, some individuals are given diverse responsibilities. Likewise, because of their close relationship, in a few cases nonexecutive directors report through executive directors to the CEO, whereas others report directly.

To avoid two management systems, one for physicians and one for nonphysician staff, the medical directorship is treated as a "staff" rather than a "line" position. It is essentially a facilitating and advisory position, and no staff members directly report to the medical director. However, the medical director has jurisdiction over the medical staff through the physician department chairpersons as well as the quality assurance and peer review committees. Assuming that the medical director is primarily responsible for the quality and availability of medical care, then there must be an advisory link, although not represented on the chart, to the executive director of operations. Similarly, the same kind of link must be established between the medical director and the directors who handle physician and allied health professional recruiting, patient and staff education, medical records, clinical research, and other medically related matters.

Managers

Managers report to directors. Managers manage and have no other actual day-to-day work responsibilities in their areas. Managers, not the nursing department, have the responsibility of running the various patient care areas. Each of the satellite offices has its own manager as well. Managers may call on any and all of the directors for assistance as they deem necessary. Just as it might be undesirable to have a physician-dominated administrative structure, it is also undesirable to have a nursing-dominated staff in the patient care areas. Therefore, few of the managers are nurses. However, the nurses and technologists write the policies and protocols and administer the technical performance standards in their areas of expertise. In the Friendly Hills model, the managers of the patient care areas and satellite offices are coordinated through the executive director of operations. The managers of departments such as the laboratory and radiology report to the director of ancillary services, who in turn reports to the executive director of operations.

Supervisors

The lowest level of management consists of supervisors. In the model, all supervisors have work responsibilities in their departments, although as "exempt" employees they are allowed some time for administrative duties. Supervisors write evaluations of their employees, devise work schedules, monitor performance standards, and report to their managers. Perhaps the most vital function of each supervisor, however, is teaching and orientation. The supervisors constitute the vital link between management and the line employees, and they play a most important role in uniting theory with practice. For this reason, it is wise to include supervisors, to as large an extent as possible, in all management programs, to train them assiduously, and to make sure that they are thoroughly familiar with the goals and mission of the company.

* * *

The Friendly Hills model is just one way of organizing a medical group. It should not be considered the only paradigm, since far different configurations have worked effectively for others. Instead, it should serve as a reminder that effective management can take many forms and that the bottom line is people. There is no chart or system that can replace open dialogue, freedom to communicate and criticize, constant effort to inform at all levels, and mutual respect. This brings us back to that ubiquitous but meaningful word, *teamwork.*

2

Strategic Planning

Judy Pierson

WHY PLAN?

It has been said that the most effective way to cope with change is to help create it. The challenge in designing strategic plans in today's health care marketplace is to create a more dynamic means of managing change. Ambulatory care organizations are emerging as the focal point of health care, with medical groups as the powerbrokers of the nineties. At the turn of the century, one might look back and say that for some the nineties were the worst of times; but for those in ambulatory care, the decade could prove to be the best of times.

As the transition in health care occurs, those groups on the leading edge will need to plan strategies that anticipate and respond to the changes. The new realities demand that each group must pursue its vision innovatively while abiding by the principles of good business management. The surviving health care organizations in this "new era" will be adaptive organizations.

Strategic planning is critical to addressing the realities of the marketplace, developing strategies for action, and then making organizational investments and changes to achieve strategic advantages. Businesses with well-designed and flexible strategic business plans will dominate the industry.

Determining the Need for Planning

One way to determine the need for a strategic planning process is to conduct a simple diagnostic audit with the organization's leadership team.

- Does the board have a defined mission and five-year strategic goals for the organization's growth and diversification?
- Does the organization have a plan for establishing a delivery network and linkages with other providers?

- Does the organization have a written plan that identifies and prioritizes new target markets, services, and programs?
- Does the organization maintain an active and effective ongoing planning process that is the basis for annual budgeting and capital planning?
- Are the decisions to prioritize the allocation of resources based on the analysis of trends and assumptions about expected outcomes for investments?
- Are educational sessions held on key issues identified as important in the industry or to the organization?
- Is there a long-range capital plan developed in conjunction with service development and growth projections?
- Have specific goals, with identified benefits to the bottom line or customer service, been set for improving the operational systems?
- Have the department heads responded to organizational objectives in developing annual budgets and staffing plans?
- Is management held responsible for achieving targets documented in the strategic plan?

If the answer is negative to any of these questions, proceed.

The approach to planning that is presented here is tailored to meet the new business demands of ambulatory service delivery systems, recognizing that they are a relatively new segment of the health care industry. Ambulatory care groups do not have to burden themselves with the cumbersome process used by large institutions. In fact, as entrepreneurs in the industry, they would do well to create and use a process that stimulates creativity and flexibility. Their need is for a process that is streamlined and that focuses on the decisions to be made and issues to be resolved, thus allowing a continued fast-paced evolution.

WHAT IS A STRATEGIC PLAN?

To understand what a strategic plan is requires understanding what a strategy is. Often the resistance to strategic planning can be traced to a lack of appreciation for strategies. Quite simply, *a strategy is a course of action that changes the basis of competition.* Organizations that do not have competition or do not need to do anything differently do not need a strategic plan.

Frequently, personality characteristics tend to influence the selection process, and the strategies chosen are really mere reaffirmations of what is being done now. The motivation for such choices is to avoid the conflict and effort required to make a change, although often this motivation is not conscious. To create the right mind set for strategic planning, the definition of strategy given above should be expanded to include the following proviso: *If a strategy is not controversial, it is not a strategy; it is the status quo.* Developing a strategic plan requires tackling the tough issues and taking the course that is best for the organization even if it ruffles some feathers.

What then is a strategic plan? There are many definitions, but one that succinctly highlights some key points follows:

> A *strategic plan is an iterative process of defining and communicating the desired future of the organization and the means to achieve it.*

The process produces the guidelines for the overall organizational development based on the organization's unique mission and desired future. A good strategic plan generates positive organizational change and stimulates improved management and organizational performance.

Strategic planning is a continuous process of making intelligent choices about the future. It must become an integral management function involving the analysis of organizational capabilities and resources in light of environmental opportunities and threats. It is a process that allows the organization to set a specific course into the future.

PRINCIPLES OF PLANNING

Strategic planning is an art, not a science. The best results are obtained when there is a balance between the entrepreneurial dreamers and the management pragmatists. Peter Drucker once said that results are obtained by exploiting opportunities, not just by solving problems; and yet, strategic planning must do both.

A strategic plan does not provide a step-by-step guide for the future development of the organization. Health care organizations, and those in the ambulatory care business in particular, are located in an environment that changes too rapidly to allow for a fixed plan. Strategic planning must be an ongoing organizational process that is revisited as frequently as needed to reassess and redefine responses.

However, too often organizations avoid setting long-term strategies based on the rationale that the industry is changing too rapidly. This rationale fails to recognize the difference between changing a long-term strategy and adjusting a short-term tactic or objective. Often participants take a nearsighted approach to problem solving that treats the symptoms of immediate management problems rather than puts forth the effort to define strategic issues that set the course for a defined business goal. Once set, the strategies will tend to be valid for several years. The strategies create the bridge between the present and the vision of the organization. Drucker often comments that strategic planning requires future tense thinking.

Part of what has made hospital planning cumbersome, for example, is the belief that planning is a bottom-up process in which everyone contributes ideas and wishes. Certainly, the planning will occur at the "bottom" of the organization as part of the development of appropriate management and resource allocation responses needed to achieve the strategies. However, strategic planning is a top-down process that is the primary responsibility of the board and the administration.

Top-down planning may sound heretical. It's not. Good leaders already have a vision and long-range strategies that they intuitively know are right for the organization. Many times all that is needed is to air these ideas, test them, and then build a consensus among the leadership team. The job of the leadership team is to crystallize a vision and translate these key values and goals into specific strategies and policy directives.

A good strategic plan will produce a vision that transcends the current marketplace indicators. Certainly, planning requires both deductive and inductive thinking applied to the strategic management of the organization. So what comes first—data or the vision? A complete data base is important for the development of a final strategic plan; it should not be a barrier to strategic thinking or a hindrance to strategic decision making. Defining the mission and vision is a visionary process that must not be bound by the limits imposed by data analysis.

One common fear is that broad strategy statements without accompanying sets of explicit directions for everyone in the organization will not be effective. On the contrary, when the mission and the broad strategy directives are communicated throughout the organization, responsible employees will seek to find ways that they can contribute to meeting those targets. Reams of detailed implementation plans communicate patronization and foster avoidance and annoyance. The strategic plan needs to stimulate creative responses throughout the organization and should not be a set of restrictive marching orders.

The strategic plan is not the most important outcome of the process. There have been many strategic plans that met textbook requirements but ended up unread on the shelf. The process is the most important outcome, at least if it has succeeded in creating a strategic management culture that is grounded in strategic, not just operational, thinking. The benefits of planning are derived from engaging in the process. As Russell Ackoff has noted, when the plan involves the key stakeholders, the change process and implementation begin before the document is off the press.

The strategic planning process educates the participants to a way of viewing the organization that is then always present when they make decisions and take action. The goal of the process then, is to integrate it into the fabric of the organization so that the periodic revisiting keeps these strategic perspectives in sight and adjusted to the changes in the environment.

DESIGNING THE PROCESS

There is no right way that will work for every organization. However, given the preceding discussion, it is clear that some things can be done to ensure success. One of the fears about embarking on a planning process is that it will take months of tremendous effort. A good plan can be developed in several weeks or less. The process should focus around issues, require a few intense planning sessions, and be outcome-oriented.

The creation of a strategic plan can occur in a short time frame if retreats are used and data are collected only to support strategic issues.

Process Design

The first step is to mobilize the leadership team. The strategic planning team needs to meet to plan the process. The team usually includes the board, the top management, and possibly key providers in the organization. The plan to plan would include the mechanics such as the time frame, goals, and objectives, as well as the level of participation by various people inside and outside of the organization.

Strategic Issue Development

The second step is to collect basic information required for the environmental assessment and to articulate the strategic issues. Information is collected from data sources and interviews with constituents conducted to solicit input on issues. The responsibility for collecting this input is best assigned to one person in the organization who can secure and analyze data from various sources inside and outside of the organization. Some organizations use consultants to do this, whereas others hire either full-time planners or interns from university management programs.

The data would be summarized as an environmental scan identifying critical success factors and strategic issues.

Strategic Framework

The third step is for the strategic planning team to develop the strategic framework and the strategic goals. One suggestion is to take the group away for two days with a facilitator to develop the strategic framework. Additionally, the team should identify what it sees as the major strategic issues for the organization in the next three years. What decisions will need to be made that will have significance to the long-term success of the organization?

Strategic Plan Development

The fourth step is to develop the strategic plan. The results from the first strategic planning retreat can be circulated to a broad base of constituents for their feedback. The data analyst would then return to the data for the purpose of developing issue papers for each of the strategic issues. Each issue paper would lay out the problem, indicate the findings and conclusions from the data, and present proposed goal and strategy statements. Groups often seem to be more productive if they respond to proposed statements rather than start from scratch.

The strategic planning team would then get together for another off-site meeting to draft the strategic plan. The order of business would include refining the strategic framework based on the feedback and reconfirming the strategic goals. Specific objectives and tactical actions would then be identified.

Management Planning

With the plan developed, the process broadens to include the management team, which will be involved in devising the management plans. The objective is to test the concepts proposed in the plan and to determine the actual changes that need to occur to solve the problems identified. This validation process may be time consuming, but it should be viewed as one of the priority activities of managers. No one questions the need to do budgeting, but still managers challenge the need to do planning. It must be an important ongoing part of their job.

Developing the management plans may require special studies to develop specific business plans or departmental plans. These studies might include feasibility studies, space studies, operational studies, or research at other facilities. With these studies completed, the management team can go back to the strategic planning team for recommendations on how to proceed. The studies need not all be done at the same time, and one study should not hold up another one.

Implementation Planning

The sixth step is to develop the annual implementation plan. With broad guidelines from the strategic planning team about when certain critical events should occur, the responsibility for the planning would be delegated to those managers who will be responsible for the plan implementation. The managers should then complete forms that include major activities, priority rating, and timing. Concurrently, they would identify the resources needed so that the information can be included in their budgets.

Review and Monitoring

The last step is to establish a mechanism for tracking the benchmarks and to identify the timing for updating the plan. Often this step is eliminated as the organization gets involved in change. However, it is very important to take the time to identify what will be measured and to make sure the mechanisms are in place to measure it over a reasonable period. Additionally, it is important to think through a typical year in light of the current budgeting cycle and to identify what planning needs to take place and when, so that the input can be timely for budgeting. If the planning and budgeting processes do not intersect, they both lose value.

Each of the steps described above will be covered in more detail below, so that the expected outcomes will be clear.

GETTING STARTED

One way to begin is to outline a set of goals and objectives for the process itself. What do you want the plan to achieve? How do you want it to be developed? Creating a brief document containing these points is an excellent way to communicate to the participants what they are going to plan and how they will do it.

The *goal* for the process might be to develop a process that will result in a clear direction for the future. The *outcome objectives* might be as follows:

- Develop a strategic framework for the organization that defines the mission, business role, values, and vision.
- Diagnose the business issues by collecting and analyzing data and interview information that will profile the external environment and the internal situation. Using this information, make assumptions about the future and indicate the implications for the organization.
- State specific attainable strategic goals to be achieved through the accomplishment of objectives that can be measured using the data collected.
- Develop strategies that will allow the organization to achieve its desired position in the marketplace. Identify more specific tactical actions for carrying out the strategies.

- Complete an analysis for the purpose of developing specific programs and marketing or management initiatives and of testing the costs and benefits of executing specific tactics.
- Establish priorities based on a set of evaluation criteria for programs and major new initiatives.
- Document the financial, staffing, and operational resources needed to carry out the plans, and integrate this information into the operating and capital budgets.
- Prepare a three-year phased tactical plan and a more detailed one-year implementation plan that identifies priority actions and responsibilities.
- Plan for the review points and the benchmarks to be measured to ensure monitoring and updating.

In carrying out the planning, the *process objectives* might be as follows:

- Be guided by the active participation of the governance and administrative leadership team.
- Encourage participation and teamwork among stakeholders.
- Provide numerous opportunities for feedback from participants not directly involved in the process.
- Use internal resources of the organizations as much as possible, augmented by consultants only when outside objectivity, expertise, or facilitation skills are required.
- Design a process that will increase the probability of its being accepted, supported, and implemented at all levels of the organization.
- Integrate other studies and projects and other management processes.
- Produce a visually intelligible document that will communicate the major elements of the plan in such a way that everyone can understand them.

DATA COLLECTION AND ANALYSIS

Data for data's sake produces data clog. To be most effective, data should be collected to support the development of strategies for dealing with specific issues. One technique is to create for each issue a position paper that incorporates data and interview results and clearly articulates the issue and the decision to be made. Issue- or decision-driven plans are much more effective in moving organizations than the traditional approach. Some of the types of data that might be analyzed are described below.

External Data

Industry Review. The purpose of the industry review is simply to have a set of operating assumptions about the future that will be the basis for change. Thus, the industry statistics should be organized into no more than a dozen key assumptions. Then, the implications for the organization should be clearly stated. Without a statement of the implications, everyone is still left to their own conclusions. For example, one assumption might be that major employers will offer fewer choices for managed care plans. The implication might be that the organization needs to be part of an integrated managed care delivery system if it is to become one of the major managed care options in the region.

Assumptions can be developed around national and state trends as well as local or regional trends. One model for the environmental scan divides variables into three categories: variables over which one has no control such as the economy and legislation; variables affecting supply and demand such as physician supply, consumer preference, and employer-union relations; and the responses of health care providers such as hospitals, managed care plans, and medical groups, to current trends. All of these are important to consider.

There is a basic set of data that are useful to have, but they are less extensive than might be expected. The external data useful for the strategic plan are as follows:

Demographic Data. Demographic data, including population size, population growth, ethnic and age characteristics, employment, and household income organized by discrete market planning areas, are useful for defining target population groups.

Provider Profiles. Again by the same market areas, it is useful on a map to identify the hospitals and other major groups or ambulatory care settings, with accompanying charts on size and services of each, in order to identify networking candidates or competitive gaps.

Managed Care Plan Profile. Collect information on the HMOs and PPOs that are active in each of the market areas (including which groups and hospitals they contract with, if the data is available) in order to identify target plans and to assess market share.

Employer Base Profile. Identify the major employers in each market area by size and type of industry, including contracts each may have with industrial clinics and managed care plans.

Internal Data

The internal analysis is dependent upon the management information system available. Types of data that are useful include the following:

- service profile by site
- patient base profile by demographic variable
- patient origin
- enrollment trends by plan
- enrollment growth estimates based on existing and targeted plans
- utilization trends by service and site
- physician profile by site and utilization trend
- capacity analysis by provider, clinic, room, and ancillary
- space and site problem identification
- referral profile to other physicians, hospitals and other services
- staffing profile by functional area and growth estimates with enrollment or utilization increases

One of the most useful pieces of information is the use rate for every 1,000 enrollees by provider type, ancillary service, and outside referral service. These ratios can then be the basis for modeling scenarios about the impact of increased enrollment or utilization so that the impact on staffing and space can be determined.

Environmental Scan

Traditionally, reams of data are collected and presented as a SWOT (strengths, weaknesses, opportunities, and threats) analysis. Frequently, planning teams have difficulty making useful decisions based on general SWOTs. Instead, it seems to be more useful to create a SWOT for each of the major planning categories. Thus, there would be one for marketplace, enrollment, services, site and facilities, finances, staffing, physicians, and so on. Each SWOT should indicate at least one specific critical success factor around which strategies can be developed.

Critical Success Factors

Critical success factors are variables that can be altered by action taken by the organization. The identification of critical success factors will help uncover the tactics required to increase the probability of achieving a desired strategy. The test of whether or not something is a critical success factor is this: (1) If it is not changed, will it affect the future of the organization significantly? (2) Can a change be caused by an action taken? Variables that the organization has no control over are not critical success factors, but external variables. Strategies need to respond to variables to enhance the organization's response or decrease its vulnerability.

Strategic Issues

As with many problem-solving processes, the art is in asking the right questions. If the right set of strategic questions can be asked, the development of the strategic plan is usually easy.

Using the same planning categories that gave structure to the SWOT, the strategic planning team would ask a set of questions to be addressed in the process. Examples of issue statements for some of the planning categories follow:

- Physician Development: What number and type of physicians are needed for the anticipated enrollment and patient volume levels in the next three years?
- Contracting: What managed care plans should be targeted and what is the expected impact?
- Services: Should additional diagnostic services be added in response to the anticipated enrollment or utilization?
- Network Development: Should satellites, to be used as primary care feeder sites beyond the existing service area, be planned?
- Market Positioning: Is there a demand for industrial services in the service area as a secondary strategy for large employers?

The test of whether the right question is being asked is whether or not the answer would give the board the direction it needs in making decisions about investments or changes that would effectively alter the course of competition.

SETTING THE STRATEGIC FRAMEWORK

The most important role of the leadership team in the planning process is to set the strategic framework that clearly articulates the mission and vision of the organization. This framework is the skeleton around which the rest of the plan is built. It is the foundation for all policy formulations and decision making.

Essentially, the framework answers the questions of: What business is the organization in? Where is it going? What type of organization does it hope to be? The framework has four key elements: the mission, vision, values, and role statements.

Mission Statement

The mission statement defines the unique and distinctive purpose of the organization. The first sentence should present the core of the mission so that it can be used on its own. Ideally, anyone in the organization should be able to say "Our mission is to . . . ." Clearly, if the mission statement is long and convoluted, no one will be able to repeat it. Likewise, if the mission statement is too lofty, people will feel uncomfortable repeating it.

In addition to being brief, the mission statement should communicate what is different about this organization. How many hospital mission statements claim that the mission is to provide high-quality health care services that meet the needs of the patients in the area while maintaining the financial viability of the organization? That statement describes most of the nonprofit hospitals in the country.

Attorneys have rightly warned against making lofty statements, claiming, for example, that the mission is to provide the "highest" quality services in the region. Consider the patient who feels he or she did not receive the highest quality care and uses that statement to take the organization to court.

Developing the mission statement will be the most difficult part of the planning process. It will take many attempts at wordcrafting to fashion the succinct statement that feels right. Herein lies the art and not the science of planning.

What should the mission statement include? One place to start is to identify the type of organization. Is it a medical group, a primary care medical group, a regional health care system, or an ambulatory care center? The next step is to find the right verb. Is the mission to deliver, coordinate, or organize services? What types of services are they and to whom are they provided? Is the mission to provide primary care, a full range of care, or ambulatory care? Will the recipients be anybody in a defined geographic area or only enrollees in managed care plans? Finally, what distinguishes the organization?

Two sample mission statements are provided for illustration:

> Our mission, as an integral part of the ABC regional system, is to be a primary care medical group network that delivers and coordinates quality medical services that are both affordable and appropriate.

> Our mission is to be a full-service regional health care delivery system that has the status of preferred provider for the contracted and capitated market in the XYZ region.

Role Statement

The role statement describes what type of business the organization intends to pursue, for whom, and in what geographic service area. The role statement describes the activities the organization will carry out in the marketplace. In some ways, role statements are public commitments to the type and level of responsibility the organization will assume. The role statement usually includes a series of sentences. The main role might be "to work directly with insurers and employers to design affordable health care programs" or "to serve the residents of ABC service area."

Vision Statement

The vision is the desired future image of the organization. In the vision statement, the future should be described in an operationally meaningful and inspiring way. The vision is the dream that may or may not ever be achieved, but it is a target to strive for over time. The vision should be a "stretch" for the organization, while still having some basis in reality. For example, one client once articulated the vision of being the best hospital in the world. This statement was so far from reality that it lost all meaning. Some organizations have catchy one-phrase vision statements, whereas others use a series of sentences that gives a more detailed or comprehensive picture. The vision is just that—a picture painted with words. Its function is to inspire and motivate.

Values Statement

Values are the beliefs that govern management decisions and guide actions. Mission statements used to be long, convoluted statements that incorporated the values as well as the mission of the organization. Lengthy statements lose meaning, so it is generally recommended to have a succinct mission statement and to set down separately a set of values or principles. Both types of statements then have more impact.

Values define the culture. The culture is the set of principles that are passed from generation to generation or, in the case of an organization, passed along to all new employees.

From the board and management perspective, the values define the management style. Will the board allow a dictatorial management style or does the belief system mandate a participatory style of management? Will decision making occur only at the top or will it be filtered down into the organization? These are the types of issues that the values dealing with management should address.

From the employee perspective, the values are a set of commitments from the board about how they can be expected to be treated. Will the organization be an equal opportunity employer? Will wages and benefits be competitive or exceed the area averages? Will the organization support professional growth and development? What type of environment is the organization willing to create for employees?

From the patient perspective, the organization should also have a set of expectations. These serve two functions. One is to communicate to patients what level of care and respect they can expect. The other is to communicate to staff the type of attitudes and behaviors that are expected of them in dealing with patients and families. Will families be included in the caregiving process? Will there be a wellness or health perspective? Will patients be passive or active participants in their care planning? In other words, what is the philosophy of patient care?

The last set of principles functions as guidelines on how the organization will do business. Will there be encouragement of innovation and problem solving by all employees? Will continuous improvement of the quality of care be the responsibility of everyone? Will innovative methods be explored to deliver cost-effective care? Will the measurement of outcomes be the basis for improving cost and utilization management?

Values, then, are the beliefs that define the culture of the organization and can be organized into sets of principles relating to management, employees, patient care, and business practices.

DEVELOPING THE STRATEGIC PLAN

With the framework in place, the strategic planning team now returns to the set of strategic issues and begins to develop specific strategic goals and objectives as well as enabling strategies and tactics.

Strategic Goals

Goals are end results to be achieved in order to carry out the organization's mission. Goals are based on where the organization is now and where it needs to be in the future. Strategic organizational goals are defined for basic business functions such as growth, financial performance, services, physician development, and marketplace position. Strategic management goals are defined for functional areas such as governance and management, human resources, contracting, marketing, facilities, and operational systems. The organizational goals dictate the management goals.

Objectives

For each strategic goal, there are several objectives. The objectives are measurable changes that are expected to be achieved when the related goal is achieved.

Objectives can be viewed in two ways. The traditional way is to view objectives as targets to be achieved. Correspondingly, objectives can be viewed as measurements of what will be different when the goal is met. They describe how the change will benefit the organization. In reality, both these statements are true—each represents a different side of the same coin.

For example, if the goal is to establish an integrated regional delivery network, then one objective might be to increase market share. Thus, increased market share is a desired change, but it will also be a measure of the change that will occur. Thus, tracking objectives as benchmarks is an excellent way to monitor the success of the plan.

Essentially, the goal describes "what" will be achieved, and the objectives describe both "what" needs to change and "why" in terms of the measurable consequences for the organization. The key differentiation of objectives is that they can be measured or the changes clearly observed.

Strategies

Strategies are broad initiatives to be undertaken to meet organizational goals. They are the means to reach the goals.

A strategic plan has two sets of strategies. The most commonly known strategies are those that describe the courses of action vis-à-vis the market. For example, one strategy may be to become the low-cost managed care plan for the region. The other set of strategies consists of management strategies. For example, one strategy might be to contract for ancillary services rather than investing the capital to provide those services directly.

Tactics

Tactics are particular courses of action designed to carry out a strategy. The strategy directs the tactics. The key element in tactics is *action,* so many people simply say "tactical actions" to indicate clearly what tactics are.

For any one strategy, there are several tactics. For example, if the strategy is to extend the service area to a new geographic area, then one tactic might be to buy a primary care group practice in that area, and another tactic might be to build a central ambulatory hub facility on one main site.

Strategies are the how-tos to achieve goals, whereas tactics are the what-to-dos to achieve objectives.

Phased Tactical Plan

It is often useful to develop a phased tactical plan. This is a graphic summary of the key achievements to be accomplished in the next three planning periods. One technique that works well is to select a catchy phrase that characterizes each planning period (e.g., "On the Move" or "Changing the Way We Do Business"). Each phase would also have a focus of action and up to six key projects as well as the expected measurable outcome.

With these strategic plan elements in place, the strategic plan is essentially complete. In some cases, this is all of the documentation that needs to be broadly communicated. Thus, the entire plan might be no more than 10 pages that graphically highlight the major aims of the organization for the near future.

STRATEGIC MANAGEMENT PLANNING

The planning activity now spreads down into the organization to the managerial level so that the management plans required to carry out the strategic plan can be developed. There are three types of management plans: the programmatic business plans, the operational plans, and the implementation plan.

Business Plans

Business plans are ministrategic plans for business lines within the organization. Each provides the rationale for the development of each business component. The plans consist of the same planning elements as the larger strategic plan, but, the design of the plans must respond to the broader organizational strategic directives. It is at this point that the market needs and the profits or losses of particular business lines would be evaluated in order to make decisions about eliminating, downsizing, expanding, or just maintaining services.

Operational Plans

Each of the managers in the organization needs to develop a plan for the functional area that he or she is responsible for. Thus, there would be an MIS plan, a financial plan, a marketing plan, and so on. Each manager is charged with the task of assessing his or her functional area to ascertain what changes would need to be made in order to support the organizational change required by the strategic plan.

Implementation Plan

The implementation plan for a given strategic plan sets forth the major activities to be achieved and indicates the priorities, responsibilities, and timing. It is the schedule of the events required to achieve the tactical objectives within a reasonable planning period, which is usually one year. At the end of that time, the plan is reevaluated and a new or revised implementation plan developed. This updating is essential for ensuring flexibility and responsiveness to external changes and for evaluating activities that are not working as planned.

Benchmarks

Benchmarks are the measurable targets to be achieved within defined time frames. They are based upon the difference between the current baseline performance and the desired outcome. They are important for measuring progress toward achieving the objectives. For example, if one objective is to increase the market share by 10 percent in five years, the benchmark might be a market share of 20 percent at the end of that period based on the current baseline of 10 percent. Data would be monitored to see the progress made toward that target.

All of the data collected during the planning should be collected into a binder entitled the Data Base Planning Binder. This data base, which contains the data on the baseline figures for tracking change, will be a valuable reference document for specific planning during the year.

The Expected Benefits

Strategic planning is not an academic exercise that a "good" organization should do. Strategic planning ensures consistency in decision making regarding the business development of the organization and the allocation of resources to support the changes required. Equally important are the benefits derived from the process itself, including an enhancement of the ability of the organization to make the right decisions at the right time. Additional important benefits include the following:

- An enhanced awareness of the organization's business in relationship to the marketplace.
- Access to a comprehensive data base upon which to make sound business decisions on vertical or horizontal integration, service development, financial management, and marketing.
- Unification of the board, the management, and the staff in their perception of the future and the rationale for the course taken.
- The ability to make quicker decisions about things that "come out of the blue" because of the strong foundation of consensus already built.
- A focusing of the entire organization on a clear set of goals.
- An increased commitment to the strategic plan based on the perception that it is "our" plan.
- Facilitation of the implementation of strategies, because resistance to the plan is reduced if not eliminated through the process of developing it.
- Formation of alliances built through teamwork, which often creates bonds among disparate groups.
- Enhanced organizational effectiveness based on having a guide for basic business processes such as budgeting, performance appraisal, and management.
- Achievement of efficiency by avoiding false starts and scattered, unfocused use of energy and time.
- Cost savings due to maximum use of internal resources—people, time, facilities, and equipment.

Essentially, the strategic plan itself is a clear statement of what the organization is and where it is going. The strategic planning process is a mechanism for unifying the organization around a set of common goals.

In spite of the need to document the strategic plan, it should be emphasized that the plan is not necessary for informing people of what has been done during the planning process. In a participatory process, they will know what was done and will already be busy doing what they can to implement the plan.

Committing the strategic plan to paper demonstrates the seriousness of the planning effort. The plan becomes the reference point for decisions and action throughout the organization. Thus, the plan must be "user friendly." That is, it must be easily understood by those who participated and those who did not.

CONCLUSION

The development of an effective strategic plan cannot occur in a vacuum. Both the leadership team and key staff members must contribute to the process in order for the plan to be accepted and implemented. The process should take on unique characteristics of the organization as it becomes a part of the culture. The process should be practical and stimulating so that it challenges the leadership team to address strategic issues and set priorities.

The planning process should be focused, intense, and outcome-oriented. Planning needs to be an iterative process that identifies issues and problems to be solved as well as opportunities to be acted upon. Today's environment does not afford the luxury of a lengthy and cumbersome planning process that produces useless reams of paper. The stakes for ambulatory care groups in today's competitive environment are too high for opportunities to be lost because the organization was unprepared to act upon them. What is needed is a highly iterative, participatory, decision-oriented approach to planning.

In order to be effectively adopted throughout the organization, the process should have these characteristics:

- It should clearly articulate the mission, vision, and strategic directions.
- It should be structured around strategic issues in functional areas.
- It should be based on sound data and cogent data analysis.
- All stakeholders should participate so as to build consensus and develop understanding.
- It should result in organizational learning and strategic management.
- It should be a basis for assignments and accountability.
- It should be reality tested so that reasonable implementation targets are set.
- It should be presented graphically for ease of understanding.

Developing a strategic plan can provide the stimulus for innovative and creative thinking without exhaustive studies and interminable meetings. The effort will be one of the best investments the organization can make. As the White Rabbit said in *Alice in Wonderland*, "If you don't know where you're going, any road will do." No organization in the health care industry today can afford to not know where it is going.

3

The Role of the Medical Group Administrator

Robert A. Nelson

The dictionary definition of *administrator* is "a person who administers or manages affairs of any kind." A medical group practice administrator could then be described as a person who manages the affairs of a medical group practice. That description aptly defines a significant portion of the nonphysician manager's role in such an organization. In many cases, the definition is complete; in others, it falls short. In every case, the job of the manager is molded to the culture and governance characteristics of the group the manager serves.

The role of the medical group administrator has evolved over the years to keep pace with the medical marketplace. Because the medical field has undergone rapid and significant change during the past 10 to 15 years, encompassing the role of the medical group administrator in one definition may miss the mark without some expansion of the term. This chapter will trace the role of the administrator from its earlier models to its present day variations and will describe the role in modern ambulatory practice.

HISTORY

Although this book concerns health care management in the 1990s, a look back at the history of the medical group administrator will help bring some perspective to the role of the present-day "administrator." Over the years, until approximately 1975, medicine was a very stable, slowly evolving profession that typically produced a comfortable income for its practitioners. Terms such as "the business of medicine" or "the medical industry" were foreign to the profession. The profession was entrepreneurial, however, in the sense that each practitioner typically preferred to practice independently in a private office setting, attracting additional clientele through good service and word-of-mouth referrals by satisfied patients. The management of the physician's office rested with the physician and his or her small staff of nurses and receptionists.

48

Beginnings

Until relatively recently, the vast majority of physicians in the United States practiced as solo practitioners. Although group practice had existed since the late nineteenth century, most notably with the formation of the Mayo Clinic by the Mayo brothers, it did not become a dominant form of medical practice until the late 1970s. The result was a relatively small cadre of people who held full-time business manager roles in medical groups. A reflection of this may be found in the enrollment of the Medical Group Management Association, which has a 1991 membership approaching twelve thousand group practice managers but had a membership of less then one thousand in 1970.

Until the mid-1970s, medicine was a fairly sedate and uncomplicated profession. Patients selected their physicians based on the recommendation of family members, friends, or neighbors. The number of physicians in practice was such that from a provider perspective, an adequate ratio of patients to physicians existed. The result was that competition for patients was understated and gentlemanly. The physicians provided services to the patients in accordance with their view of the existing needs. The physicians charged their patients fees for the services rendered. The fees could be almost anything the physicians wanted to charge, although they were fairly consistent in each community.

The patients were held responsible for paying these fees and were billed directly. The physicians or their staff would assist patients who had insurance in billing their insurance companies by either offering a billing service for the patients or providing the necessary information so the patients could make out their own bills. The insurance companies paid their agreed-upon portion of each bill, and the patients were expected to pay the difference between the insurance payments and the physicians' fees. The patients usually paid that difference.

Medicine was a respected profession. Physicians were highly regarded members of the community. They were perceived as healing and caring people. Their income was recognized as being well above average, but the source of that income was shielded from patients by the significant contribution of insurance in the payment of their fees.

As time went by, physicians found that practicing alone had disadvantages. Being on call every night was a hardship and affected the physician's physical status and his or her family life as well. Managing the office staff was trying at times and interrupted the physician's concentration on the clinical aspects of practice. The physician also found that keeping abreast of the latest technology was almost impossible when practicing alone. Moreover, accounting and finance were not subjects covered in the medical school curriculum.

More and more physicians began forming or joining group practices to solve these problems. Becoming members of a group allowed them to share the burdens of the business side of medical practice while continuing to enjoy the more traditional clinical benefits. Except for being on call, the burdens of the practice seemed to be mainly administrative such as the management of personnel, the maintenance of proper accounting books, the oversight of fee billings and collections, the selection and operation of billing systems, the arrangement of finances for needed equipment or facility enhancements, to name a few. The solution was to employ a medical group administrator who had the background and training necessary to take these burdens from the physicians' shoulders.

Medical group administrators before the 1970s did not typically have special training. Although there were baccalaureate-level degrees available in hospital administration and public health, no college-level offerings were available in ambulatory medical practice management. Since the business aspects of medical practice were fairly straightforward in those earlier years, in-depth specialized training for managers was not considered essential. That is not to say that managing of a medical practice did not have its challenges even then. Certainly, not all patients paid their bills on time. Revenue received did not automatically exceed expenses, if the expenses were not properly managed. And personnel management was as critical a need then as it is now. Therefore, medical groups looked for individuals with management and financial skills earned primarily through education and experience.

Many administrators were staff members of long service who had been promoted. They were hardworking bookkeepers or front office supervisors who had demonstrated an ability to handle problems and lead people. This was particularly true in smaller groups, where stronger management skills, such as in finance, were not as necessary as good hands-on supervision. If the position was not or could not be filled by a current staff member, it was often filled by someone known to the physicians of the practice. Sometimes the individual had managerial skills that had already been observed (e.g., an accountant from an accounting firm or a branch manager from a bank used by the practice). Rarely did the selected manager have a hospital administration degree, since individuals with this degree were usually bent on a career in the hospital industry.

Whatever background the medical group administrator had, the job was to administer the business operation of the practice. The focus was inward. The administrator's role was to ensure the practice was operating efficiently and effectively. An outward focus, for all practical purposes, was not essential to the well-being of the practice. The medical delivery system and the financing of medical care had changed very little over the years. Even the introduction of Medicare in 1965 was basically an extension of the existing system; all that occurred was the addition of another, albeit very large, insurance carrier, the government, whose purpose was to insure the elderly. Change was not something that medical organizations needed to watch for or fear.

Was an outward focus needed to attract patients? Of course, the practitioners did want to attract and retain patients, but that was done almost exclusively by offering good service and depending on referrals by satisfied patients, reinforcing the inward focus of management. Therefore, the administrator, as the only active manager of the practice, was charged solely with the task of administering. Physician managers were nearly unheard of. Except for the time devoted to the governing body, rarely did physicians actively participate in the management of the group. As a result, one could generally describe the role of the medical group administrator, until the 1970s, as the manager of the internal operations of a medical group practice.

Transition

During the late 1970s and early 1980s medicine went through a phase of rapid change. The traditions that had been depended upon by all medical practices for so many years came to a quick end. Physicians and hospitals were asked to assume risk. An influx of new physicians, as a result of the expanded output of U.S. medical schools and the increased entry of foreign-trained graduates, changed the patient-to-physician ratios. The cost of health care came under careful scrutiny by government, insurers, and employers. New three-letter combinations reflected vast changes in the medical system. DRGs, PPOs, EPOs, IPAs, and HMOs upset the former tranquility. Blatant marketing of medical practices, after years of being considered unethical, became customary almost overnight. The inward focus of most medical practices would no longer suffice. Change was everywhere. Opportunities abounded for the venturesome. The one practice form best positioned to take advantage of these awesome changes was the medical group practice.

Medical group practices had distinct advantages in the new setting if they were prepared to respond. Most of the three-letter options being offered to physicians fit groups better than individual physicians acting independently. Most of the three-letter options required more and better management as well. Medical group practices were in the right position—if they shifted their focus outward quickly enough. Medical groups had numbers of physicians acting as one. Medical groups had the management staff in place. The only question was whether the groups, and their management, were ready and willing to adapt to the new world of medicine. Many were. Many weren't, but would make the necessary changes in order to adapt. Some still aren't ready.

The centerpiece of the new world of medicine was management response. Remembering that medical practice management was inwardly focused, with management centered around the administrator, changes often were well underway before managers, or the medical group physicians, realized that their world was altered. In fact, initially only a few saw the change clearly. Most didn't see it coming, or waited, hoping the change was only a momentary aberration that would soon go away.

The new styles of practice required medical practices to make changes totally foreign to their fundamental principles. Practices in the past had never been asked to discount their fees in order to attract or retain patients. But now, as preferred providers, they were required to charge lower fees for enrollees. Practices had never been asked to assume financial risk for the medical care they provided. Now, as members of IPAs and HMOs, they were assuming risk. Practices had never been asked to control the number of days their patients spent in the hospital. Now Medicare and the HMOs, through the use of DRGs and prospective payment, were pressuring them to do just this. Practices had never been asked to select which specialists they would refer their patients to based on cost. Such selection was now required by the IPAs and HMOs. Practices had never been asked to select outside specialists based on their participation in specific health plans. Now they were, by PPOs, IPAs, and HMOs. Practices had never been asked to compete for patients based on the cost of health care. Now they were. Practices had never been allowed to market their services. Now they were. Practices had never been asked to organize their management and decision-making processes to respond to outside influences. This also was now necessary.

The problem most medical groups faced was that, although management power was held by the medical group administrator, the expectation was that the administrator would merely manage internal operations. The administrator's traditional job was not to be outward looking and in the lead of a changing marketplace. In particular, the administrator was not expected to assume the role of changing the fundamentals of the practice with regard to marketing, risk taking, discounting, and cost-controlled medical practice, even though these factors vitally affected the livelihood of the partners or shareholders. The result was a period of confusion as to the role of management, particularly the role of the medical group administrator.

As in most times of confusion, managers attempted to adapt to the culture and organizational structure of their companies. Some continued to function in their roles as previously defined, blindly ignoring the changes occurring outside, satisfied that they were performing their defined jobs well. Others launched into the new world without the specific authority of the physician-owners, recognizing that no one else was stepping forward to fill the perceived need. Still others became confused as to the role they should assume and what the group expected.

The key to the dilemma was the role the governing board and physician leaders took in the leadership of their group. The role of the medical group administrator was changing, but so also was the role of the physician leaders. Suddenly, the term "physician-manager" came into common use. The concepts of team leadership and team management were being introduced. The medical group administrator, working closely with a physician manager and devoting at least some time to management in the role of board chairperson or president of the organization, began to evolve.

The process was not without controversy. Hardcore medical group administrators challenged the Medical Group Management Association when it proposed that there was a place for physicians in the association and formed the Society of Physicians in Administration (SPA). They argued that physicians didn't have the proper training or education to assume these roles. At the same time, some physicians argued that lay administrators should be replaced with physicians, since a medical practice was, after all, a physician enterprise. As time has passed, the importance of each team member's role in group practice management has come more clearly into focus. But there still is not universal agreement. The concepts of physician and nonphysician management are in transition in many groups even today (see Chapter 4).

DUTIES

There are few administrative jobs more complex than managing a medical group, which is one of the few types of business that provide goods or services to one party and expect the payment for those goods or services to be made by another party. It is also one of the only types of business that agree to accept a statistical average compensation for goods or services provided, a very sophisticated method of payment. At the same time, a medical group uses highly trained professionals as production workers, professionals who have never been educated in fundamental business practices.

The need for strong management is evident. But strong management does not consist of independent actions by individual physician or nonphysician managers. The management of a medical group in the 1990s must be a team effort, and the role of the medical group administrator is to be a part of the management team. That role will vary, however, depending on the size of the group, the location of the group, the practice makeup of the group, and how the group is compensated for the services it provides.

A medical group is often defined as a practice in which three or more physicians form together to practice as one, distributing their income under some agreed compensation formula. The range in size of groups is great. Over 70 percent of the groups in the United States are practices of fewer than 10 physicians who typically are all in the same specialty. Large multispecialty medical groups, however, are found throughout the United States, with staffs ranging from 25 to hundreds of physicians. These large groups are increasing in both numbers and size.

Where does the administrator fit in the spectrum of practices? When should a group employ a full-time administrator? Obviously, large medical groups need and have administrative staffs to deal with their significant management needs. In such groups, a midlevel manager may direct a department staffed with 50 to 100 employees, and with that experience the manager would probably be qualified to fill the position of administrator for a smaller group.

In the sophisticated and complex medical marketplace of the 1990s, there is probably no medical group that should not have at least one full-time administrator. Each administrator should be skilled in business and finance. Medicine is no longer simply a profession of service to patients in which only simple supervision is required. A medical group is no longer a business that can be casually run by the "front office" staff and survive. The role of the administrator is to bring business and finance skills into the practice. Some groups may still be located in regions where the challenges of managed care have not yet reached, but it is just a matter of time before outside influences will be pressing in upon these groups as well. No matter where a practice is located, the time has come for outward looking management to be in place.

The job description of the medical group administrator will vary depending upon the group size and the degree of physician involvement in the management of the group. The responsibilities of each management team member need to be well defined in order to minimize conflict and duplication of effort. The following is a recommended list of responsibilities defining the administrator's role:

- Overseeing the daily operations of the medical group and working with the line department heads to develop and refine the efficiency and effectiveness of each of the departments in order to promote excellent operational systems.
- Studying and understanding all programs and plans that have been adopted by the board of directors.
- Overseeing the preparation of operational budgets, ensuring that all operational budgetary elements are addressed in the group's overall budgetary process, and ensuring that appropriate accounting systems are in place to furnish data on all financial matters.
- Developing operational staff plans and directing the filling of all operational staff positions.
- Developing capital equipment plans for new programs and ongoing operations and overseeing the acquisition of the necessary equipment.
- Developing operational space need plans for ongoing operations and new programs adopted by the board of directors.
- Observing daily operations and identifying areas where modification of policies or procedures will improve patient care.
- Developing sound billing and data retrieval systems and overseeing the claims-processing and collection systems to ensure timely cash flow.

- Ensuring that claims, complaints, and inquiries from patients are handled courteously, capably, and promptly.
- By working through the line departments, ensuring the regular training of personnel so they develop the knowledge and skills needed to perform their jobs and encouraging individual employee development so that future needs of the group are adequately met.
- Evaluating the objectives of the group from an operational viewpoint and in light of the changing medical delivery environment and making recommendations to the board of directors concerning changes that may be appropriate given the group's objectives.
- Reporting regularly to the board of directors regarding significant operational issues, including plans for change, staffing issues, and operational problems.
- Attending regular meetings of the board of directors and shareholders meetings and offering advice and recommendations concerning issues under consideration, particularly as they may affect operations.
- Representing the group, as the administrative delegate, at various community meetings where such representation is appropriate.
- Studying and negotiating agreements and contracts with health plans under which the group provides medical care, then advising the board of directors of the outcome of such negotiations and reporting any difficulties that the agreements or contracts may pose.
- Keeping current on all developments in the medical arena on local, state, and national levels and educating physician leaders and staff so that they can proactively respond to the various threats and opportunities.
- Performing such other management duties as may be assigned from time to time by the board of directors.

This list of duties is operationally focused but may be expanded to include responsibilities beyond the actual operation of the practice, depending on the responsibilities of the physician managers. Following are examples of responsibilities that the administrator of today will often assume or share with the physician managers:

- Exploring and appraising the local health care market on an ongoing basis to ensure a full understanding of the health care needs of the population as well as the responses of competitive providers.
- Exploring and appraising various means to position the medical group to better serve the health care needs of the population. For example, there may exist opportunities to acquire or merge with other medical practices or facilities, open satellite offices in underserved areas, or add new medi-

cal capabilities. The administrator would present all viable alternatives to the board of directors for consideration and oversee the implementation of approved programs.

- Working with the board of directors to develop and update, as appropriate, the strategic plan of the medical group. This plan shall establish both short- and long-term goals and set measurable objectives and schedules for accomplishing the established goals.
- Directing the development of new business opportunities related to the medical group practice and the delivery of health care. The administrator would negotiate appropriate contracts and agreements with organizations offering new business alternatives and oversee the implementation of these programs.
- Overseeing and guiding the public relations and marketing programs of the medical group.

Coordination of the responsibilities of physician managers and the administrator is essential. Typically the responsibility of the physician managers is mainly to set goals, objectives, medical standards, and group policies. The medical group administrator then focuses on operationally achieving the goals and objectives in accordance with standards and policies that are in force.

TRAINING

Given the role of medical group administrators, what training and education will assist them in advancing their capabilities and fulfilling their responsibilities? As noted earlier, the educational opportunities of years past centered on the hospital manager. During the 1980s, nearly every "hospital administration" curriculum broadened its course content to include ambulatory care courses and was retitled "health sciences administration." Accompanying this trend came the opportunity to acquire a Masters of Health Administration (MHA). This brought about a change in the source of medical group administrators. Whereas 20 years ago administrators came from within practices or from outside the field of medicine, today the primary supply is provided by the health administration curriculums offered at universities throughout the United States. The graduates of these programs will typically join medical groups as mid-level managers. Then, with experience, they may move up to higher management positions or take similar positions in other medical groups.

Continuing education and management networking is essential for managers if they are to keep abreast of the business complexities of modern medicine. Appropriate educational opportunities need to be sought by administrators to increase their expertise in medical group management. Various associations offer a broad spectrum of educational seminars and courses of study. The primary association aimed at the medical group administrator is the Medical Group Management Association. This national association offers between 50 and 75 educational programs each year aimed at almost every level of experience. The most fundamental topics, such as credit and collection, are covered, and there are also sophisticated planning and leadership symposiums designed for physician and nonphysician team development. For personal development, the American College of Medical Group Administrators offers uniquely focused and challenging educational opportunities and assessment tools. Other associations such as the American Group Practice Association also offer excellent educational opportunities for the administrator.

CONCLUSION

The role of the medical group administrator has grown to new importance in the operation of the medical group practice. During the transitional years, there were those who feared that the role of the administrator was in jeopardy. This was never really true. The role just required redefinition as the administrator began to work with the physician members of the medical group management team.

In the decade of the 1990s, medicine will continue to evolve. The changes experienced during the 1980s will not stop. The demand for better management skills and teamwork has never been more imperative. The medical group administrator was described at the beginning of this chapter as "a person who manages the affairs of a medical group practice." Although the "affairs" now include external matters such as marketing and relations with third-party payers, the definition is still valid. Every administrator needs to explore that definition, understand the role to be played, and be prepared to fulfill the heavy responsibilities that come with it.

4

The Role of the Medical Director

Albert E. Barnett

The major duty of the medical director in an ambulatory group practice can be simply stated: to direct, supervise, and coordinate the professional and medical activities of the organization to ensure that patients receive the highest quality of medical care. To perform this duty, the ideal medical director must possess an amalgam of abilities, including clinical acumen, administrative expertise, people skills, and political prowess. The leadership qualities of honesty and fairness and the ability to command respect are also of great value. The position of medical director almost defies description, for it encompasses responsibilities that are among the most diverse of any position in the medical organizational galaxy.

A CHANGING ROLE

Virtually every organization redefines the position of medical director to meet its needs, if not to suit the talents and strengths of the individual filling the role. In fact, the title Medical Director has not been adopted by all those holding the position. Other titles include Executive Director of Medical Affairs, Physician Executive, and Physician Manager. Some of the myriad tasks performed by the medical director are necessary even in a solo practice. Quality standards must be met, credentialing maintained, and regulations adhered to. But as the number of practitioners expands in a group practice, the position begins to assume greater significance. In the large multispecialty group practice, having a single medical director may be insufficient, despite a large nonphysician support staff, and an assistant medical director may need to be added for certain specialized tasks.

In the past, physicians elected or appointed to the role of medical director had virtually no background in management or administration. In small or emerging group practices, such individuals might have been group founders who desired to cut back on their clinical duties. Rather than being referred to as

58

medical director, they were often entitled Managing Partner or President of the professional corporation. Often they were older physicians who had benign personalities and were unlikely to interfere. Their main responsibility was to interact with the nonphysician administration in order to maintain physician prerogatives and autonomy and to help arbitrate conflicts among the professional staff members.

Today, the role of medical director is dramatically different, especially in large group practices and in groups with a large stake in prepaid managed care. Guy McKhann (1989), of Johns Hopkins University School of Medicine, comments in a recent paper that "the role of a director has been modified considerably in recent years. Changes in medical policies and priorities . . . mandate that much more time be spent on administrative-managerial activities than was formerly the case. For better or for worse, directors must now be managers of increasingly complex organizations that would be challenging even to a well-trained business executive" (p. 779). This shift to managerial and administrative functions for the medical director has caught many groups off guard, leaving them forced to contend with physician managers who possess the wrong or inadequate skills in an increasingly competitive arena.

TRAINING

Health care providers in today's environment are being asked to combine the highest quality of care with the most effective cost containment. The accountability for meeting these demands rests on the physician manager. Tabenkin, Zyzanski, and Alemagno (1989) studied physician manager characteristics in various types of organizations. They found, not surprisingly, that physician managers in small primary care practices spent significantly more time in patient care and less in management than physician managers in HMOs. Their data also showed that there were wide discrepancies in training. Approximately 19 percent of the respondents had no training in management, 57 percent had some to moderate training, and only 24 percent had a graduate degree in management. The results revealed that physician managers in HMOs have significantly more management training than those in other groups. The American Medical Association's Physician Masterfile, a few years ago, listed over 14,000 physicians whose primary professional activity was administration. However, in a survey sample of this group, only a very small percentage reported MBA or MS degrees obtained within the past 8 to 11 years, recent enough to include the more current management training. Grebenschikoff and Kirschman (1989) reported on data from 1,200 respondents from the American College of Physician Executives; they found only 3 percent had MBAs. Again, a higher proportion of HMO physician executives were working toward a MBA than physician executives in group practices. This statistic has grave implications for those organizations competing with the larger prepaid entities or with the sophisticated management teams of the major insurance companies. Although advanced formal education in business is just one factor contributing to successful management, it seems evident that possession of a recent advanced business degree would be useful and desirable for the medical director of a modern and progressive group practice.

Another area of training to be considered in hiring or promoting an individual to the position of medical director is specialty board certification. Certainly, in dealing with utilization review and peer review problems, as well as maintaining credibility among the specialist physicians of one's own organization, excellent credentials attesting to clinical knowledge are desirable. They would similarly be valuable in negotiating with or evaluating the work of outside contracted providers as well as maintaining the respect of the medical directors of contracting HMOs and other payers.

On the other hand, especially if the organization has a heavy involvement in prepaid managed care, a medical director who is too academic or highly specialized could be a liability. Such an individual may have a tendency to be overly demanding in his or her utilization of laboratory and radiologic procedures and may produce clinical guidelines of care that are too esoteric to be cost-effective. The question of board certification, then, might be ideally resolved by selecting an individual who has board certification and good clinical acumen in a broad field, such as internal medicine, emergency medicine, or even general surgery. Such an individual should be an asset in the areas of utilization review, peer review, quality assurance, and risk management.

Of course, the attaining of management degrees or clinical specialty board certification only means that at some point in the past the individual went through a rigorous training program and passed an examination. The medical director must keep abreast of the *latest* information, evaluate it, and implement it if the organization is to have any chance of achieving and maintaining a high quality of clinical care. Being able to access data and pertinent publications as well as obtain information from outside colleagues and organizations is of utmost importance. The medical director must have the desire and initiative to continue his or her training and education by utilizing reading materials, seminars, and courses of study so as to be able to keep up with developments in medicine and medical administration and to access information and data quickly and accurately.

Particularly if the practice has a large stake in managed care, specific characteristics should be sought in recruiting a medical director. Allan Fine (1990), of Witt Associates, summarizes these as follows:

- Knowledge of utilization review—i.e., current practices, protocols, issues, and trends.

- Experience in product development and a penchant to new and innovative ideas.
- Aggressiveness in developing and implementing more rigorous protocols and guidelines in the practice of utilization review.
- Board certification in internal medicine or general surgery (other specialties, however, can be considered).
- Evidence of support for the marketing department in generating prospects for new business and making attempts to retain business.
- Experience in a managed care organization—e.g., HMO, PPO, IPA, utilization review firm, or insurance carrier offering managed care products along with traditional indemnity plans.
- Strong understanding of and sensitivity toward physician problems and concerns.
- Excellent verbal and written communication skills and ability to address audiences of all sizes.
- Strong decision-making and negotiating skills.
- Ability to interpret data and offer recommendations based on characteristics unique to an organization.
- Pro-activeness not only in planning but also in implementing new programs.
- Intensity and tenaciousness in keeping abreast of the latest trends and in projecting the future directions that utilization and managed care may take. (p. 37)

To the above list should be added *vision,* for the medical director will be very active in planning the strategy and direction of the entire organization.

DUTIES

Depending on the size of the organization, its involvement in managed care and prepaid medicine, and other factors, there are numerous areas of involvement for the medical director. Among many key responsibilities would be the following:

- Developing and implementing policies, plans, and procedures to achieve and maintain high professional standards.
- Ensuring that the organization and its physicians comply with all medically relevant licensing and regulatory bodies.
- Keeping current on technical and medical advances and innovations that might be of value to the practice.

- Monitoring and evaluating quality assurance, utilization review and risk management activities.
- Assuming a major advisory role in the organization's educational programs, including continuing education programs for physicians, nurses, and other professional personnel.
- Ensuring adequate physician coverage to meet patient needs and assisting with the physician selection, recruiting, and retention activities of the organization.
- If nonphysician allied health care professionals are utilized in the practice, ensuring that their professional requirements are met and assisting in establishing their requisite protocols.
- Acting as principal liaison between the physician staff and the nonphysician administration and management.
- Facilitating professional and cordial relationships between the organization and other organizations such as HMOs and other payers.
- Establishing and maintaining relationships with outside physicians and provider groups, assisting in contracting for their services when advisable, and ensuring the quality of care of these outside providers.
- Providing regular input into the planning and resource allocation processes of the organization.
- Assisting in the monitoring and evaluation of all physicians and allied health care professionals for performance, compensation, and other purposes.
- Interacting with and responding to patient surveys and patient grievances regarding quality of care.

POLITICS

Because of constant interactions with physicians, many of whom may be partners or shareholders in the organization, the medical director must have a keen sensitivity to changing political scenarios. Besides cordial relationships with members of the executive committee or governing board of directors, the medical director must maintain a good rapport with department chairpersons and indeed all members of the physician staff, especially those with ownership interests.

In some organizations, the medical director is considered "just" an administrator and is not invited into the ownership circle. Exclusion from ownership is often rationalized as a means of keeping the medical director "out of politics" and therefore more objective in his or her dealings with physicians. The medical director, on the other hand, interprets this exclusion as an indication of the organization's valuation of administrative and management services—if not an indication of outright greed. This can create a mindset of "us and them" among physicians and administrators and thus interfere with the collaborative functioning of the practice.

Another argument for allowing the medical director a chance to acquire an ownership interest is that ownership provides the medical director the stature to deal with owner physicians as an equal. Indeed, many well-trained and qualified medical directors work in large organizations that provide stock options or similar access to equity and are reluctant to accept a position in an organization that does not provide such an incentive.

FAILURE

It should be obvious by now that the medical director's duties and responsibilities are formidable indeed. It is small wonder, then, that many fail and that the average time of service of a medical director with a particular organization is but a few years. Aside from the diverse areas of accountability, there are often significant differences in the problem-solving methodologies taught to managers and physicians.

Certainly there is a vast difference between the immediate response to problems surgeons are taught to have and the patient, collaborative, analytical response professional managers are taught to have. In a paper entitled "Why Physician Managers Fail," McCall and Clair (1990), of the University of Southern California Graduate School of Business Administration, state that "the doctor manager is the epitome of the oxymoron, for never in the history of language have two terms been so utterly opposed." The authors go on to list the 10 deadly flaws that cause physician managers to fail:

1. Insensitivity and arrogance
2. Inability to choose staff
3. Overmanaging (inability to delegate)
4. Inability to adapt to a superior
5. Fighting the wrong battles
6. Being seen as untrustworthy (having questionable motives)
7. Failing to develop a strategic vision
8. Being overwhelmed by the job
9. Lacking specific management skills or knowledge
10. Lacking commitment to the job (p. 9)

The above list can also be utilized for assessing the suitability of a prospective medical director. In understanding failure, the seeds for success often can be visualized and nurtured.

THE FUTURE

The position of medical director, so long a part of hospital organizations, has dramatically entered the ambulatory health care arena. The role, although rapidly evolving, is still somewhat confusing. But as time goes on the outlines of this new breed of health care executive are becoming more discernible. Armed with a recent advanced business degree and with good clinical credentials, the medical director can provide leadership and expertise and act as a liaison to all members of the ambulatory health care organization.

In a 1987 issue of *Healthcare Forum,* Mark Doyne concludes a discussion of the role of medical director by stating the following:

> Whether a hospital, an HMO or PPO, or a corporate giant, the healthcare provider that can forge meaningful and creative alliances with physicians will likely be numbered among the survivors in the competitive years ahead. Who better to serve as liaison, facilitator, communicator, negotiator between medical staff and management than one who understands both sides and speaks both languages? Neither faction can succeed without the other, therefore, new partnerships and collaborative efforts must be created.

REFERENCES

Doyne, M. 1987. Physicians as managers. *Healthcare Forum,* September-October.

Fine, A. 1990. New challenges for medical directors. *Physician Executive* 16 (March-April): 36–37.

Grebenschikoff, J., and Kirschman, D. 1989. Getting the third degree. *Physician Executive* 15 (March-April): 27–28.

McCall, M., and Clair, J. 1990. Why physician managers fail. *Physician Executive* 16 (May-June): 6–10.

McKhann, G. 1989. Clinical department director: Manager or scholar? *Annals of Neurology* 26 (December): 779–781.

Tabenkin, H., Zyzanski, S., and Alemagno, S. 1989. Physician managers: Personal characteristics versus institutional demands. *Health Care Management Review* 14, no. 2: 7–12.

5

Physician Recruitment

Mary Jo Littlefield and Steve Daily

WHY RECRUIT PHYSICIANS?

Most observers agree that in the cost-conscious decade to come, multispecialty medical groups will provide the most efficient and economically viable model for large-scale delivery of health care. At the same time, the wave of the future—and in some parts of the country, the present—is a rapid move away from fee-for-service payment systems and toward some type of capitation or discounted fee structure. Today, these two trends move forward in lock step: As more patients enroll in managed care plans, more physicians join multispecialty group practices.

From the viewpoint of administration, one primary consideration is a group's ability to provide the broadest possible range of services to an increasing patient base. As managed care enrollment increases, so does the importance and economic feasibility of offering additional medical specialties and services in house rather than utilizing outside contracted physicians, who generally charge the group on a fee-for-service basis. Controlling these outside referrals is extremely important to the financial viability of a group with a predominant prepaid practice. A major driving force behind physician recruitment, then, is simply this: In order to grow from a small, less efficient group practice to a large multispecialty ambulatory care provider, more doctors with a greater array of specialties must be brought on board.

A LITTLE BIT OF HISTORY

In mid-twentieth century America, physicians were at a premium in most parts of the country. When Dr. Jones completed his residency, he went to his friendly hometown banker and easily obtained enough credit to hang out his shingle as a private practitioner. The traditional fee-for-service payment system was the rule of the day. Doctors didn't move around much, tending to become fixtures of the community. In the medical world, the terms "competition" and "cost control" had not yet been heard.

Today, it's much more expensive to establish a private practice. Soaring malpractice rates, staff costs, physician time required for management tasks, intricate third-party payment systems—all these make going solo a daunting proposition for the young, freshly minted physician. Additionally, the availability of credit to young physicians to establish independent practices is now much more limited. Our late-twentieth century Dr. Jones has clear-cut options: Join a staff-model HMO, join a large medical group that contracts with HMOs, or join two or three established doctors in an existing practice. Even older physicians in fee-for-service private practice for years are not immune to the forces of the marketplace. Many of them are finding it necessary to join large groups, just like their young counterparts. All of this means that, as a group, physicians today are subject to the same kinds of forces that affect people in other walks of life; they have to job hunt. It is the task of the physician recruiter to find them, facilitate their hiring, and help retain them in their new positions.

WHOM TO RECRUIT

The physician candidate of today may well become the group's senior partner or major stockholder of tomorrow, so it behooves recruiters to evaluate candidates not only on their skills but also on their compatibility with other members of the group and with the group's long-term goals. In general, efforts of recruiters may be applied to two categories of candidates: physicians nearing completion of residency programs and physicians already in some form of practice.

Recruiting Residents

Many recruiters devote a large portion of their efforts to new doctors: senior residents just preparing to strike out on their own. Several studies indicate that the vast majority of residents finishing training will start out in a group or HMO. It is not surprising that this is so. The average debt of a new medical school graduate is considerable. Few have the resources or the credit to establish themselves in private practice. These "new generation" doctors are also looking for a more family-oriented and relaxed life style than their predecessors, a life style many will find difficult to achieve except in a large group practice. Practicing with others also provides young physicians with a continuation of the collegiality and support of other physicians they became comfortable with in their years of training.

Frequently, however, physicians directly out of training present difficulties to the recruiter and the group practice employer. In the first place, residency programs usually end in July, so if physicians are needed by a practice at other times on an urgent basis, a resident may not be a reasonable choice. For a fee-for-service practice, young residents may not have developed the "marketing" skills and self-confidence to attract and retain new patients. In the prepaid practice setting, a new doctor's insecurities may result in overutilization of expensive studies, unnecessary follow-ups, and lengthy patient visits. Excessive patient advocacy, together with rigid and overly stringent standards of care, can likewise be costly in prepaid medicine. Young physicians are also sometimes criticized by their older colleagues as not willing to put in the long hours of patient care that they originally had to expend to build the practice.

There are other difficulties in recruiting residents as well. Unless the recruiting group is located near a training center, is affiliated with it in some way, or already employs physicians with residency program contacts, recruiting residents can be a highly competitive endeavor. The very largest groups and HMOs, with their national advertising, slick brochures, and images of programmed financial security, seem to enjoy a significant edge. These large employers utilize numbers of professional recruiters. For a small or medium-sized practice to send a recruiter to distant locations or arrange for site visits for new physicians is usually prohibitively costly. Finishing residents receive many job offers and are often ambivalent and unrealistic in their expectations and desires, which presents further difficulties to the recruiter.

Recruiting Practicing Physicians

But residents aren't the only physicians available for recruitment. As noted above, many currently practicing doctors, including older physicians in small practices, are now entering the job market. These experienced doctors may be especially desirable for certain leadership positions, and they can often form the backbone of entire new departments. Personal and professional relationships with these physicians often facilitate their recruitment. Moreover, their expectations regarding compensation, work schedules, and benefits are often far more realistic than those of residents. They are usually experienced professionals who know how to do the job.

Difficulties in hiring practicing physicians, however, often arise in dealing with their existing office leases, equipment, and accounts receivable. They frequently are endowed with an entrepreneurial spirit that is difficult to quench in a large group setting; it is not easy for them to surrender control of staff and administration. And it can take many months of discussion and negotiation for them to decide to give up their private practice. Entering a prepaid environment for the first time, many find it difficult to abandon old habits of high utilization in favor of more cost-effective practice guidelines.

Recruiting Other Health Professionals

There exist many types of professionals who are playing an ever-expanding role in the provision of health care. For example, there are non-MD doctors such as chiropractors, optometrists, and podiatrists. There are also allied health professionals such as nurse practitioners, physician assistants, certified nurse midwives, and certified registered nurse anesthetists. With efforts at cost containment dictating work redesign for highly compensated MDs, these professionals are assuming increasing importance in group settings. A system of physician recruitment should include these highly skilled midlevel practitioners. The recruitment process is the same, and in some cases the services of these professionals are more difficult to obtain than the services of physicians.

WHEN TO RECRUIT

One of the earliest decision points in recruitment occurs when it is determined a physician is needed for the practice. In a fee-for-service setting, this point is generally reached when the work burden of the practice exceeds the time the existing physicians are willing to spend. Since acquiring a new physician necessarily produces a reduction in individual net income, the decision is largely an economic one. Retirement, death, and disability are, of course, other reasons for obtaining the services of new practitioners.

In a largely prepaid practice organization, the decision point for acquiring additional help is not as easily identified. One of the most objective ways to make this determination is by the measurement of access times. With more and more HMOs concerned with quality, assessing access times is often a requirement. These differ among the various HMOs and among the different specialties. In some fields such as neurology, an access time of six weeks for an elective consult might be reasonable, whereas in family practice an access time of three days might be considered too long. Access times, of course, vary from day to day, but if they consistently exceed established guidelines, additional physician help may be required.

Another area to monitor in a prepaid group practice is the number and cost of referrals to outside specialists. Obviously, if this cost exceeds the cost of hiring the requisite specialist, a recruitment effort may be indicated. Reliance on objective data in making recruitment decisions is extremely important. Otherwise, if the decision is left to department chairpersons, physicians may be recruited simply to fill out tight call schedules and with little regard to the financial impact on the entire organization. It must also be kept in mind that the average time needed to recruit and bring on board a new physician is 90–120 days. It is important to plan long range in the recruitment process.

HOW TO RECRUIT

There are two basic options available to the individual designated as the recruiter: (1) to utilize an outside agency that specializes in physician recruitment and (2) to build an in-house recruitment capability. Typically, growing medical groups start with the former and move to the latter as their needs and experience increase. But even when utilizing an outside agency, it is important to have one person designated as liaison with new and prospective staff members. Although that person can be a physician, as demand for new physicians increases, physician recruitment will become a full-time job.

Recruitment Agencies

Many physician search and consulting services offer professional resources for physician recruitment. There are two basic types of agencies: retained search and contingency recruiting. Both types are simple to use: All they need are the specific physician requirements of the practice.

With a retained search firm, a financial investment, in the form of a retainer fee, is necessary in advance, with the balance of the firm's fee due upon placement of the candidate. In utilizing a retained search firm, close inspection of the contract should be made prior to signing. Many such contracts have a clause stipulating that even if the physician is hired directly by the practice, and without help of the agency, the full placement fee to the agency must still be paid. With contingency recruiting, the agency's money, rather than the group's, is at risk. The full fee is due only upon placement of the candidate. Often, the payment schedule can be negotiated, for example, with one-third due upon signing the contract, one-third on the first day of employment, and the final third at the end of the first 30 days.

In a small group, only one physician at a time may be required. In that case, the stated commission rate would generally be paid. However, if a group needs five or ten physicians annually, a discounted commission structure can usually be negotiated. Most agencies charge a fee equal to 15 percent–30 percent of the physician's first-year compensation. A contract drawn at a commission rate of 10 percent, for example, can be proposed as a basis for agency negotiations. Some agencies may decline, but in the usually competitive recruitment market many agencies will work at a lower rate in exchange for volume.

In-House Recruitment

For large groups, it makes economic sense to institute in-house physician recruitment. Even if the recruitment function is brought in house, outside agencies may continue to be used as well, especially for the scarce specialties. For practical purposes, if a practice requires at least five new physicians a year, a part-time in-house recruiter should be considered. After that point, the benefits of creating such a position should greatly outweigh the costs.

Selecting an In-house Recruiter

The selection of an in-house recruiter of professional staff can make or break the program. In a very real sense, the recruiter's personality defines the program. It takes a special type of person to do the job effectively. An outgoing personality, the ability to establish rapport with physicians and their families, a willingness to take phone calls at home after office hours, and the organizational skills to keep track of many different leads at once are just a few of the attributes that the ideal in-house recruiter should possess. In order to evaluate the suitability of candidates and guide them through the interviewing process, the recruiter should be familiar with the personalities of the physicians in each department of the group.

In a large group setting, physician recruitment is more than a full-time job. Compensation for the in-house recruiter should be based on productivity, with a defined financial incentive to perform well and meet goals. The recruiter should report to the medical director regarding issues related to staffing needs and medical qualifications and to the chief executive officer regarding the negotiation of physician compensation and other contract terms.

THE RECRUITMENT PROCESS

Marketing to Physicians

Physician recruitment has many of the same elements as marketing. First, there is the need to reach prospective candidates and present the group's message to them in a way that makes them respond. There are a number of ways to do this, including targeted direct mail, journal advertising, attendance at professional association meetings and job fairs, and physician networking. Of these, targeted direct mail is the most aggressive and effective medium. Mailing lists are available for every major specialty and region of the United States.

Direct mail programs can be targeted in many directions. As a start, two major lists might be implemented. One would designate, by specialty, residents just beginning their third year of training, and the second would indicate established, practicing physicians. The choice of targets may also be influenced by the group's unique drawing cards. For example, if the group is located in the Sun Belt, a mailing might be sent to physicians in the northern tier of states in January, when they're susceptible to the lure of warm weather. All mail should be routed to home addresses. This is especially important in the case of doctors who are currently employed elsewhere, since discretion is an important part of an effective relationship with candidates.

An initial step is to develop a direct mail marketing piece. This "teaser" mailer should briefly inform the physician about practice opportunities, and invite a response via an attached business reply card. On the card, the candidate will be instructed to supply specific information about specialty, undergraduate education, medical school, dates of residency, years in practice, type of practice, and current medical license status in the state of the recruiting group. When responses are returned, they should be followed up with a glossy image brochure that might focus on both the high-tech professional aspects of the practice and the equally important family and life-style issues, together with a professional staff application. Also included in this second mailing might be a benefit sheet and a cover letter from the medical director. Splitting the mailings into two phases ensures that the candidates who receive the more expensive package of detailed information are well qualified and are indeed looking for a position.

Responding to Inquiries

When responses to the teaser mailing are returned, the recruiter, medical director, and department chairperson can select likely prospects based on the furnished information. The criteria for determining the priority of a prospect vary on a case-by-case basis, but every inquiry should get a personal letter from the medical director. If the group cannot place a candidate at the time, he or she should be politely informed that the particular position has been filled.

Credentialing

A system for checking credentials is crucial to the recruitment process. After the formal application is returned, the candidate's state license, DEA, references, and residency training must be verified before an interview takes place. If board certification is required, that too should be verified prior to spending time and money on interviewing.

Building Rapport

After the initial credentialing process, the recruiter should call the candidate to set up a mutually convenient time to come to the facility for a tour and an interview. This may involve a trip, with expenses for plane fares and overnight accommodations.

This type of call is best made to the candidate's home rather than the office, where sensitive conversations can be overheard. It is especially valuable in finding out about the candidate's personality, family, and life style. The goal is to establish a warm, friendly, and comfortable relationship between the recruiter and the candidate. It should be kept in mind that not just the candidate but the entire family unit, with all of its various agendas, is being recruited. The everyday concerns of the spouse and children will play a major role in the physician's decision to accept or decline a contract offer. To build rapport, the recruiter should have a good grasp of these concerns. Where will the family live? Where will the children go to school? What are the recreational and shopping opportunities? The spouse may also have a career and be interested in employment opportunities.

Interviewing and Evaluating Candidates

The most crucial phase of the courtship is the actual face-to-face interview. The recruiter should act as guide for out-of-towners and as official escort for all candidates. This includes coordinating interviews with the medical director, department chairperson, and administration representative, taking the candidate and spouse on a tour of local attractions, and investigating housing options.

The candidate will get a great deal of salient information during that first site visit—available benefits, compensation levels according to specialty, availability of partnership or stock options—and a good grasp of what working at the facility will be like. The majority of the information should come from the recruiter. In particular, the recruiter, with support from the CEO, should be the only person to discuss compensation with the candidate. This minimizes later misunderstandings regarding crucial monetary issues or ownership opportunities. During the interview day, the recruiter will guide the candidate from one interview to another and will check back with the interviewing team for their appraisals before the candidate leaves the premises to determine whether an offer should be made. The recruitment team, including the recruiter, medical director, department chairperson, and administration representative, must accurately evaluate the candidate's clinical skills, interpersonal skills, and team attitude.

Making an Offer and Getting Acquainted

In most organizations, the medical director has the final word on a candidate's suitability and should inform the recruiter whether to make a contract offer. The recruiter should have a contract ready in case an offer is made. The principle of closing the sale is much the same here as it is in an automobile showroom: The desirable candidate should not be allowed to leave the premises without a contract in hand. Putting a time limit on the duration of the contract offer ensures a timely response.

It is at this point that the recruiter should urge the candidate to call him or her at home if there are any questions. If the recruiter has performed well and established a relationship with the candidate, the candidate will call. The recruiter represents the organization and should be approachable, easy to talk with, understanding, and helpful. If the candidate feels comfortable with the recruiter, there may be several phone calls before signing.

The candidate's spouse might not participate in the first visit, allowing the candidate to concentrate on the interview. Once a contract has been offered, the candidate may then want to return with the spouse and together investigate the housing market and check out educational opportunities for the children. Once a contract offer has been made, it is very helpful to invite the candidate and spouse to dinner with a member of the department. If the interviewing physician has not previously met the candidate, the recruiter should also be present at the dinner. Social contact with prospective colleagues in the department will encourage acceptance of the offer and help the candidate and family to adjust to their new surroundings more quickly. If the candidate declines the contract offer, then the response should be supportive and professional. The candidate may have another offer, and a supportive response leaves the door open to renewed negotiation if the other offer falls through.

Signing the Contract: It's Only the Beginning

For most salespeople, a signed contract signifies the job is done. But in physician recruitment, when a candidate physician accepts a contract, the paperwork is just beginning. The paper trail starts with the signing of the contract. Additional credentialing, as well as additional personnel forms, must be completed. The appropriate staff members must be notified of the new physician's arrival so that space is available and appointments are made. Since recruitment is national in scope, many candidates are from out of town. Over the weeks or months that elapse between the first interview and the physician's first day at the group, the recruiter should stay in touch by telephone, smoothing the transition by acting as a friend and helpful resource for both physician and family.

When the new physician arrives to begin work, an orientation program should be provided. The orientation should give the physician the opportunity to learn the history of the practice, discuss the particulars of the benefit package, and meet the key administrative people as well as fellow physicians.

Follow-Up and Physician Relations

During and after the orientation period, the recruiter should follow up to make sure the doctor and family adjust to their new environment with a minimum of problems and should also continue to be a resource for any concerns that may arise. Large groups frequently have a physician advisory committee to help with ongoing physician relations. Whether utilizing agencies or recruiting in house, physician recruitment is a very expensive and time-consuming process. Retention of these professionals is extremely important for economic reasons as well as for good patient relations. Discussions of practice problems between the newly hired physician, his or her colleagues, and high-level administrators should be facilitated.

CONCLUSION

How the process of physician recruitment is managed depends in large part on the size of the organization and its rate of growth. But unquestionably the process of finding, attracting, and retaining quality physicians and other professional staff will continue to be of primary importance in the group practice environment. Quite simply, the handling of physician recruitment issues will help determine the composition and character of the group for years to come.

6

Physician Compensation

Susan Cejka

Physician compensation continues to be one of the most hotly debated topics in group practice. The changes in health care economics over the last 20 to 30 years have only exacerbated the controversy. The growth of subspecialty medicine, the proliferation of third-party payment mechanisms, and the variations in practice style all have contributed to obsolete compensation plans. In a relatively short period, physician practices, which used to be mostly simple businesses dominated by solo practitioners, have evolved into complex, often unpredictable corporate entities.

The object of this chapter is to bring order to the current debate about compensation alternatives. It provides a framework for analyzing an existing plan and developing a compensation plan that meets the test of fairness and appropriateness. The chapter is divided into four major areas of discussion:

1. the goals and limitations of compensation plans
2. the role of strategic planning in developing a compensation plan
3. key issues in evaluating compensation plan alternatives
4. managing a compensation plan review

THE GOALS AND LIMITATIONS OF COMPENSATION PLANS

Before sorting out the issues, it should be understood that there is no perfect compensation plan. All plans, no matter how carefully crafted, include biases that favor one physician or specialty over another. This is true of all group practice environments. Each organization makes decisions that reflect its own biases by the manner in which terms are defined, policies are structured, and rules for administering the plan are set. The key to developing a successful compensation plan is to understand how the biases that are selected impact physicians and the group practice competitiveness and to ensure that the biases do not impede the achievement of long-term goals.

The terms *fairness* and *appropriateness* will be used frequently in this chapter with regard to compensation plans. *Fairness,* in this context, relates to the rewarding of physicians financially in accordance with their contribution to the organization's success. This contribution may be measured in a variety of ways, including production, efficiency, good citizenship, administrative effort, or any other trait the group values. *Appropriateness* refers to the alignment of the compensation plan with the goals of the organization and with the types of revenue coming into the group. If a plan does not meet the test of appropriateness, then its fairness is only academic, since the long-term success of the clinic will be in jeopardy.

Compensation plans are not static documents. Changes in the marketplace, technology, and group size and mix all generate a need to review and revise the compensation plan recommended. Therefore, developing and maintaining a "good" compensation plan is an ongoing process. The process should facilitate discussion and education regarding compensation issues and alternatives as well as improve overall group financial performance. A successful group makes frequent although incremental changes to the compensation plan to reflect changes in its strategic plan and the health care environment.

The compensation plan must be easily understood. This means as few "moving parts" as possible and simple, direct calculations. The compensation plan is meant to motivate behavior. If the plan is so complex that few physicians can understand how the algorithm works, then there is little chance the plan will have this effect. Typically, plans become complicated in the name of fairness, but it is hardly fair to anyone if the average physician cannot predict and/or understand how actions relate to income.

Finally, physicians exhibit great concern over the way the pie is divided. More often, the problem is the size of the pie. No matter how fair or simple a compensation plan is made to be, if the total distributable dollars are not sufficient to allow physicians to meet their personal income targets through hard work and responsible behavior, they will soon be heard from.

The ability of the group to achieve long-range goals and objectives is inextricably linked to the structure and content of the compensation plan. Compensation issues will play a significant role in how involved the physicians become in group practice issues and in implementing key strategies. The compensation plan can motivate physicians to work toward the common goals of the group, modify physician behavior with regard to practice style and efficiency, and increase communication flow among the specialties. A compensation plan can build group culture; but, more realistically, it can shape or influence group culture.

Although the method a group uses to determine income is important, the plan itself cannot be expected to be a substitute for strong group leadership and a consistent management team. It does not replace culture, values, or morals, although it may affect them. The compensation plan cannot make a physician practice "good" or "bad" medicine. It does not replace long-range planning or the institutional mission. The plan cannot make everyone equal; it cannot erase inequities between specialties that have existed for many years. Finally, the compensation plan will not cause or cure a serious case of terminal greed.

In the aggregate, the primary objectives of the compensation plan should be as follows:

1. The compensation plan should enhance the ability of the organization to achieve its long-term goals. Specifically, it should function
   - to ensure the financial viability of the practice (this includes a defined program to retain earnings)
   - to promote harmony within the group
   - to take account of the competitive environment of the practice
   - to enhance the organizational environment of the practice
   - to enhance the organization's ability to recruit and retain physicians
   - to encourage the efficient and effective practice of medicine
2. The compensation plan should also distribute available cash fairly and appropriately. Specifically, it should
   - distribute income in accordance with effort and contribution to the practice
   - distribute cash in accordance with the sources of revenue flowing into the organization
   - take adequate account of the built-in biases
   - be simple to understand

THE ROLE OF STRATEGIC PLANNING

The three most common problems found in existing compensation plans are unnecessary complexity, misalignment with long-term goals, and rigidity. As discussed above, the major benefit of a well-designed plan is that it motivates desired behavior. When a compensation plan is so complex that physicians are unable to determine how specific actions will impact compensation, this benefit is lost.

Complexity is frequently related to weak group leadership, the absence of a strategic plan, conflicting long-term goals, or a cultural bias toward making special deals as a way of placating the most vocal members of the group. Misalignment with long-term goals is often related to the evolutionary nature of compensation plans and the lack of a structured planning process. Finally, many plans eventually become rigid because compensation debates in group practice tend to revolve around subjective assessments of the value of each specialty rather than more objective issues such as achievement of group goals and the motivation of desired behavior. A formal strategic planning process that includes review of the compensation plan issues will lead to a more simplified plan, alignment with group goals, and a more flexible approach to compensation issues.

The first step in ensuring that the compensation plan works in concert with the strategic plan is to review the organization's long-term goals and identify the behaviors required to achieve the desired outcomes. The annual strategic plan review should also include a review of the key policies and provisions of the compensation plan to determine if the two plans are in harmony.

The ability of the compensation plan to accommodate changing reimbursement patterns has become one of the most critical issues in compensation plan discussions today. In this regard, it is essential that the distribution methodology reflects the various types of revenue that flow into the organization. Fee-for-service revenue varies with the volume of services provided and the charge structure of the practice. Conversely, prepaid revenue is a fixed stream of revenue that is designed to cover a predicated level and scope of service for a given population. Motivating physicians to increase service volume within a prepaid charge structure will eventually lead to financial losses.

Table 6-1 provides some examples of how the compensation plan might be structured to support typical group practice goals.

Table 6-1 Compensation Plan Structured To Support Group Practice

If the Goal Is . . .	The Compensation Plan Should . . .
To be the top-quality provider, dominant in the area	Result in income levels that attract and retain the highest quality physicians
To encourage collegiality	Pay for good citizenship, maintaining open communication, and teamwork (this typically implies discretionary bonuses)
To be the managed care leader	Motivate increased capacity, manage for quality outcomes, and regulate the use of outside services (the plan must recognize physicians who manage care appropriately)
To be the low-cost provider	Motivate efficiency and cost control (full cost accounting is required)
To grow rapidly	Stimulate productivity, but not pay out all net income (funds are needed for growth, which requires, in effect, a retained earnings policy)
To diversify the practice	Pay to attract physicians of different specialties capable of working together and building departments (the plan must balance teamwork and individuality)

It is important to review the organizational goals to eliminate any conflicting goals. A poorly drafted or out-of-date compensation plan can undermine the financial stability of the organization. Symptoms of a compensation plan that no longer supports the strategic plan are listed in Table 6-2.

Any of these issues should raise a flag about the fairness and appropriateness of the current compensation plan.

A final point to remember when reviewing the existing plan for fairness and appropriateness is that all compensation plans contain subsidies. Subsidies are neither good nor bad but simply a fact. The key to designing fair subsidies is to understand the goal of the subsidy and to ensure each subsidy is in agreement with the overall culture and goals of the group. Some accepted ways of paying subsidies are given in Table 6-3.

The key to developing a fair and appropriate compensation plan is to make conscious, informed choices. The level of trust and open communication among physician leaders sets the tone for examining the issues. Success is enhanced if the group appoints a compensation review team that includes a wide spectrum of views.

COMPENSATION PLAN ALTERNATIVES

Most compensation plans today are based on one of three major compensation philosophies:

1. Production Formulas
   - Individual production formulas are designed to reward physicians in direct relationship to the revenue they produce.
   - Equal share formulas split the excess of revenue over expenses among the group members evenly. These plans are designed to build group culture, values, and teamwork.
2. Salary Formulas
   - Indexed salary plans rely on comparisons to standard benchmarks for a prescribed scope of work, with annual increases linked to merit or time of service.
   - Market-based salary and bonus plans seek to balance the stability of a salary with incentive payments to stimulate desired behaviors. The plans often include some elements of a production formula.
3. Capitation Formulas
   - Capitation formulas assign the responsibilities associated with meeting the goals of managed care contracts to the physicians directly.
   - Gatekeeper formulas assign the main task of managing care to the primary care providers.

Table 6-2 Symptoms of a Failing Compensation Plan

Issues	Possible Areas of Concern
The practice continually needs to borrow to cover operating deficits.	There is a fixed payout percentage without overhead incurred. There is no cost accounting for compensation or management of resource utilization. A production-based compensation formula is being used in a fixed revenue environment. The plan has not kept up with changes in payment sources.
Physician turnover is increasing.	Compensation is not competitive. The pay plan discriminates against particular specialties. The culture is undermined by the pay plan.
The practice is unable to recruit the quality and quantity of physicians needed to meet demand for services.	Compensation is not competitive. The plan is complex and not easily understood. The link between effort and compensation is unclear. The group is not clear about goals.
Arguments among physicians are frequent and heated. Disputes may revolve around the use of resources, time off, referral patterns, call coverage, etc.	Biases and subsidies have resulted in physicians exploiting the system. The goals of the organization have not been clearly discussed and integrated into the plan. There is no accountability for costs incurred by individuals.
Overhead appears to be uncontrollable.	There are hidden subsidies. There is no accountability for costs incurred. There are too many special deals. The organization's long-term goals are unclear. Growth is uncontrolled.
Physicians have become apathetic and do not take part in clinic meetings and decision processes.	The plan is not clearly understood. The plan is not perceived to be fair or appropriate. The goals of the organization are unclear. Special deals are made outside the context of the plan.
There is increasing pressure on the administrator to craft special deals.	The plan is too complex. The plan is not fair. The goals of the organization are not understood.

Table 6-3 Accepted Methods of Paying Subsidies

Goal	Subsidy Mechanism
To lessen the overhead burden on specialties with lower charge structures	Application of one overhead percent to all or allocation of overhead on the basis of revenue as a percentage of total revenue
	Some portion of equal share compensation
	Retain earnings based on revenue percentage
To give support to producers who carry significant discounts and allowances	Share in the discounts and allowances equally
To support physicians who handle large amounts of charity care	Share in bad debt equally
To show appreciation for longstanding members of the practice	Seniority pay
	Age-related adjustments to call schedule
	Equal share salary
	Guaranteed minimum salary
	Additional paid vacation tied to years of service
	Sabbatical policies
To encourage physician participation in administrative affairs	Hourly rate or annual salary compensation for administrative time

- Department or individual capitation formulas assign a specific scope of risk to each physician involved in the delivery of care.

While each methodology in its purest form was designed to meet the needs of specific practice settings, today there are numerous variations and permutations of each. In a fee-for-service environment, production-based formulas are most prevalent and appropriate. A salary and bonus system, which is heavily influenced by production, can also be successfully used in a fee-for-service environment.

As discounted medicine and prepaid care contracts increase, salary systems and capitation formulas are essential to ensure financial stability. In the prepaid environment, the goal is to encourage physicians to move beyond the standard provision of medical services toward managing the use of physician services and health care resources, including hospitalization, ancillary services, and specialty and subspecialty services outside the practice group.

Production Formulas

Production formulas have their roots in the solo practice arena, where each physician is an entrepreneur managing his or her own small business. The net practice income (excess of revenue over the expenses associated with running the practice) is exactly what the physician receives in compensation. The higher the collections and the lower the expenses, the greater the level of earned compensation.

The individual production formula is suitable not only for solo practice but also for multispecialty groups with a large fee-for-service revenue base. In a group setting, each physician is compensated on the basis of individual production. Any physician capable of generating a larger revenue base is compensated accordingly.

The benefits of using an individual production formula are as follows:

- Physicians are most familiar with this system of compensation and understand what is required to achieve the desired level of income.
- It keeps physicians focused on productivity and meeting the demand for service.
- It accommodates life-style choices. The trade-off of time for income is clearly understood and the formula allows individual decision.
- It can be customized for variations in practice style through cost accounting. If a physician needs more space or technical staff to support the practice, cost accounting allows this choice without penalizing others in the group.
- It is flexible and can be adopted to support the organizational goals by assigning a production credit to each activity that the group wishes to encourage.

On the downside, the individual production formula is criticized for the following shortcomings:

- It may not promote group culture and communication.
- The lower income producers are subsidized and higher earners are penalized if cost accounting is not used.
- Overhead costs may rise out of proportion if some form of accountability is not applied.

Variations in production formulas typically result from the way revenue and expenses are defined. Income to physician shareholders should be determined in the manner outlined in Exhibit 6-1.

Exhibit 6-1 Income to Physician Shareholders

Gross revenue (or bookings) less discounts and allowances = net collections

Net collections less direct and indirect expenses = net operating income

Net operating income less retained earnings = distributable income

Although most compensation discussions revolve around ways to divide the distributable income, groups are advised to focus first on understanding revenue and expense issues and to discuss the importance of retained earnings in achieving long-term goals.

Revenue Issues in a Production Formula Environment

Revenue, in a production formula, is appropriately defined as net cash collection *after* discounts and allowances have been subtracted. It is inappropriate to pay physicians based on bookings or charges. In today's environment discounts and allowances are too significant. Determining physician compensation on bookings alone can result in paying out substantially more than is actually collected by the practice. Payment to physicians should be made only after the collection effort is completed.

Bad debt can be handled as either an adjustment to revenue for the individual physician, similar to discounts and allowances, or as an overhead expense item. The argument for treating bad debt as an adjustment to revenue is that each physician has an impact on uncollectible accounts and should be responsible for the first-line collection efforts. By assigning bad debt as an adjustment to the revenue stream, physicians are motivated to work for a better collection rate.

Those who prefer to treat bad debt as an overhead expense point to the fact that patient and third-party payments are applied in the business office to outstanding accounts according to a policy that maximizes group collections. The individual physician has little to say about this policy. Likewise, if the group has a goal of providing a certain level of charity care, bad debt expense is typically dealt with by the group and is treated as an overhead expense. Bad debt may be handled as a strategic or operational issue. Either method is technically correct, although the former is more expensive in bookkeeping and accounting time.

Expense Issues in a Production Formula Environment

On the expense side, there are also choices that impact individual income in a production formula compensation plan. The simplest way to share expenses is to apply a standard overhead percentage to all production. This method results in the higher producers paying a larger dollar amount of the overhead, which may or may not be in accordance with usage. As the levels of production diverge, the inequities grow. What is gained in simplicity is lost in fairness, causing many groups to turn to cost accounting.

Cost accounting principles hold that each physician should bear the burden of the expenses over which he or she exercises control. There are many choices to be made in determining how to assign costs fairly. The discussion here is limited to simple departmental accounting of direct costs and three methods of handling indirect costs. Direct costs are defined here as those expenses that can be traced directly to the delivery of a unit of service or that are controlled by the individual physician in the practice setting. Indirect expenses are those costs that cannot be traced to a unit of service or physician but are required for the operation of the practice. Examples of direct and indirect expenses include the following:

1. direct expenses
   - nursing and physician assistant salaries and benefits
   - office and examining room space
   - medical supplies and drugs dispensed
   - marketing or advertising directed to individual physicians or specialties
   - equipment
   - professional liability expenses
2. indirect expenses
   - practice administration expenses
   - business office expenses
   - data processing
   - general insurance expenses
   - building occupancy expenses
   - legal, accounting, and purchased services
   - equipment repair
   - recruiting and training
   - general marketing

Direct expenses are either assigned to the department and shared equally among the physicians or are assigned directly to individual physicians. The decision to track by department versus the individual physician is usually made based on (1) the group's ability to identify the costs by individual and (2) the expense of implementing a more precise accounting mechanism.

One of the more recent controversial issues in regard to direct costs is when and how to account for physician extender revenue and expenses. The term *physician extender* refers to those professionals who perform services under physician responsibility such as physician assistants, nurse practitioners, nurse midwives, and certified nurse anesthetists. Although groups vary greatly in their approach to using physician extenders, the accounting rule of thumb is that if the revenue generated by the extender is credited to the physician, then the total cost of that extender must also be assigned to the physician. In this matching of revenue with expenses, the total cost of the extender includes the salary, benefits, supplies, space, and overhead associated with the revenue produced by the extender.

Additional controversy exists regarding the allocation of indirect expenses. The simplest method of handling indirect expenses is to allocate total indirect expense on the basis of the percentage of net collections accrued to each department or physician. Use of this method may result in the high producer carrying a disproportionate share of the indirect overhead. However, this bias is lessened to the degree that direct costs have been identified and properly assigned.

Another method of allocating indirect overhead is to identify the fixed portion of indirect overhead (e.g., the administrator's salary, building rental, etc.) and share this portion equally among the physicians. The remaining overhead is considered to be the variable portion and is allocated on the basis of net collection percentage. Although this method lessens the burden carried by the higher earners, some groups feel this begins to erode the practice culture.

Still another method of allocating indirect overhead is to aggregate costs into separate pools on the basis of head counts, patient visits, invoices generated, procedures completed, and so on. Each pool of overhead expense is then allocated to the appropriate department or physician based on the accepted "use" assumption. Naturally, this method is more precise, but ease in computation and simplicity are traded away. Cost accounting methodology itself is very complex and expensive. It can be easily extended to the point of absurdity, by applying it, for example, to patient parking and other questionable areas.

Before turning to equal share formulas, there is one final divisive issue to consider in deciding upon a methodology for allocating practice expenses. Many surgeons and subspecialists with high procedure fees and low office volume feel their expense allocations should be low, since much of their work is hospital-based and does not increase group expenses. On the other hand, primary care physicians, especially family practitioners and general internists, feel their own expenses should be shared by surgeons, since their productivity is what generates the surgical cases. This array of potential conflicts, many on a very emotional level, makes the use of production formulas anything but simple.

Equal Share Formula

An equal share formula is a variation of the production formula. Distributable income, as calculated above, is divided equally among the shareholders. Revenue is defined as the net collections of the practice; expenses are subtracted from the net collections to arrive at the distributable income. This method of determining physician compensation is typically found in small single-specialty groups where the culture, values, and scope of practice are similar. The primary motivation for the equal share formula is to build group cohesiveness and promote the steady growth of the practice in a market where demand exceeds supply.

The major risk associated with this formula is that, over time, differences in scope of practice and life-style needs grow and the variations in production become material. The production issue is often camouflaged in discussions of subspecialization, life-style needs, or call coverage. Typically, the problem is exacerbated when there is a large difference in the ages of the partners or when several physicians are nearing retirement at the same time.

A group adopting an equal share compensation formula must develop policies addressing seniority, contributions to administrative work, vacation time, call coverage, and subspecialization. More than any other system, this methodology demands strong group culture and trust among the partners. A periodic review of common understandings is just as important for this system as it is for the more complex systems.

Production Formula Limitations

Production formulas are appropriate for distributing income on fee-for-service revenue in both single-specialty and multispecialty settings. However, in the current environment, where the shift of payment is moving steadily away from fee-for-service to prepaid revenue associated with managed care plans, organizations must be aware of the problems a production formula can create.

When a group begins to take on prepaid contractual obligations, a production formula becomes a serious liability because it motivates the wrong behavior. It motivates physicians to increase production by increasing patient visits and performing a large number of costly procedures rather than managing care for the appropriate level of use. When a production formula is used in a prepaid environment, the physician who benefits is the one who most actively works against the spirit of the prepaid agreement, thereby creating a shift of income away from the cooperative physician. This can result in a substantial increase in overhead or a need to shift patients to urgent care centers. The group might also find it has inadequate capacity to meet the terms of the contractual agreement. Physician compensation under a managed care contract is appropriately determined by either a salary or capitation formula.

Finally, when a group has a production formula in effect, any review of the formula should including the following:

1. A complete examination of the sources of revenue and expenses. Verify that compensation decisions are based on actual cash collected. Do not use bookings as a means of determining compensation.
2. A review of the handling of expense allocation and an evaluation of the alternative methods for allocating both direct and indirect expenses. Use actual expenses to determine compensation. Do not use a fixed payout percentage in the compensation formula.
3. A review of managed care obligations. As managed care revenue increases as a percentage of total revenue, the group must begin to move away from production formulas and instead pay physicians for the work associated with the prepaid contracts.

Salary Formulas

Salary-based compensation systems are found in small and large practice settings and can be structured to respond to fee-for-service and prepaid revenue streams. The major advantage of a salary and bonus system is that is can be crafted to reflect the specific goals, culture, and values of the group.

On the downside, salary and bonus compensation plans are more difficult to manage. The subjective nature of these plans may be cause for considerable debate and manipulation. A strong department structure and stable, trusted leadership are prerequisites for success. Management of physician productivity, efficiency, and effectiveness is a major issue under this form of compensation.

Salary systems typically fall into one of three major categories: straight salary, salary with production bonus, and salary with discretionary or merit bonus. Bonuses need not be monetary. In many groups, they take the form of stock or stock options, partnership shares or other equity, or a combination of these elements. Base salary may be set using numerous criteria, but it is typically related to (1) market rates by specialty, (2) expected productivity, and/or (3) equal share.

Bonuses can take numerous forms. A production bonus is typically associated with individual or department net collections or is related to achieving specific targets in the following categories:

- hours of clinical availability
- visits per patient per year

- average ancillary charge
- procedures performed
- patient visits per time period
- average charge per visit
- hospital consults
- management of hospital length of stay

Other bonus criteria frequently used for a discretionary bonus include the following:

- patient management
- efficient use of referral resources
- good citizenship and committee participation
- administrative contribution
- seniority
- profitability
- patient satisfaction
- physician peer group rating

When several different factors are used to determine the bonus portion of compensation, a point system is the most objective method. The group goals should be used as the foundation for designing the point system, with qualitative factors accounting for no more than 10 percent of total pay.

Although salary and bonus systems are the most flexible form of compensation, the key factors for successfully developing and administering a salary compensation system include a strong organizational culture and strong leadership. The group must have

- a clear understanding of and agreement on a limited number of goals
- a stable, educated leadership
- a system for managing physicians (typically a departmental structure with clear lines of task assignment and authority) and a strong medical director
- a predetermined evaluation criteria for physicians
- an individual or office with the responsibility to administer the compensation plan

Trust, clear lines of communication, and a structured decision-making process are essential for administering salary and bonus compensation plans. The ultimate decision making often rests with one person or a very small executive team. Ideally, this compensation committee should review the performance of all physicians in the group and match it with the previously established performance criteria. Careful attention should be given to the opinions of the pertinent department chairpersons in this process, since it is sometimes difficult for the chairpersons to manage day-to-day operations without this leverage. As the group practice increases in size, the departmental leadership becomes critical to the successful administration of a salary system. The above factors are the keys to success whether the salary system includes production bonuses, discretionary or merit bonuses, or simply straight salaries.

Typically, the group practice with a successful salary system has a corporate culture dominated by the founder or is motivated by a clearly defined institutional mission.

Although salary and bonus systems address many of the problems associated with physician compensation in group practice settings, there are still issues that must be monitored and evaluated in any review of the compensation plan. For example, the compensation plan should

- enhance physician productivity
- optimize the use of resources
- identify the optimal point for adding to the physician staff
- build leadership ability within the organization to accommodate future needs

Nevertheless, a well-administered salary system with a review process and proper incentive bonuses is generally considered ideal for most multispecialty groups if they receive any significant percentage of revenue from prepaid capitation.

Capitation Formulas

In response to the growing volume of managed care systems, capitation as a method of compensating physicians has also evolved. A capitation system compensates the physician for both managing care and providing direct patient services. In general, under a capitation compensation plan, the physician receives a fixed sum of money, on a monthly basis, for each patient under the physician's care. The monthly payment is computed actuarially, based on specialty, the expected use of a defined scope of services, information relating to patient age and sex, and the area's prevailing charges. The physician agrees to accept the capitation payment for providing and managing health care for a defined period of time.

In many respects, the capitation payment is comparable to net collections in a production-based compensation system. Revenue is generated against which the physician or practice incurs the costs of providing services. The more patients under a physician's care, the greater the revenue received. Whether to cost account or pool expenses is decided on the same basis as is used for production compensation plans. Direct costs are allocated to the individual physician and indirect costs are shared on the basis of revenue received as a percentage of the total or a general overhead percentage is applied to all physicians.

A key difference between fee-for-service collections and capitation payment is the scope of service the physician is responsible for providing. Fee-for-service collections represent payment for services rendered at a given point in time. Capitation is payment for physician management of patient health care needs, including evaluation of the most efficient and effective combination of treatment and services, provision of those treatments and services as appropriate, and coordination with another physician when referral is required.

Using a production incentive compensation formula in a prepaid environment will encourage the physician to be less concerned about the appropriateness of the levels of health care services provided. The production formula will reward a physician for upcoding or churning patients and performing unnecessary procedures, which can lead to financial losses in a prepaid environment.

Additionally, a production formula in a prepaid practice will ultimately result in "crowding out" of fee-for-service patients, because the prepaid patients will be spurred to consume as much medical care as possible (see Chapter 7).

The major risks for managing patients in a capitation compensation system are borne by the total group. In the aggregate, the group must be able to

- manage patient demand so it is appropriate for the level of prepaid revenue
- control patient dumping through a carefully designed set of medical policies and protocols, a strong utilization review process, and a quality assurance committee charged with evaluating patient outcomes and issues
- negotiate with providers of services not available inside the practice to provide these services at a reasonable cost
- manage the use of outside physicians and ancillary services
- control the use of hospital services

Two basic types of capitation compensation systems are in operation today: The gatekeeper system and capitation by specialty. In the gatekeeper system, the primary care physician receives the full professional capitation payment and is responsible for providing or subcontracting all of the professional services needed by the patient. The gatekeeper capitation rate, in addition to covering primary care services, typically will cover all ancillary services, all specialty and surgical services, and hospital consults. The primary care physician becomes a gatekeeper who must sometimes focus on the management of other health care providers. Groups with effective gatekeeper systems have developed extensive protocols and utilization review systems to keep patient care moving smoothly between the primary care provider and specialty physicians.

Capitation by specialty, within a group practice, can take the form of individual capitation or departmental capitation depending on the patient base to which the capitation payments are applied. The key to success in this form of capitation compensation is clear definition of medical policies, procedures, and protocols relating to specific situations and referrals between specialities. Specialty capitation will vary from group to group depending on the population enrolled, the economics of the market, and the scope of services covered. Each group must define what it believes to be the appropriate timing and conditions for a handoff between physicians in order to avoid patient dumping and disputes over patient care. Utilization review and quality assurance committees must meet frequently to address individual situations that are not clearly covered by established medical protocols.

In any capitation system, the cost of referrals to physicians outside the group becomes a major potential liability to the group. Volume, cost, and quality of outside services must be monitored closely to control the impact on the group's financial performance. The selection of competent providers, access to services in a timely manner, and quality outcomes are important goals to achieve if a capitation system is to work efficiently. Access to services can become an issue if the group has a cumbersome utilization review process or insufficient physician resources to meet normal demand.

Most capitation compensation plans include bonus pool payments to physicians who manage care efficiently and effectively. In addition, the hospital risk pool payment is a bonus given to those physicians who have managed hospital stays with efficiency and have had positive outcomes. Bonus pools may also be used to achieve other goals such as committee participation, administrative contributions, and patient satisfaction.

A capitation compensation plan benefits groups with a substantial prepaid revenue in the following manner:

- The plan keeps physicians focused on group goals. Servicing managed care contracts requires coordination.
- The plan assigns risk to those who can best control it. Physicians are at financial risk for managing service delivery appropriately.
- The plan eliminates churning and upcharging, two behaviors that undermine the success of managed care contracts in other modes of compensation.
- Departments are given an incentive to take an active role in defining and rewarding standards of care and high-quality medical results.
- The plan is a production-based system with regard to panel size. Physicians understand production-based compensation and quickly adapt to this new twist on the old philosophy of pay for effort.

- Physicians are motivated to devote a maximum amount of time to treating and monitoring patients with real medical needs.

As might be expected, capitation plans are not without risk. A group practice must be prepared to assess and control a number of risks when this compensation methodology is accepted, which include the following:

- Inequities among physicians may materialize if the panel of patients is too small to project accurate capitation rates.
- If the practice does not have access to accurate production data, developing capitation rates will be costly and may require several adjustments in the early years of the plan. This may undermine group harmony if not understood at the outset.
- Physicians who are unwilling to accept risk or take an active role in educating patients about managed care services may leave the group if a capitation plan is implemented.
- If the group culture is not strongly biased toward quality issues and patient satisfaction, access and quality problems will increase.
- Without control over practice resources, physicians may be frustrated in their attempts to structure their time for maximum return. Cost accounting is essential in a capitation plan designed to deliver cost-efficient service.

Both gatekeeper and specialty capitation plans are successfully in operation in practices throughout the country. However, as with production-based and salary-based plans, there is no "canned model" that may be purchased and installed effortlessly. Each group must work through the issues in a structured process in order to adapt the basic capitation model to its goals, cultures, and specialty mix. The process is neither quick nor without pain, but the outcome is an efficient, financially sound organization with physicians and group practice goals closely aligned.

COMPENSATION PLAN REVIEW

Annual Review

The annual review is a minor review and has a limited scope. The object is to make certain that small problems do not go unresolved. Its purpose is similar to an annual physical. Typically, the outcome is peace of mind, but occasionally a problem is identified at the early stages of development.

1. Objectives
   - Confirm the plan is aligned with practice's long-term goals.
   - Make minor technical adjustments to the plan, as appropriate.
2. Scope
   - Review the long-term goals.
   - Review average compensation by specialty to ensure competitiveness.
   - Review individual outliers to ensure fairness.
   - Review practice financial issues.
   - Make technical adjustments, as appropriate.
3. Review Process
   - Institute a review team of three or four key physician leaders.
   - Hold two or three short focused meetings.
   - Issue a summary report to shareholders.

Major Review

The major review is a significant intervention and must be managed with care to ensure the treatment is not more devastating than the disease. After the following outline, some of the key factors for a successful major compensation plan revision are discussed in detail.

1. Objective
   - Make major revisions to the plan to address substantive issues that have been identified by the executive committee.
2. Scope
   - Develop a full understanding of alternatives.
   - Develop a computer model that projects individual compensation under two or more compensation algorithms.
   - Select a methodology and modify it as necessary.
   - Educate physicians regarding issues, alternatives, and the option recommended.
3. Review Process
   - Institute a review team of six to eight physicians representing a broad cross section of views.
   - Hold biweekly meetings over a period of two to three months in order to research and summarize issues.
   - Discuss recommendations one on one with physicians once they have been determined.

- Provide shareholders or partners with a summary document and a discussion of the issues.

Successful compensation revision project teams typically have few members but include representatives of diverse views. Stacking the compensation review team so it reflects only one point of view will ultimately lead to an unbalanced compensation plan. By including all points of view, selling the final plan will be an easier task.

If a major compensation review process is indicated, the first step is to identify the global issues of concern:

- Is there agreement regarding the long-term goals of the practice group?
- Are the goals congruent and attainable?
- What behaviors should the compensation plan motivate?
- What behaviors should it discourage?
- Where can efficiencies be realistically achieved?
- How can service quality issues be addressed more effectively?

The team will need to isolate issues that require physician understanding and support in order to achieve successful implementation. If major organizational or departmental changes are required, a special effort will be necessary to implement them.

The team should then examine specific compensation issues:

- Does the plan accurately reflect the revenue streams flowing into the practice?
- Is the practice's compensation plan competitive with the plans of other groups in the marketplace?
- Are risk and reward properly balanced?
- Which specialties are subsidized by the plan and why is this appropriate?
- Is revenue a function of individual actions or centrally negotiated contracts?
- Are individual production levels appropriate given the market, the mix of specialties, and the mix of payers in the system?
- How are costs monitored and controlled?
- Are physicians as a group sensitive to the issues?
- How successful were prior efforts to revise compensation?

The review should conclude with a summary of the strengths and weaknesses of the current plan, along with an evaluation of alternative compensation policies that might be considered. The issues involved in the success or failure of prior efforts to revise compensation should be noted by the project team.

The next step is to review alternative types of compensation plans and project how compensation would change under each of these plans:

- Who would the change affect most?
- How would behaviors and attitudes change?
- What resources would be required to support the change?
- What fallback positions are possible that would keep the process going in the right direction?
- What would be the financial cost to the group?

Structural changes of any type carry the risk of failure, and compensation plan revisions are not exceptions to this rule. The compensation review team should incorporate risk assessment and minimization strategies into the work plan.

Some techniques for minimizing the risks associated with the change include:

- using financial modeling with a what-if capability to examine potential problem areas
- holding educational sessions to discuss the changes and the reasons for the changes
- setting a limit on the amount of actual change experienced by any one physician, positive or negative, during the first year of the new plan
- defining a period for phased implementation

Once the preferred revisions are selected by the review team, a projection of physician compensation should be prepared for each physician and the group as a whole. There are no shortcuts here. A one-on-one physician discussion is required to address the issues that have necessitated change in the compensation plan.

The potential outcome of the plan revision must be made clear to the entire group of physicians. The task of selling the solution is second only to developing the plan itself. In selling the plan, unless the leadership is extremely strong and relatively invulnerable, it may be wise to utilize the services of a highly regarded consultant or accounting firm in order to present the changes in the most positive light. The importance of keeping the plan simple and maintaining a link to group goals and culture will be fully appreciated during this last phase of the revision process.

CONCLUSION

The issue of physician compensation will continue to be hotly debated. No plan is perfect. Even effective plans require some review and change over time. Physicians and administrators who are committed to excellence will encourage discussion of compensation issues in an open forum and work to keep the focus on group goals, fairness, and appropriateness.

7

Merging Fee-for-Service and Prepaid Medicine

Albert E. Barnett

INTRODUCTION

If the title "Merging Fee-for-Service Medicine" had been used in the early 1970s, the first question asked might have been, "Merging it with what?" As recently as two decades ago, virtually all medicine practiced in the United States was fee-for-service. The few alternative prepaid models that had arisen, such as Kaiser-Permanente and Ross-Loos in California and HIP in New York, were held in wary regard. And even these few early plans were not originally fee-for-service but were established from the outset in a prepaid format. They were considered by most physicians as outside the "mainstream" of American medicine, suitable perhaps for certain industrial or low-income patient populations, but only for these. The free choice of a physician was felt to be the inalienable right of every citizen and the watchword of organized medicine. How present-day medical groups may evolve effectively from the dedicated fee-for-service mode of health care delivery to one that also encompasses a significant prepaid component is the subject of this chapter. This orderly transformation is vital to the future success of most medical groups, yet it is not an easy one.

The decade of the 1980s saw a great spurt in the growth of group practice in the United States. But most medical groups did not arise in order to practice managed care or participate in prepaid contracting. They emerged, rather, for the sake of convenience—to facilitate time off, make call schedules easier, and pass off unpleasant administrative duties to lay managers. Of those groups that did venture into the prepaid waters, most only intended to get their toes wet as a defensive measure "just in case."

Many group practices were totally unprepared for what happened next. In geographic areas as divergent as Minnesota and California, the popularity of prepaid medicine and the rise of HMOs caught provider groups totally by surprise. Persistent annual growth rates in outpatient visits of 20 percent to 30 percent created vast administrative problems and enormous tensions among the group physicians, accustomed as they were to a very orderly and consistent practice style. Some groups made an irreversible decision to forsake prepaid medicine entirely, considering it too risky, too unmanageable, and too likely to cause a diminution in income. Others plunged forward, although poorly prepared for the difficulties to be encountered.

By the beginning of the 1990s, a number of groups had already worked through many of these problems and made an irreversible decision not only to "tolerate" a prepaid component but to focus on it. Often the change in emphasis was accomplished with considerable success. Using insights gained from past experience, this chapter presents some of the problems associated with the merger of fee-for-service and prepaid practice. It describes successful strategies that medical groups have employed to alleviate many of the tensions and pitfalls often created by this merger.

PREPAID MANAGED CARE

Establishing Suitability

Although the practice of prepaid medicine, in the present competitive medical climate, would seem beneficial for any medical group, not every physician or group is suited to that mode of care. Some, because of years in practice and a relatively stable clientele, might choose to "ride out" slowly shrinking patient volumes in anticipation of retirement. Others might feel that their particular specialty, because of its market scarcity or esoteric nature, will insulate them from change. In addition, access to suitable prepaid plans is not universally available throughout the United States. The only access to prepaid medicine for solo practitioners or small specialty groups is usually through an independent practice association (IPA) of similar arrangement on a discounted fee-for-service basis. However, discounted fee-for-service care is not really prepaid managed care in the full sense (at least it is not so considered in this book). In any case, all those who seriously consider entering a true prepaid environment must make the decision in the light of their own strengths and weaknesses.

To be successful in prepaid medicine, a physician must

- enjoy collaborative endeavors
- be a team player
- work cooperatively with administration and staff
- be able to adapt (especially to medical guidelines, regulatory requirements, and imposed performance standards)
- be able to work without needing to be motivated by short-term financial incentives

- be efficient and be able to manage a large volume of patients effectively
- possess business and negotiating acumen
- be able to think logically and focus on goals
- be innovative
- be aware of weaknesses and be able to access help
- practice with confidence and without relying on excessive ancillary support
- be sincerely committed to cost control
- be sincerely committed to quality care
- be sincerely committed to service to patients
- be attentive to risk management

A medical group that wanted to achieve success in prepaid medicine would begin with a collection of physicians of the type described above. It must also, however, be prepared to deal with the following issues.

Service Area

Are there financially strong HMOs available? Are the products they market suitable for group practice? Many HMOs are primarily suitable for an IPA and have a methodology that is not easily adaptive to multispecialty group practice.

What are the patient demographics? Areas and populations that are not generally suitable for prepaid medicine include farm areas lacking major employers and areas that are very affluent.

Physician Commitment

Of all the factors involved in choosing to enter a prepaid mode of practice, physician commitment is probably the most important. Probably more groups make relatively uninformed decisions to enter or escape from prepaid medicine on the basis of political maneuvering to preserve an existing compensation structure than for any other single reason. Group politics, leadership, and dynamics are discussed elsewhere in this book.

Primary Care Orientation

Since prepaid medicine requires efficiency in patient care, the emphasis in practice must be on patient volumes and not on procedures. Although the utilization of RBRVS has leveled the playing field somewhat in fee-for-service medicine, the fact remains that in no other style of practice is the primary care physician as important to the success of the enterprise as in prepaid medicine. Because of this requirement, the salaries of primary care physicians and procedural subspecialists are relatively close together in prepaid practices. Since no one elects to reduce his or her income voluntarily, it is much easier to go into prepaid medicine from a primary care mode than from a subspecialty mode, where income reductions may be necessary.

Organization and Leadership

See Chapters 3, 4, and 11 for discussion of the group administrator, the medical director, and the organizational strucure of medical groups.

Staff and Administration

The staff of a prepaid managed care practice differs in content and emphasis from the staff of a fee-for-service practice. In nursing, for example, skills in telephone triage replace skills needed to stimulate office revisits. In the business office, ICD-9 coders give way to prepaid coordinators. The adaptability mentioned previously as a necessary characteristic for physicians becomes equally important for the entire staff.

Nowhere in the organization is there more necessity for a different level of skill than in administration. Prepaid contracting is complex and arduous. The accounting methodology differs greatly from that used in fee-for-service medicine. As the prepaid component of a combination practice grows, thresholds are reached that may require the hiring of new people with skills and training that are not possessed by current employees. Another strategy commonly used is to employ consultants, but this is an expensive option, especially when plan enrollment is low. Therefore, it is important to consider the human resources available within the group's administration, not to mention the administrators' commitment and willingness to learn, before moving too rapidly into prepaid medicine. Fortunately, adaptability and the willingness to learn are generally at least as common among administrators as among physicians.

Physical Facilities

Major considerations regarding outpatient office space for a prepaid population include facilitating a larger patient volume. Since productivity is always dependent on patient enrollment, the ability to provide care for large numbers of patients is essential. In contrast, many fee-for-service offices are organized around procedure-dependent subspecialists utilizing few exam rooms and much private patient consultation space. The prepaid office also requires more support staff areas, and functions such as enrollment, patient eligibility review, and utilization review all require increased administrative space that is accessible to patients (see Chapter 35).

Hospital Relationships

Despite the emerging dominance of outpatient treatment in the total spectrum of patient care, the hospital component still accounts for a great percentage of health care spending. Therefore, in order to control this element of costs, it is absolutely necessary to have satisfactory hospital relationships. Multiple hospitals in the service area enhance competition for the prepaid book of business, especially if the hospitals' census rates are low. In order to obtain a low capitation rate from a hospital, the hospital usually requires some assurance of an overall increase in utilization.

However, in order to take full advantage of this sort of competitive situation, the group physicians must be willing to move as a unit to a different hospital. Politics, medical staff positions, referral patterns for fee-for-service patients, and preexisting financial and investment interests all conspire to make this sort of mobility difficult for many group practices, and indeed these factors may serve to increase divisiveness among the involved physicians. Many fee-for-service physicians will also be reluctant to change hospitals if they think that their patients will be disinclined to accept the new hospital.

Because of these factors it is usually difficult to get the necessary physician consensus to change hospitals until the portion of group income derived from the prepaid component has reached a certain size. Paradoxically, one of the factors that may induce a hospital to offer a low per diem rate to a prepaid plan is that the physician group will also admit a large percentage of fee-for-service patients. The greatest leverage in obtaining a desirable rate is, therefore, present when the prepaid enrollment is relatively low. That takes us back once again to the question of commitment. To make the successful transition to prepaid practice, the physicians must understand that they must surrender short-term gratifications for long-term success and stability.

Professional Relationships

Professional relationships constitute another extremely sensitive area, but a vital one, in which to attempt to effect change. Unified Medical Group Association statistics in California show that the percentage of the total capitation that a typical large group spends on outside physician providers of medical care exceeds 16 percent. Many of the same factors that were considered in the previous paragraphs apply to professional relationships as well. The greatest leverage in obtaining good contracts for the provision of services outside the group practice occurs when the fee-for-service component of the practice is still sizable enough to entice the subspecialist. But as in the case of hospital relationships, the group physicians must be willing to disrupt old and comfortable referral patterns. The best contract for prepaid patients may come from the specialty group that does not provide the best holiday parties or other secondary gains. So once again, the ability of a group practice to act together as a unit directly translates into improved chances for success in prepaid managed care.

HMO Relationships

In any geographic service area in which prepaid practice is contemplated, there must be available financially solid HMOs that have payment formats that are suitable for group practice. These HMOs must also provide a payment structure and subsequent contract and capitation that permit the group to practice high-quality medicine. Such HMOs may have certain negotiating advantages in dealing with a medical group just getting started in prepaid medicine. These might include negotiating and administrative experience or bids from competing providers. Elements that increase the leverage that the medical group can exert vis-à-vis even a strong HMO include

- geographic dominance
- name recognition and reputation
- the potential for providing access
- strong and longstanding patient relationships

Dominance in the group's geographic area provides a strong negotiating lever. Usually a dominant group has little organized competition among the other providers in its neighborhood. Its strength in the area enables the group to take the necessary risks and undertake the needed administrative costs to enter the prepaid marketplace. The HMO commits itself to an expensive marketing effort to expand into a given area. It does not wish to compound that administrative expense by undertaking time-consuming negotiations with countless solo and small group providers. Thus, a medium or large group with a powerful geographic presence has a distinct negotiating advantage.

Name recognition and reputation are also an advantage in negotiating. Although it may seem that contracting mostly revolves around financial issues, there is no question that when selling the plan to employer groups, the HMO must be cognizant of perceived quality of care. It is much easier to market a plan to employers that includes well-known and respected groups and clinics, and those groups with a good reputation have a negotiating edge.

Another important factor in positioning a group to enter prepaid medicine is its ability to provide access. Again, the HMO commits substantial funds to its marketing efforts and does not wish to deal with a group that may cut off access through its inability to service the large volumes of patients that may seek enrollment. Of course, to provide access requires availability of capital for land, buildings, equipment, and staff. So once again, genuine commitment on the part of the physician owners is essential, since otherwise the group would be unable to provide or borrow the capital needed for investment.

A solid patient base is another asset that eases contractual negotiations with an HMO. If, when a plan is offered by an employer, a considerable number of employees are familiar with that medical group or are patients of that group, enrollment is greatly enhanced. Most patients would rather stay with their own physician and change health plans than seek a new physician. Furthermore, a strong patient base not only provides negotiating strength vis-à-vis the HMO but also enhances the growth of enrollees in the medical group. Increased enrollment helps both the HMO and the provider group, because the larger the enrollment within the group, the less the risk of adverse selection of patients and the more efficient the administration and provision of care.

Entering the Prepaid Marketplace

There are two basic methods a physician group can use to become involved in prepaid managed care. One is to originate a pure prepaid practice from scratch, and the other is to evolve into a prepaid practice from a fee-for-service base. Both strategies have advantages and disadvantages.

Starting a New Prepaid Group

Originating a new prepaid group is a strategy that has been employed with varying degrees of success in the past. Staff and group model HMOs, such as Kaiser-Permanente and FHP, utilize this method almost exclusively rather than purchasing existing fee-for-service groups and converting them to the prepaid mode. Additionally, there have been private physicians and administrative people who have put together groups for the sole purpose of providing care under prepaid contracts.

One of the major advantages of entering the field in this manner is that the prepaid contract can already be negotiated, evaluated, and put in place prior to the start of operations. With appropriate analysis of the contract projections of enrollment, budgetary issues and the size and type of staff can all be thoroughly considered before the first patient signs up for care.

With a group practice designed for prepaid medicine, experienced administrative personnel can be brought on board early. It is particularly vital to have experienced personnel in the areas of contracting, coordination of benefits, and claims payment, and to have an experienced medical director.

The design of the facilities also differs in important respects from the design best suited for a fee-for-service office (see Chapter 35). A prepaid practice must be organized to accommodate large patient volumes, and thus the need for patient exam rooms is great. On the other hand, the need for elaborate private physician consultation and office space is minimal. Parking requirements are generally greater. Extensive administrative space in patient care areas is a must because of the need to verify eligibility, register large numbers of new patients, and take care of referrals and utilization issues.

The profile of the employee staff is different in a prepaid practice, since more people are necessary to coordinate benefits and respond to grievances. Prepaid patients are under contract and cannot walk away if dissatisfied with medical care or service. But, conversely, a pure prepaid practice does not require the billing skills and coding expertise that is at a premium in a fee-for-service setting.

Finally, the physician staff can be selected on the basis of their suitability to practice in a prepaid environment. The essential physician characteristics mentioned earlier can be more realistically sought. The hired physicians would not have their compensation predicated on the number of years spent accumulating a large fee-for-service patient base. Physicians with an established track record have generally acquired a high sense of entitlement in the area of compensation. Instead, physicians recently out of residency programs can be hired thus effecting a considerable savings in physician costs.

In spite of the number and magnitude of these advantages in starting up a new prepaid group, there are significant offsetting disadvantages. To begin with, even if a medical group has a contract in place, it will generally not be designated on the printed material the HMO sends to employers prior to actually beginning operations. This is understandable, since the HMO must be assured the group has adequate capacity, appropriate management systems in place, and physicians and staff with proper credentials before offering the group's services to its clients. Even when the new group finally appears in the HMO's brochure, there is a further delay. Open enrollment periods for employees usually occur annually, thus further delaying the arrival of patients to the clinic. The time that elapses between the opening of a new clinic and the arrival of significant capitation checks is often at least a year.

For these reasons the need for working capital, whether borrowed or contributed by individuals, is very great. Many lending institutions have difficulty understanding and evaluating prepaid medicine and refrain from making loans to these entities. Consequently, in order to accommodate its extensive capital needs, the new prepaid group must often seek the help of a financial partner. The joint venture partner might be a venture capitalist, a hospital, or an HMO. In any case, acquiring a partner generally involves surrendering considerable control of the enterprise. The intense capital needs of a new prepaid medical group—and the major difficulties in successfully addressing these needs— almost invariably make it impractical to start up a group from scratch.

Evolving into Prepaid Medicine

A gradual evolution from fee-for-service care to prepaid care is by far the most common strategy selected. The major advantage is that large amounts of capital are not required in advance. Because the fee-for-service practice is already a "going concern," there is an income base to support the prepaid start-up costs. Furthermore, since the decision to get involved in prepaid care in the first place is usually the result of declining fee-for-service patient volumes, the group generally has considerable incremental capacity for the new line of business. In the early stages of low enrollment, capitation checks are looked upon as money found, since very little additional effort or expense has been involved in obtaining them. It is also at the time of early involvement in prepaid medicine that the medical group has its greatest leverage in obtaining beneficial contracts with hospitals and outside physician providers. Because of the massive leverage exerted by the big fee-for-service referral base, contracting with outsiders is greatly facilitated.

The cooperation of the group physicians is also easier to obtain in the early stages of evolution. They generally do not perceive at this point the changes in practice style and compensation formulas that are impending further into the process. Because their present patient base and income stream may be shrinking, the prepaid option is looked upon as something worth trying. At the present time, because of the uncertainties in the fee-for-service universe, it is usually not difficult to make the initial decision to enter prepaid medicine. The advantages, especially in the early stages of evolution, are generally apparent. The disadvantages to the physicians of evolving toward prepaid medicine are perceived a little later on in the process and can often produce considerable conflict within the group when they are perceived.

The disadvantages involve the basic organizational and administrative core of the practice. Certain issues related to the evolution start to become important when the group receives upwards of 30 percent of its income from capitation. At that point, the decision to continue in the prepaid venue becomes irrevocable, since the potential loss of revenue, if the contracts were canceled, would devastate the group. Up to that point, there may exist ambivalence toward the new book of business, and the physicians might still harbor the fantasy of returning to a lucrative unadulterated fee-for-service practice. Furthermore, physician compensation, up to that point, usually requires little tinkering, and the leadership and organization of the group may appear to be little affected. But after the benchmark of 30 percent revenue from prepayment, the issues of commitment, compensation, leadership, and organization must usually be confronted. At that point, it generally becomes apparent that the current political and organizational situation is not conducive to a successful transformation into prepaid medicine.

Of the major issues that arise, physician compensation is paramount. The "high producers" in the fee-for-service arena become the most costly practitioners in prepaid medicine. As the group enters the Alice-in-Wonderland world where more is less and less is more, confusion and conflict rage—and become focused on physician compensation (see Chapter 6). And although the winds swirl around compensation, important leadership problems also arise. The kindly, benign individual who so often fills the position of medical director in a fee-for-service practice is usually not suited to play the powerful role required of a prepaid practice medical director. In a fee-for-service practice, the individual physician is usually only responsible for his or her own income. In a prepaid practice, each medical decision financially impacts the entire organization. And, as mentioned previously, since productivity in a prepaid practice is dependent on the number of enrollees the practice is able to accommodate and not on the number of expensive procedures performed, the division of income must change accordingly.

It is unrealistic to expect all group physicians to change their outlook at any given point in time. Many will cling to a fee-for-service mind set well past the 30 percent income stage. Using phrases like "better patient care" and urging more individual patient advocacy, these physicians will continue to resist managed care, some of them for their entire careers. Others with a more progressive outlook (and possibly lower compensation) are able to adapt themselves to the prepaid managed care methodology much sooner.

Failure to resolve the political and organizational problems will cause physicians to want to reenter the fee-for-service environment and may result in the demise of the group. HMOs, as has been stated, need dependable and unlimited access, and once the relationship with a provider group has been breached, it may be difficult to reestablish.

Compared to the compensation and leadership problems, the administrative problems are easily resolved. Experienced personnel can be hired and consultants utilized. Appropriate MIS programs must be implemented. The fee-for-service mode requires an emphasis on billing procedures and coding. Prepaid medicine requires an emphasis on operational controls, so physicians and staff can track costs and expenses by department and by physician. The physical plant must usually be adapted and expanded to accommodate the larger new patient base. But all these changes can usually be implemented in the time frames that are available during the transformation.

Some of the other problems that occur during the evolution of a prepaid practice are directly related to the small enrollment present at the outset. Two areas deserving of mention are risk and costs. The smaller the enrollment with a prepaid plan, the greater the risk, since a catastrophic case would not be fully offset by the capitation income. As greater numbers of patients enroll, this risk becomes less and the actuarial predictability becomes more accurate. One method of guarding against the expensive case is to buy reinsurance, either from the HMO itself or independently from an outside carrier. However, to protect itself, the medical group would ordinarily begin with a low attachment point or deductible, and this makes reinsurance an expensive commodity during the start-up phase of prepaid operations.

Other costs are also greatest when there is a small enrollment. For example, specialized administrative and support staff must be hired for the prepaid segment, and their salaries must be covered by a relatively small capitation income. Prepaid medicine increases staffing in many areas. Additional MIS requirements to support a prepaid practice contribute to the expense, as does the reconfiguring of certain facilities. Advice, legal counsel, and consulting services must be purchased on the outside if enrollment figures do not warrant bringing these important services in house.

Contracting leverage with the HMO itself is also weakest when enrollment is low and before the group can prove that it is adept at controlling costs. Full-risk contracts, for example, where the potential for significant profit may be greatest, are usually neither advisable nor obtainable until the group can prove it can contain costs and reduce hospitalization. It is paradoxical that at the same time that a predominantly fee-for-service practice has the greatest leverage with its outside providers and hospitals, it has the least leverage with an HMO in securing a financially attractive contract.

But, again, perhaps the greatest cost is found in the practice habits and patterns of the physician staff. Prepaid medicine must be of a very high quality, not only to benefit the patients but also to ensure financial success. Quality medicine requires much discipline and much introspection regarding practice habits. Adherence to guidelines of patient care, based on outcomes research, must replace individuality. Physicians who fail to accept the disciplines willingly will not only be unhappy in a prepaid setting but will seriously retard the success of the entire practice. Which raises this important question: Can a physician practice in accordance with two standards of medical care? When caring alternately for fee-for-service patients and prepaid managed care patients, can a physician reasonably make the transition from selling services to controlling costs?

Unfortunately, most physicians seem unable to make frequent switches and can only comfortably practice one style of medicine. Therefore, somewhere during the evolution of the practice the transition to cost-effective medicine must take place. Changing compensation formulas, going to salaries, and accepting direction from administration may all help, but old habits die hard. The commitment must be there for a medical group to make a successful transition, and this commitment must include the learning of new practice patterns and the acceptance of technology and methodology assessments. If this commitment cannot be made early, preferably prior to searching for the first HMO contract, then the group will probably not be a viable candidate for prepaid managed care.

CONCLUSION

This chapter has discussed issues that a medical group needs to consider before attempting the very difficult and costly process of entering the prepaid practice arena. The evolutionary format that most groups select is perilous both at the outset and at junctures along the way. Not all groups will satisfactorily complete the process, or even survive it. But at the same time, prepaid managed care provided by multispecialty medical groups seems to be the direction in which the country's health care system is moving. Merging fee-for-service into a basically prepaid practice can be done successfully with proper planning, advice, and physician commitment.

8

Motivation and Morale in Health Care Organizations

Michael E. Kurtz

"I just don't understand why people act like they do!"

"Why are people so negative sometimes and why can't they get along with each other?"

"Professionals should be able to manage themselves, so why do I have to constantly solve 'people problems'?"

"Why aren't people motivated? How do I get people to do what they're supposed to do?"

These are the most common questions asked when a discussion of motivation and morale takes place in an organization. They are not unique to health care, for they are raised in all types of companies operating today. These same questions were probably asked by the pharaohs of ancient Egypt as often as they are today by most supervisors and managers.

Are there answers to these questions? Is there even any set of answers that might provide the "recipe" for producing a high degree of motivation and morale for individuals as well as employee groups?

The answer is no. There is no set of answers or recipe book that will effectively address these questions for all types of organizations and situations. The issue of motivation is multifaceted and requires input from many different perspectives on topics such as human behavior, organizational dynamics, the psychosociology of leadership and management, and organizational structure and design.

The one thing that is known is that people's behavior in any organizational setting will be dependent upon the environment, the organizational climate and culture, and the leadership style and philosophy developed and practiced by management.

AN HISTORICAL PERSPECTIVE

Current leadership thinking, theory, philosophy, and practice have all emerged through an evolutionary process during this century, and, in turn, concepts about what motivates people have shifted and flowed with the thinking of the times. A review of this evolution shows that a major shift in thinking and style has taken place approximately every 10 years since 1930, and these shifts correlate with major national, social, political, and economic changes (see Figure 8-1).

From 1900 until 1930, the dominant school of management practice was the "scientific school," which propounded a hard-nosed, authoritarian philosophy and insisted that power be centralized at the executive management level. Very little, if any, power was delegated downward in the organization, and management perceived its primary role as one of setting goals, planning activities, and controlling and directing the behavior of others.

This school of thought was firmly entrenched in management thinking and was directly reflected in leadership behavior up until the Great Depression of the 1930s. Because of its longevity, the doctrines of the scientific school became firmly entrenched in American management philosophy and practice.

Most American medical schools were founded during this period and, in accordance with the teaching of the time, structured themselves using the scientific school model. This model of organization imposed a pyramidal hierarchy, multiple supervisory layers, and extensive compartmentalization and departmentalization.

In turn, hospitals organized and structured themselves in like manner, primarily because of the close interface required with the medical schools. The allied and ancillary health care professions and disciplines then followed suit because of their interdependent relationships with both medical schools and hospitals. As specialty and multispecialty medical group practices developed, they used this same organizational model, since it was the one with which they were most

Scientific	Motivational	Sociotechnological	Human Relations
1900	1930	1940 Sciences Technologies	1950 D. McGregor
Theory X		*Theory X*	*Theory Y*

Participative	Collaborative-Team	Collaborative-Team-Futuristic	Integrative
1960 F. Herzberg	1970	1980 Technologies	1990
Theory Y		*Theory Y*	*Beyond Theory Y?*

Figure 8-1 Historical Development of Management Philosophy and Practice

familiar. By the 1940s, the scientific school's philosophy of organization and management practice was deeply entrenched throughout the entire health care industry. Some group practices are still trying to use this type of organizational structure and management practice today.

In the 1930s, management thinking and practice moved away from an authoritarian or autocratic approach toward a more supportive model that used job security and employee representation as motivators. The change was encouraged by the rapid development of unionization at the same time, which most likely took place as a reaction to the severity of the scientific school.

In the early 1950s, the single greatest shift in management and leadership thinking took place when Douglas McGregor introduced the "human relations school" based on his work and research at the University of Michigan and the Massachusetts Institute of Technology. Until that time, people were thought to be lazy, self-centered, indifferent, and disdainful of work. The primary motivator was thought to be money: People only worked to make money in order to buy themselves pleasure outside of the work situation. For management to accomplish organization goals, close supervision of the work force was required, and the emphasis was placed on controlling and directing the behavior of others.

It was during the early 1950s that McGregor introduced his concepts of Theory X and Theory Y, which identified two antithetical sets of assumptions. He felt that each of us, as a human being, walks around in the world carrying a certain set of beliefs about others—who, why, and what other people are. We behave toward others based on our belief system and these assumptions that have been developed through our educational and work experiences.

According to the Theory X set of assumptions, people are basically lazy and self-centered. Theory Y assumptions, on the other hand, included the belief that people are not lazy and disinterested but rather derive pleasure and satisfaction from work. Theory Y held all adults have a need to work in order to be able to demonstrate competency and capability to others, which is how they develop and obtain confirmation of their sense of self-worth and value. The "work" may be formalized in a job or it may be informal, such as volunteer work, housework, community service, and so on. Theory Y proposed that people could be self-directed and self-motivated as long as the nature of the work and the values of the organization were consistent with professional, social, and personal values.

Today, this concept has been widely accepted by most organizations, and major changes in management and leadership thinking have taken place. Much of the research in the behavioral and social sciences during the 1970s and 1980s supports this concept. The 1990s will undoubtedly see a further defining of the role of management and leadership as basically supportive and facilitative in nature. The main purpose of management will be to integrate the goals of the organization with the personal and professional needs and goals of the employees.

THE NEED FOR NEW THINKING

The integrative and collaborative-team approach to management is currently dominant. American health care organizations have become more future-oriented, since they realize that the health care industry is changing more rapidly than ever before. For example, many experts anticipate that almost all health care in the United States will be provided in multispecialty group practices within the next 5 to 7 years, most often in ambulatory prepaid care settings. Insurers and buyers of health care will be making greater demands for the demonstration of cost-effectiveness, sound fiscal planning, and efficient management of human resources. A realistic balance between quality and cost containment must be developed for success, and ways must be found to help all employees work more productively (while enjoying greater satisfaction) during the organizational restructuring and redesign that will be required. Constant evaluation and modification of individual, group, and organizational performance will be required.

We are experiencing an evolutionary and revolutionary stage in leadership thinking. Organizations are reinventing themselves, and many new organizational forms are being tested. The traditional adversarial structures of the past, exemplified by the dual power structures of the medical and administrative staffs, are being demonstrated to be less than desirable and in some cases actually destructive. Collaborative team management and leadership at all levels of the organization are mandatory if health care organizations are to survive these turbulent times.

CURRENT CONCEPTS AND THEORIES

Theory X and Theory Y

Douglas McGregor stated that the conventional concept of management's task in harnessing human energy to achieve organizational goals could be stated broadly in terms of three propositions. To avoid a label bias, he called this set of propositions Theory X:

1. Management is responsible for organizing the elements of productive enterprise—money, materials, equipment, and people—for the purpose of achieving economic ends.
2. With respect to people, this is a process of directing their efforts, motivating them, controlling their actions, and modifying their behavior to fit the needs of the organization.

3. Without this active intervention by management, people would be indifferent, or even resistant, to organizational goals. Therefore, they must be persuaded, rewarded, punished, and controlled—their activities must be directed.

Based on his research and experience, along with the research findings of other behaviorists, McGregor believed that the propositions of Theory X were untrue. He thought that modern organizations required a different theory of management based on more progressive assumptions about human nature and human motivation. He referred to this new set of propositions as Theory Y:

1. Management is responsible for organizing the elements of productive enterprise—money, materials, equipment, and people—for the purpose of achieving economic ends.
2. People are not by nature indifferent or resistant to organizational goals. They have become so as a result of past experience in traditional organizations (in which Theory X is the basic management philosophy).
3. The motivation, the potential for development, the capacity for assuming responsibility, and the readiness to direct behavior toward organizational goals are all present in people; management does not put them there. It is instead the responsibility of management to make it possible for people to recognize and develop these human characteristics themselves.
4. The essential task for management is to arrange organizational conditions and methods of operation so that people can achieve their own goals best by directing their own efforts toward the achievement of organizational objectives.

According to Theory Y, the object of management should be to create opportunities, release potential, remove obstacles, encourage growth, and provide guidance. Such management is what Peter Drucker called "management by objectives" in contrast to "management by control." It does not involve the abdication of management, the absence of leadership, the lowering of standards, or the nonpresence of many other characteristics usually associated with approaches based on Theory X.

Motivation Theory

McGregor based his Theories X and Y primarily on the research findings of psychologist Abraham Maslow. Maslow proposed that there is a "hierarchy of needs" operating for people and that an unmet need creates tension that, when converted to energy, provides impetus and direction for behavior (see Figure 8-2).

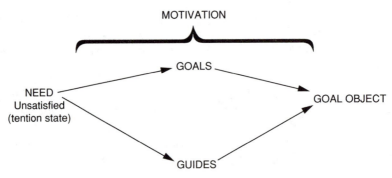

Figure 8-2 The Role of Unsatisfied Needs in Motivating Behavior. *Source:* Reprinted from *Work Motivation Inventory and Style of Leadership Survey* by Jay Hall and Martha S. Williams with permission of Teleometrics International, The Woodlands, Texas, © 1967.

Maslow presented an argument that a human being is a wanting animal: As soon as one need is satisfied, another takes its place, and this process is unending.

Maslow presents human needs as organized in a series of levels—a hierarchy of importance (Figure 8-3). At the lowest level, but preeminent in importance when they are thwarted, are physiological needs. Humans live for bread alone, when there is no bread. The need for love, status, and recognition are inoperative when a person is hungry, but when meals are regular and adequate, hunger ceases to be a motivator. At that point, shelter from the elements has priority.

A satisfied need is not a motivator of behavior! This, both McGregor and Maslow believed, is a profoundly significant fact that is regularly ignored in the conventional approach to the management of people. A good example of this is the human need for oxygen: Except as we are deprived of it, oxygen has no appreciable motivating effect upon our behavior.

Whereas Maslow approached the question of human motivation from a very general perspective, Frederick Herzberg, a researcher at Case Western Reserve University, took Maslow's concepts and expanded on them. It was Herzberg who adequately translated these concepts into organizational settings, and it is Herzberg's work that most current motivational theory is based on.

In Herzberg's version, the physiological needs identified by Maslow become the primary need for satisfaction of the "basic creature comforts."

Safety needs, which are on the next higher level, are expanded to include "security" (the need to know that one is protected from harm and is provided with job and financial security). Job protection, fringe benefits, and retirement security are all needs at this level. Since every employee is in a dependent relationship, safety and security needs may assume considerable importance.

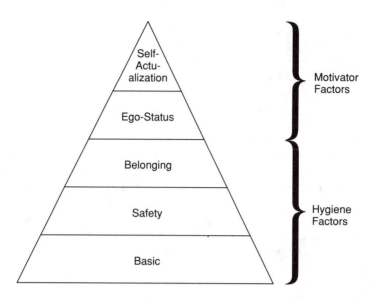

Figure 8-3 Maslow's Hierarchy of Needs. *Source:* Reprinted from "Leadership Styles" by M.E. Kurtz in *A Primer on Management for Rehabilitation Medicine,* P. Maloney (ed.), *Physical Medicine and Rehabilitation: State of the Art Reviews,* Vol. 1, No. 2, pp. 197–212, with permission of Hanley & Belfus, Inc., © 1987.

Arbitrary management actions, behavior that arouses uncertainty with respect to continued employment or that reflects favoritism or discrimination, and the unpredictable administration of policy can make employees at every organizational level feel the need for security with special intensity.

When these safety and security needs are satisfied and there is no longer a fear about physical and personal welfare, "social or belonging" needs—needs for belonging, for association, for acceptance by others, and for giving and receiving friendship and love—become important motivators.

On the next highest level are the needs of greatest significance for the purposes of management. These are the "ego-status needs," and they are of two kinds:

1. Needs that relate to a person's self-esteem: needs for self-confidence, independence, achievement, competence, and knowledge.
2. Needs that relate to a person's reputation: needs for status, recognition, appreciation, and for the deserved respect of colleagues.

Unlike the lower needs, these higher needs are rarely satisfied. People seek indefinitely for more satisfaction of these needs once they have become important to them.

Finally, at the top of the hierarchy are the needs for self-fulfillment and self-actualization: the need to realize one's own potentialities, the need to continue to self-develop, and the need to be creative in the broadest sense of the term.

The work of McGregor and Herzberg demonstrates that the conditions imposed by conventional organizational theory and by the traditional approach to scientific management have tied people to limited jobs. These types of jobs fail to utilize the full capabilities of employees, discourage the acceptance of responsibility, encourage passivity, and eliminate meaning from work. It would seem that people's habits, attitudes, and expectations have been conditioned by their experience working in such jobs. Unfortunately, they thus become accustomed to being directed, manipulated, and controlled in most organizations and are forced to find satisfaction for their social, egoistic, and self-fulfillment needs away from the job. This is as true of managers as it is of workers.

Those who accept Theory X place exclusive reliance upon the external control of human behavior, whereas adherents of Theory Y rely heavily on self-control and self-direction.

Herzberg found that in most modern organizations the needs for basic safety and security were well provided for, and most (but not all) of the belonging needs were met through organizational identity and membership. It was the higher level of belonging needs and especially the ego-status and self-fulfillment needs that were being thwarted; therefore, they were identified as the motivators managers should be concerned about.

The task then becomes one of assisting the manager or supervisor in developing behaviors that are consistent with the role of facilitator and supporter rather than controller and director. This new focus requires a shift in philosophy, attitudes, and traditional leadership practice.

MOTIVATION AS A FUNCTION OF LEADERSHIP

Leadership Styles

There is no one "right way" to be an effective manager. There is a full range of leadership styles that are available (Figure 8-4), and one of the most important things for a manager to learn is to recognize all the different options and the consequences (both positive and negative) of selecting one over another. It is also extremely important for a manager to be able to analyze a situation objectively so that the most appropriate style for that situation can be chosen.

In the "continuum model" which was first developed by Robert Tannenbaum and Warren Schmidt, a style can be assessed by measuring the amount of power and influence maintained by the manager or leader versus the amount shared with the group or team or with subordinates. Each style can be described as

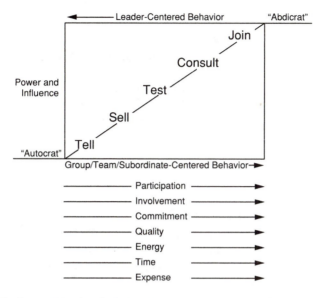

Figure 8-4 The Range of Leadership Styles. The seven outcomes listed below the model increase with each step away from authoritarianism (left) toward shared responsibility (right). *Source:* Reprinted from "Organizational Behavior" by M.E. Kurtz in *The Physician in Management,* R. Schenke (ed.), with permission of American Academy of Medical Directors, © 1980.

being more "leader-centered" or more "group- or team-centered." In Figure 8-4, the available styles are identified as "tell," "sell," "test," "consult," and "join." Not included in the range of styles is the "autocrat" and the "abdicrat" (an individual who simply abdicates all responsibility for coordination and facilitation), since in modern organizations there are too many checks and balances in place to allow anyone to be a total authoritarian or to totally abdicate all responsibility. The range of leadership styles between these two extremes is what needs to be understood.

As a manager moves up the scale from "tell" toward "join," more power and influence are shared with the group or with subordinates and different dynamics come into play. The dynamics that occur with each more participative choice are critical for the manager to understand. The primary dynamics are as follows:

1. Participation by group members increases.
2. The psychological and physical involvement of group members increases.
3. Personal commitment is maximized.
4. The quality of decisions increases.

5. There is greater expenditure of energy (physical and psychological).
6. There is a greater expenditure of time.
7. There is increased expense due to the increase in manhours.

It can be demonstrated that the above consequences will occur as the leader moves each step toward the "join" or shared responsibility end of the scale (see Figure 8-4). Employees react and respond differently as each style choice is brought into play:

1. As employees are allowed to engage in problem solving and decision making, their active participation in the process increases correspondingly.
2. As active participation increases, psychological and physical involvement in the process increases.
3. Through participation and involvement, employees develop a stronger commitment to decisions and problem solutions. A strong sense of "ownership" and "vested interest" is developed.
4. Through the participatory process, more resources are identified and used. The result is increased quality through the dynamic of "synergism."
5. Active participation and involvement consume more energy than passive observation. Assuming available energy to be finite, less energy is then available for other tasks.
6. It takes much more time to allow active participation in group settings than to make independent decisions (usually 9 to 12 times more time).
7. As more people are involved and allowed to participate, the number of manhours used increases, which translates into an increase in money expended.

It's obvious that different styles of management will be needed at different times and in different situations depending on what outcomes are desired or required. If all that is needed is a quick one-time response, a "tell" approach will be effective, but if a long-term commitment to a decision is required, the leader will have a better chance of obtaining it through the initiation of consensus building. A fire in the wastebasket doesn't require a team meeting to figure out what action to take, but a major personnel policy change that will affect a majority of the group will require support and commitment.

Experience has shown that most individuals and groups intuitively know what leadership style is most appropriate to a given situation, and employees will respond in a positive way as long as the leader's choice of style is consistent with their intuition. It is when the leader's choice is inconsistent and considered inappropriate that resistance is encountered. Because of previous experience, poor role models, or lack of training and education, some managers become "locked in" to thinking that there is only one style that is appropriate and will try to use it under all circumstances and in all situations.

Behavior is reciprocal; the behavioral reactions demonstrated by employees and colleagues depend on the behaviors exhibited by the management group in the organization. A manager who consistently uses a "tell" or "sell" style will most likely become frustrated with the negative reactions and resistance constantly encountered, even though the resistance is a result of that manager's own behavior.

Forces

In addition to understanding the range of styles an individual has available, there are three primary sets of forces operating in all settings that must be understood:

1. the forces operating personally in the leader or manager
2. the forces operating in the manager's group, team, or set of subordinates
3. the forces operating in the organization or in the situation itself

It is also critically important that the manager be able to evaluate these forces objectively, because this evaluation will help in determining what style will be most appropriate.

The evaluation of one's own personal forces should be part of the initial step in developing self-awareness. As a manager, what are your orientations, behavioral styles, wants, needs, and philosophies? What are you comfortable with and willing to accept? What training and preparation have you obtained to help maximize your effectiveness as a manager or supervisor? In short, where are you now?

The evaluation of forces operating in others requires that the manager develop an awareness, understanding, and appreciation for individual differences. People do not behave in certain ways because we want them to; they behave according to their life experiences. Traditional organizational structures have led people to believe that the "tell" and "sell" approaches are standard and that there are few or no other options. Comfort with more participatory and group-centered leadership styles must be developed through team development training or team-building experiences.

All health care organizations are similar but also unique. Every organization has a life style of its own. It has a history, a philosophy, and values and norms that must be understood and appreciated. As an organized entity, it will be made up of purpose, people, power and influence, and philosophy. The executive management group will determine how power is to be used to accomplish purpose through and with other people dependent on the philosophy it espouses. Executive management, through its policy-setting responsibility, clearly sets the tone and climate for the rest of the organization and provides role models for the management and supervisory staff. Motivation starts at the top of the organization. If it is perceived that executive management values the authoritarian use of power, is obsessed with the "bottom line," and attempts to lead by telling or selling, subordinates have no other choice than to behave in similar ways or leave the organization.

These forces are the basis for what is termed "organization behavior," and they operate in every situation, in every organization, and in every group at all times. They determine whether effectiveness, productivity, and satisfaction will be achieved or whether the manager will encounter resistance and low productivity, resulting in low morale and high turnover. Therefore, it is evident that motivation is a function of leadership behavior in combination with organizational philosophy.

MOTIVATION AS A FUNCTION OF ORGANIZATIONAL DESIGN

The current structure of most health care organizations is based on the pyramidal hierarchy propounded by the scientific school of management. This structure reinforces the traditional concept that management's primary role is to control and direct the behavior of others. It implies that all power and influence is centralized at the top of the organization and thus has a restricting effect on communication. In this structure each management level expends a great deal of energy protecting its position and power base in the organization rather than devoting its full attention to the work of the organization. It often results in high competition for individual attention and rewards rather than fostering an atmosphere of collaboration and teamwork.

Open, direct, and constructive communication is also hampered by this traditional model. Most often communication flowing downward from the executive level focuses on what is wrong. As each negative message passes down through the management levels, it tends to gain strength, so that by the time it reaches the employee level, the negativism is usually blown far out of proportion. As a result, subordinates perceive the management levels above them as concentrating on mistakes, showing disapproval, and punishing.

As communication flows upward from the employee level to management, negative information tends to be watered down or discarded at each higher level, so that executive management may be totally unaware of problems, employee dissatisfactions, or issues that may significantly jeopardize organizational effectiveness.

This traditional organization model usually specifically separates functions from each other. Figure 8-5 shows a definite separation of business functions (administration) from clinical functions (the medical director and department chairperson roles) and implies that the functions are unrelated to each other. In reality, these functions are highly connected, and their management should be a collaborative effort. To keep them separated creates an "us versus them" attitude and reinforces the traditional adversarial positioning between administration and clinical services. It can also create a feeling that one group is inferior to the other. The size of the organization dictates what structure and organizational design will be most effective and efficient, but the less hierarchical and compartmentalized the organization can be made, the better.

Figure 8-6 shows the design of a typical small group practice where business concerns and clinical concerns are integrated as a management function. In this model, the administrator and medical director operate as a team, and the interdependence of all organization functions required for success is clearly taken into account.

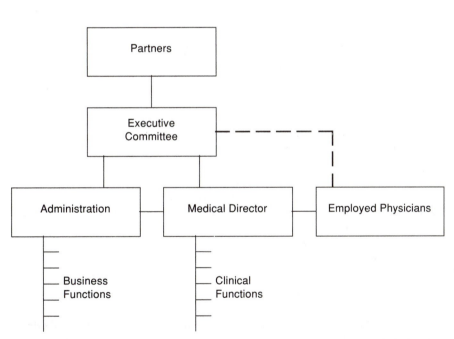

Figure 8-5 Traditional Group Practice Organizational Structure. This structure reinforces the traditional pyramidal hierarchy, centralizes power at the top, restricts communication, and implies that business functions and clinical functions are unrelated.

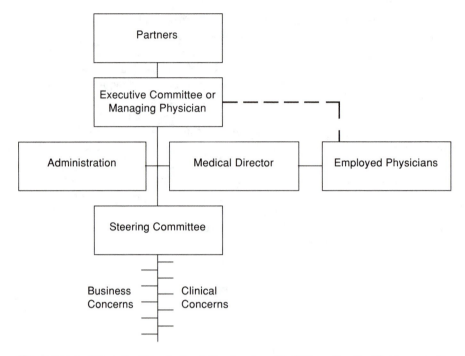

Figure 8-6 An Alternative Organizational Structure for a Small Group Practice That Incorporates a Steering Committee Design.

As already mentioned, there is a need to increase the participation, representation, and involvement of employees. One way of doing this in a small group practice is to create an office steering committee or advisory committee. The membership of an office steering committee should include a physician partner or shareholder, a nonphysician executive, and at least three employees elected by their peers (including employed physicians). This committee is charged with the task of monitoring and evaluating all matters concerning practice efficiency and effectiveness and recommending to the governing body solutions to identified problems.

To be effective the committee must be empowered by the governing body and formally authorized by the physician owners. The nonphysician executive is usually the designated chairperson, but this can vary in different organizations. Committee members suggest agenda items as well as solicit agenda items from their peers. The agenda is posted so that all members of the organization can see it, and approved minutes of the committee meetings should be published and distributed to all employees and physicians.

In a large group practice, the administrative and clinical functions may need to be separated because of the group's size and complexity (Figure 8-7). Even when this is the case, the chief executive officer and medical director should be charged to work in collaboration by the governing body. Most often an assistant administrator or chief operating officer is required. This individual collaborates with both the medical director and the person responsible for business functions.

The use of a steering committee, or of several steering committees, can be built into this model. A divisional steering committee may be appropriate, as well as departmental committees, depending on the size of the organization. In

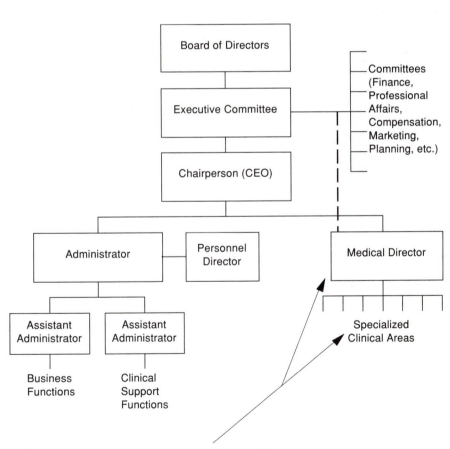

Build in divisional and departmental steering committees

Figure 8-7 An Alternative Organizational Structure for a Large Group Practice That Incorporates a Steering Committee Design.

this model, the persons responsible for the business and clinical support functions would be included in the division steering committee, and a member (or members) of the division steering committee would be included in the departmental committees.

CONCLUSION

Just as there is no one right way to manage or provide leadership, there is no one right way to provide motivation. Motivation is multifaceted and is a result of the interaction of human behavior, organizational dynamics, organizational structure, and leadership and management.

People will support that which they help create. Therefore, it is imperative that all members of the organization participate, in one form or another, in formulating the mission statement, establishing organizational goals and objectives, and planning activities for implementation. Collaboration and teamwork should be the overriding goal.

Behavior is reciprocal: The behavioral reactions of employees and colleagues depend on the behaviors exhibited by the managers of the organization. If the managers establish an environment of support and facilitation rather than one of overcontrol and top-down direction, employees will respond with support for the management and the organization.

Part II

Legal and Financial Issues

9

Contracting with an HMO

Thomas P. McCabe

INTRODUCTION

Although the term *health maintenance organization* was not coined by Dr. Paul Ellwood until 1970, prepaid group practices have actually existed for almost a century. They began at the turn of the century in the Northwest in order to provide medical care for the large numbers of itinerant workers in the lumber and gold mining industries. More formal prepaid arrangements were developed in the 1930s by Drs. Donald Ross and Clifford Loos, who founded the Ross-Loos Clinic in Los Angeles. In the 1940s, Henry Kaiser developed a health care program in the San Francisco Bay area to care for the thousands of shipyard workers needed for the war effort. This plan, called the Permanente Health Plan, survived and thrived, and it is today the largest HMO in the United States. In 1973, with the passage of the HMO Act, these organizations became a keystone of federal health policy and precipitated the explosive growth in HMO plans that has continued to the present day.

HMOs, by definition, have a very distinguishing characteristic: They all have a prepaid compensation mechanism called capitation, from the Latin *per capita* (per head). In this system, regular monthly payments are made in advance to the health care provider based not on services rendered but on the number and composition of the patient population enrolled in the plan. It is this characteristic that distinguishes the HMO system from the long-prevailing fee-for-service system and that has aroused such deep and emotional hostility from the forces of organized medicine. In more recent times, the competition for patients has caused many physicians to take a much closer look at the realities of the HMO successes. These physicians have come to realize that HMO plans do have long-range viability and that the wisest course might be to develop at least some measure of participation with them.

By today's standards, capitation schemes in the 1970s were simplistic. They were usually based on the type of subscriber enrollment such as single party, two party, and family. Some payers experimented with male, female, and child capitation systems, while others attempted straight per member per month payments. In contract negotiations in those early days, the two sides typically treated each other as "friendly adversaries." Neither payers nor providers had much experience with the new payment system, and meaningful data were scant. But as more employers accepted the government mandate to offer HMOs to their employees, and as provider groups recognized that an increasing portion of their income was derived from HMO payers, more sophisticated contracts evolved. Present-day contract negotiations require review by attorneys, actuaries, and consultants to protect the interests of the involved parties. But even before actual contract negotiations commence, a physician or group practice, here termed the "provider," must make a thorough evaluation of the proposed prepaid plan.

EVALUATING A PLAN PROPOSAL

The evaluation of a provider contract is a complex process. It begins with an evaluation of the company presenting the HMO plan contract itself. What is the financial strength of the company? If the plan is new, an assessment should be made of the competitive environment in which it is attempting to establish itself. It should be apparent that there is much greater risk inherent in contracting with an unstable HMO or one that has a very low market share. It is also unwise to contract for physicians' services if neither the provider nor the HMO has a good hospital contract in place.

The administrative capabilities of the plan are similarly important. Can it adequately process eligibility information? Does it have the systems to pay claims accurately and promptly? Does it have a sensitive patient relations staff and capable marketing personnel? The items discussed below should be examined carefully during the evaluation process.

The Plan's Financial Statements

Copies of the plan's balance sheet, income statement, and cash flow statements should be requested and examined. If it is a new plan, its pro forma financial statement can be perused. Does the plan have the assets to pay claims? What is the extent of its liabilities, both medical service liabilities and nonmedical items such as mortgages and long-term debt? What is the projected margin of profit on the income statement? A one or two percent margin is common. What is the percentage of revenue spent on administration and marketing? A mature HMO should only require 14 to 16 percent for these items, whereas a new plan might need 20 percent because of startup costs.

The Billing Process and Billing Experience

Does the plan bill negatively or prospectively? Negative billing sends the employer last month's bill for employee premiums, thus leaving to the employer any adjustments for employees added or deleted during the month. This process can result in premium payment delays and can affect the plan's cash flow, even impacting provider capitation payments. If billing to the employer groups is not prospective, or in advance of services, the plan may fail to control its premium collections. This may result in countless retroactive adjustments to the providers and waste much administrative time.

Eligibility Reporting and Verification

This element of an HMO contract can have a significant financial impact on the provider. If the provider does not have timely information identifying plan members, valuable resources will be consumed providing care to patients no longer eligible, whereas those who do qualify might be turned away or have services delayed. Eligibility reports should be delivered to the provider no later than the third working day of each month, either by printout, on magnetic tape, or on diskette. Most plans have an eligibility verification system to enable providers to get up-to-date assurance of a patient's eligibility, especially for more costly items such as hospitalizations and surgery. Such a system may involve simply telephoning the plan, but this is usually time consuming. A better method is to have an on-line system, which, if available, should be installed at the plan's expense. These systems are also necessary in order for the provider to collect from the plan under the eligibility guarantee clause discussed later in the chapter.

The Plan's Data Collection Requirements

Most plans are required to collect encounter information, with various facets of patient care itemized. It may be acceptable to provide this information in the form of routine billing statements, or the information can be submitted on tape-formatted input. Information on patient visits to outside contracting providers is also usually necessary. Because of this, providers must have clauses in their contracts with outside specialty contractors that require them to submit complete billing statements to the primary providers who can then forward them to the plan.

Stop-Loss and Reinsurance Coverage and Its Costs

Information and policies regarding stop-loss and reinsurance coverage should be carefully evaluated, for these policies define the financial risk of the provider. Plans vary greatly in the levels of stop-loss and reinsurance coverage that they offer, as well as in the cost of these policies to the provider. A new plan should have low attachment points for both types of coverage. Mature plans will have higher levels available, but these should be accessed only when the provider has achieved enrollment levels sufficient to justify the increased risk.

The cost of stop-loss and reinsurance coverage also varies dramatically between plans. The plan should be able to furnish on request its experience with these programs over a three-year period. It is also important to know whether the plan is purchasing the protection or is self-insured. A new plan that is self-insured can become bankrupt by a few serious and expensive medical problem patients. It is also possible for provider groups to purchase reinsurance directly from outside insurance companies, thus saving the markup on these policies that plans sometimes attach. Medical groups in California, for example, have developed a program through Unified Medical Group Association to purchase reinsurance through Lloyd's of London, with considerable savings in cost.

The Plan's General Liability Insurance Concept

It is usual for a plan to want each of its providers to indemnify it and to name the plan as an additional insured on the provider's liability policy. It is certainly reasonable, therefore, for the provider to be named as an additional insured on the plan's general liability insurance policies. This concept may be discussed prior to actual contract negotiations.

The Plan's Growth Strategy

The plan's strategy of growth in the provider's service area should be discussed. The plan's strategic business plan can be requested and reviewed. What is the plan going to accomplish in the next three to five years? What are its goals? What are its intentions regarding contracting with competing providers such as hospitals, IPAs, or other providers? This information is necessary for the provider to forecast enrollment growth, plan for appropriate access for patients, and plan for capital needs. Few plans do a good job of forecasting enrollment growth, and most are frequently off target. The plan and the provider must work together in this planning process so capacity is available to service the enrolled patients. Because of antitrust implications in this area, especially regarding geographic exclusivity, discussions of competition must be limited and legal advice is recommended.

The Plan's Benefit Packages

HMOs often listen attentively to their marketing staffs, sometimes creating myriad benefit packages. Individual HMOs can have over 50 different benefit packages for their various groups of enrollees. Variations in benefits geometrically increase the administrative burden on providers, unless they have available the sophisticated computer equipment necessary to adequately service them. A plan with myriad benefit options and few enrollees in each option might be a plan to be avoided.

Résumés of Management Personnel

The résumés of the plan's key management personnel should be carefully reviewed. What experience do they have in prepaid health care? The prepaid environment is competitive and demanding and requires experienced and intelligent management. What is the management training and educational background of the executives of the plan? Is their experience in hospitals or in the ambulatory care sector? Do they know the local market or has their experience been in other geographic areas?

References

As in the initial stages of any significant business relationship, due diligence should be practiced. References should be sought from other providers. Questions should specifically address timeliness of capitation payments, grievance handling experience, dispute resolution techniques, eligibility verification, provider relations department capabilities, and marketing success.

Summing up, there are strategies that can be successfully employed to reduce the financial risk to a provider in contracting with HMOs. These include selectively choosing HMO partners and contracting only with strong groups and insurers, coordinating a strategy for contracting with hospitals, and strengthening the provider's utilization and peer review mechanisms. The next critical element is to carefully evaluate the terms and conditions of the actual contract.

THE CONTRACT

After it has been determined that the plan has the necessary positive characteristics, the contract itself is ready to be studied. The "Definitions" section of the contract is of crucial importance, especially the definitions of such terms as *emergencies, service area, covered services, members, dependent, eligible enrollee, capitation, shared risk, out of area,* and *stop-loss/reinsurance program.* The definition of *medically necessary and reasonable* can have a great impact on an HMO-provider relationship, which can also be affected by whether the HMO or the provider is the one that determines medical necessity and reasonableness. The interpretation of each of these terms can involve many thousands of dollars in the course of a few years. A highly experienced consultant or counsel is recommended if clarification of terms becomes difficult.

Provider Obligations

Since the HMO contract is prepared by the plan, it is only natural that the duties and obligations of the provider section will always be many times longer than the duties and obligations of the payer section. Particular attention should be paid to the "Provision of Covered Services" clause. The provider should ask for an attachment or matrix that precisely defines which services are the responsibility of the payer, the hospital, or other participants such as the reinsurance carrier. The proper credentialing of providers is a major requirement of most payers, and the credentialing responsibility now generally extends to outside providers and contracted physicians as well as outside ancillary service providers. A legal counsel's advice may be required in this area because of issues of confidentiality and requirements for reporting to state or federal data banks.

Another area of concern is the administrative obligations of the provider in quality assurance (QA) and utilization review (UR) systems. All plans have requirements for providers to participate in or develop and implement a QA and UR program. It is recommended that in the contract negotiation process the plan be required to submit in writing its QA and UR plan for review. The provider must be fully aware of what will be required with respect to quality audits and utilization reviews. The administrative costs to the provider could be significant and should be assessed when analyzing the adequacy of compensation and the amount of risk assumed. Regardless of whether the plan or the provider is responsible for the QA and UR program, the provider should insist on a clause specifying that the plan will indemnify the provider for QA and UR proceedings and their outcomes. For reasons of confidentiality, it is not advisable to allow payer representatives to attend QA meetings. Rather, the payer may be allowed to review a summary of the minutes of each meeting that does not mention the names of patients or physicians.

Payer Obligations

Plan Administration, Premium Collection, and Enrollment

The plan should spell out all administrative functions it is responsible for performing, including marketing, billing and collecting premiums, and furnishing the provider with accurate eligibility reports. It should also precisely spell out its QA and UR responsibilities.

Distribution of Benefit Information to Enrollees

This is a function that many plans handle poorly. Usually benefit interpretation and dissemination falls to the provider, so it is essential that the plan's operations manual be clear, concise, and complete. No changes affecting provider risk assumption, nor any change in benefits to enrollees, should occur during the term of the contract without prior approval of the provider. An approval process would also be needed for the purpose of negotiating compensation for taking on additional benefits as covered services.

Distribution of Experience Reports to the Provider

The collection of data and the timely distribution of meaningful experience reports based on those data are also obligations of the payer. Plans require the submission of encounter data such as the number and type of patient office visits. By the same token, providers should insist on receiving meaningful and timely experience reports comparing the provider's utilization statistics with the statistics for the plan as a whole. It is important that the provider knows, for example, the status of its hospital utilization on a monthly basis. Since the plan pays claims that are then charged against the provider's hospital pool, timely reporting allows the provider to verify the accuracy of these claims and to make sure that negotiated discounts are being implemented. Were all the patients eligible at the time of service? Was the hospitalization authorized and directed by the provider? Was it within the provider's service area? These reports also enable the provider to track patients who may exceed the reinsurance attachment point to ensure proper credit under the reinsurance policy.

Enrollment and Eligibility Information

The plans must report eligibility information to the provider within the first few working days of each month. There should be a structure for notification and verification of eligibility such as membership cards or, preferably, an on-line data system. It is important to have an enrollment guarantee clause in the contract that requires the plan to pay the provider for services rendered to a patient who was perceived to be eligible but later proves to have been ineligible for care under the plan. The provider must make a reasonable effort to verify eligibility such as checking current eligibility reports, and attempt to bill ineligible patients directly, before the guarantee system is invoked. Retroactive additions and deletions of enrollees by the plan should be limited under the contract to a maximum of three months in order to conserve the administrative and financial resources of the provider.

Marketing

A significant portion of each premium dollar will be retained by the plan to pay for marketing. It is the obligation of the plan to take reasonable steps to procure enrollment for itself and its providers through advertising and other marketing activities. The provider should be kept informed of the marketing strategies of the plan so it can anticipate projected growth and add the necessary facilities and personnel to accommodate additional enrollees.

Administrative Assistance for the Provider

Plans vary greatly on the issue of furnishing administrative assistance to their providers, and providers vary in their need for such assistance. However, any plan should be prepared to assist the provider in managing the administrative aspects of participating in the plan, especially early in the relationship. Some plans may even agree to place a representative at the provider's facility to deal with patient questions, orient the provider's staff, and resolve problems as they arise.

Payment Methods

Various payment methodologies have been used by payers, including discounts from charges, per diem for inpatient care, RBRVs, capitation, or any combination of these. Since capitation is the most generally utilized method for HMOs and appears to be the most cost-effective, it is important to see how the capitation figure is derived.

In the late 1980s, many plans changed their system of capitation so that providers received a percentage of the premium charged to enrollees or employers. This method is usually perceived by providers as basically fair, since their capitation payment is raised whenever the plans raise their premium. A drawback to this method occurs in a competitive marketplace, where plans may hold the premium down in order to "buy" market share. Since a provider is at risk under a capitation payment scheme, HMOs may have little difficulty holding premiums down in order to sell the plan to employers. Another objection to percentage-of-premium contracting is that inflation in the cost of medical services has usually outstripped the inflation in administrative costs. Thus it can be argued that the provider should actually get an increasing percentage of the premium as contracts are renewed.

Other forms of capitation are beginning to appear, including use of an age and sex table of rates. This method recognizes that the cost of medical care varies with age and sex. For example, a woman of childbearing age has a greater potential for health care needs than a male of the same age. Also, a 64-

year-old male will generally have more health care needs than a teenager. Many employers, moreover, are now asking for statistics on the health care costs of their particular employee groups. If their employees are requiring less health care, they want that fact to be reflected in the premium charged by the HMO. Evaluating these differing forms of capitation is a complex task, and the provider may need to hire an actuary to act as a consultant.

Risk Sharing

The concept of "risk sharing" is common to virtually all HMOs as well as other types of managed care plans of other types. In a risk-sharing system, both the provider and plan share in the risk of providing certain services, including perhaps hospital and pharmacy services, among others. Under this scheme, a pool of money or a budget is set aside by the plan to cover the expected expense. If the services do not consume the entire budgeted amount, the provider shares in the savings with the plan. If the budget is exceeded, the plan and the provider share the additional cost. Often risk sharing has only an upside potential for the provider—it can share in savings but losses are the sole responsibility of the plan. The issue of risk sharing is a major area of negotiation in contracting with HMOs.

In the case of hospital services, it is essential that providers know how the risk-sharing budget is developed and which services are covered within it. A service matrix delineating precisely which services are covered under professional services capitation and which are charged against the hospital budget should be an attachment to the contract. The agreement should specify the method by which surpluses and deficits are calculated and what portion of either will be charged against or paid to the provider. Settlement of the shared risk pool should occur at least annually. Most plans have a three- to four-month "runoff" to accumulate charges for services that were incurred prior to the cutoff date but where the bills were not received until later. Incurred but not received (IBNR) charges can be expected to be negligible after the three- to four-month runoff period. Some plans allow for quarterly advance payments of surpluses in the shared risk pool in order to motivate providers and help them with cash flow. It is recommended that providers receive monthly budget calculation reports as well as monthly utilization and claims paid reports so that they can track their progress under the risk-sharing arrangement and, if necessary, reserve funds for any predicted deficits.

Termination

Termination clauses in HMO contracts can be difficult to construct and interpret, and it is advisable to have counsel review them. The section on *termination for cause* should specify the events under which either party may terminate the contract; these would include bankruptcy, loss of licensure, and failure to perform. The section on *termination without cause* should be constructed to protect both parties. The plan will want to include a phase-out time period in order to protect its enrollees and find a different provider. The provider will want to ensure that the plan does not severely damage its practice by suddenly withdrawing a large number of patients and the attendant capitation cash flow. If the plan exercises its termination-without-cause provision, the provider should insist on a hearing and possibly arbitration. The provider will usually have a contractual as well as ethical obligation to continue providing care for a period of time following termination of the contract. It is recommended that the contract specify the conditions and length of time this obligation covers as well as the method of compensation during this period.

Grievance Procedures

How the provider participates in plan grievance policies and procedures is often not well spelled out in the contract. Since patient complaints and grievances could have an adverse financial impact on the provider and even provoke malpractice claims, the provider should insist on representation at any proceeding involving a grievance or arbitration of a disputed claim. In addition to addressing patient grievances, the contract should identify a dispute resolution procedure for resolving problems arising between the plan and the provider. If arbitration is selected for this process, the contract should specify whether it is binding or nonbinding and which arbitration group or firm is to be utilized and where the process will take place.

Coordination of Benefits

The agreement should specify how benefits from primary payment sources will be coordinated with payments made by the plan to the provider. In a noncapitated situation, for example, will the plan make a full payment at the contract rate to the provider or will it be entitled to reduce its payment in the amount of any primary payments made to the provider from another source? It is recommended that the provider be allowed to bill and keep payments from third-party payers. Points such as these arise frequently and are responsible for the increasingly lengthy contracts now commonplace in the industry.

EVOLVING RELATIONSHIPS

As this is written, many employers have taken advantage of the cost-savings inherent in managed care and especially prepaid health plans. But they are attempting also to cut their administrative costs by reducing the number of plans available to their employees. Some employers are also realizing that they can reduce premiums by eliminating plans altogether and going directly to providers for contracts. Still others are going self-insured under TEFRA (Tax Equity and Fiscal Responsibility Act), which allows employers to avoid the HMO Act mandate. As these relationships evolve, some HMOs are beginning to perform the function of a third-party administrator (TPA), which means the plan merely administers an employer's self-directed program.

Chapter 11 describes the increased degree of sophistication that characterizes arrangements for health care provided by independent practitioners. Similarly, in the group practice arena the volatile payer-provider relationships have necessitated more complex interactions. Larger groups and networks of providers have augmented the need for specialty health care consultants and attorneys. Trade associations such as the Unified Medical Group Association on the West Coast provide a wide variety of services to their provider group members, including contract review, actuarial services, malpractice insurance programs, accreditation, and research.

As providers become larger and cover more area by virtue of mergers, buyouts, and joint ventures, they become more attractive to employers as a means of cutting the cost of the middleman, in this case the plans. Some providers are buying, merging, or joint venturing with hospitals, creating regionally based and highly integrated organizations. These can contract through plans or directly with employers for basic health care services and can establish relationships with large tertiary care centers for the more esoteric or specialized services. Now, after years of experience and the development of operational efficiencies through administrative and management expertise, these organizations have a vital role to play in the control of rising health care costs.

10

Direct Contracting for Patients

Ellen Kaufman, Edward Lipson, and Thomas Mayer

INTRODUCTION

Although the majority of contractual relationships between ambulatory care providers and purchasers of health care services are negotiated through a third party, there is a growing trend for providers and employers to deal with each other directly. Preferred provider organizations (PPOs) are the most commonly used mechanism for direct contracting. They are characterized by

- a panel of providers who agree in advance to set fees in exchange for greater patient volume
- a mechanism to monitor the quality of care provided
- a financial incentive to use network providers

The first PPOs began in California in 1979, and there is now at least one PPO in virtually every state. Most PPOs are sponsored by intermediary organizations, such as insurance companies, Blue Cross and Blue Shield plans, provider organizations, or independent vendors. This chapter focuses on the growing segment of employer groups that choose to contract directly with providers rather than through one of these intermediary organizations.

PPOs, in combination with utilization management programs, have become an increasingly important component of managed health care delivery systems. The 1989 market share for such managed care systems increased to 33 percent, whereas the market share of unmanaged fee-for-service plans fell to 18 percent. A continuation of that trend will make managed care systems the dominant group health insurance mode by the end of the decade.

CURRENT STATUS

Who is contracting? To date, most of the managed care activity has been organized and sponsored by insurance companies or management entities that package and sell HMO and PPO products to employers. Increasingly, self-insured employers have begun to contract directly with health care providers. In this way they can

- cut out the intermediary to save administrative fees
- exercise more control over the provider network
- increase provider responsiveness to employer needs
- target providers who practice health care efficiently (low utilization) and effectively (high quality)
- strengthen prior business relationships with community providers

Purchasers of directly contracted services include private employers (both for-profit and not-for-profit), employer coalitions, public entities (both federal and state), and union trust funds.

Simultaneously, health care providers are developing delivery systems with sufficient depth and breadth to both initiate and respond to employer-based managed care contracts. Health care providers are motivated to cut out the middleman in order to protect their current market share, increase their volume of patients, and improve their level of reimbursement.

Although the PPO model predominates in direct contracting, there are other types of managed care providers, including the exclusive provider organization (EPO). Administratively, an EPO functions like a PPO, but the employee is required to use an EPO provider in order to be eligible for health care benefits. PPOs, on the other hand, are offered to employees as a less expensive option, but their use is not mandatory in order to obtain health care benefits.

Health maintenance organizations (HMOs) have not been a vehicle for direct contracting between self-insured employers and providers, because they are generally structured around capitated arrangements. Self-insured employers lack the actuarial data and internal administrative systems to support direct contracting under capitated arrangements. In addition, the state and federal licensing requirements for HMOs are not conducive to the development of direct contract relationships. Consequently, this discussion focuses on contractual arrangements based upon modified fee-for-service payments that are typical for both PPOs and EPOs.

What are purchasers buying? With regard to ambulatory care services, purchasers are directly contracting for

- hospital outpatient services that might not be covered under a contract with an acute care hospital
- urgent care, laboratory, radiology, and surgical services provided by free-standing centers

- professional services provided by medical groups, individual practice associations (IPAs), and multispecialty clinics
- ancillary services such as physical therapy, home health, and durable medical equipment

As a practical matter, purchasers usually contract with hospitals and physicians for a broad range of inpatient and outpatient services rather than just ambulatory care. However, the considerations are the same regarding the qualities of a good contracting partner, the payment arrangements that are anticipated, the services that the provider is expected to deliver, and the new opportunities that a particular contractual relationship brings to the provider.

For the purchaser, the financial terms of the agreement should generate sufficient savings to at least offset the costs of contracting. For the provider, the purchaser must be sufficiently large that the patient base represents a significant potential for increased volume. Additional factors the provider needs to consider include

- other ambulatory care providers in the network
- existing relationships with contracting hospitals
- total number and specialties of network providers
- whether the other network providers are complementary or competitive

ADVANTAGES OF DIRECT CONTRACTING

Provider. With the proper contracting partners, the ambulatory care provider can preserve its patient base and develop a potential stream of new patients. The provider can market services working directly with the purchaser, who has a vested interest in channeling employees to the preferred providers. Direct contracting can help providers protect market share and establish a reliable income base.

Purchaser. In a direct contracting situation, the purchaser can select the ambulatory care providers of choice. The selection criteria include historical employee utilization patterns, the quality of care provided, and demonstrated cost-effectiveness.

The managed care network that results is customized to the purchaser's needs and priorities.

DISADVANTAGES OF DIRECT CONTRACTING

Provider. Direct contracting can be costly and time consuming and may lead to a multitude of contracts that must be managed and maintained. For physicians in particular, negotiating direct contracts with a purchaser may result in a sense of losing control of the relationships previously enjoyed with their patients. However, not contracting may ultimately mean no patients at all.

More importantly, there is a potential financial loss if the volume of incremental business does not offset the financial concessions that the provider has made to obtain the contract. A very major concern for the provider is that it is not simply discounting existing business but is simultaneously increasing patient volume.

In addition, the performance of the purchaser as a payer is potentially a major concern. The purchaser must be sufficiently large and adequately solvent to honor the terms of the contract and pay agreed amounts within specified time periods.

Purchaser. There has been considerable discussion about the liability of employers who directly contract with providers. Although there have been no definitive court cases to date, there is concern that employers who direct or financially incent employees to use specific providers may be held liable for the providers' conduct under the corporate negligence theory. Consequently, provider credentialing and quality assurance activities are becoming increasingly important to purchasers, although they require specific skills and funding to establish and maintain.

EVALUATING THE DIRECT CONTRACTING POTENTIAL

Health care providers enter into contractual relationships because they want to retain current patients, they need a source of new patients, and they believe that payment for services will be more timely. Purchasers of health care services establish direct contracts with providers to manage utilization and costs and to channel their employees to efficient, high-quality health care services. Therefore, both providers and purchasers should analyze their organizational needs and the existing local health care environment before deciding whether or not to pursue direct contracting as an organizational strategy.

Provider. Good administrative systems and management, coupled with personnel who understand and are committed to managed care, provide the foundation for successful participation in direct contracts. Therefore, organizational factors that the provider should evaluate prior to contracting include its

- structure
- ability to administer multiple contracts
- systems for tracking payment sources and monitoring accounts receivable
- current sources of patients

The provider should also assess the available forms of support for participation in managed care.

Environmental factors that might influence the provider's decision to enter into direct contracting include

- the number of major employers located in or near the provider's service area
- the employee population that would be covered in such arrangements
- the managed care environment in the community
- other providers participating in the directly contracted network
- the proposed health care benefit plan design
- the mechanism for channeling employees into the network

In view of the trend toward managed care, it is probably not in the provider's best interest to adopt a general policy that precludes direct contracting. Instead, criteria should be developed for evaluating the worth of a direct contract, and the decision to accept or reject should be made on a contract-by-contract basis.

An ambulatory care provider may independently or in combination with other providers actively solicit direct contracts with employers. Generally, any individual provider is better served by combining forces with others in order to present an attractive package that includes a broad range of services and is accessible to employees. In developing this strategy, the provider (or group of providers) should target purchasers who understand and have demonstrated a commitment to managed care.

An often overlooked area within which ambulatory care providers might initiate direct contracting is workers' compensation. The cost of the medical portion of workers' compensation has been escalating, and ambulatory care accounts for the largest segment of workers' compensation medical costs. Consequently, employers are looking to managed care systems such as utilization review, case management, and direct contracting for application to workers' compensation.

State statutory requirements that obligate employers to pay for care and, in some states, allow employers to direct employees to selected providers create the framework for ambulatory care providers to pursue contractual relationships actively. The employers are assured that care is being rendered in a cost-effective manner, while the providers know there is a commitment by the employers to use their services. That creates a strong foundation for a directly contracted relationship.

Purchaser. The purchaser should analyze the following organizational factors prior to entering into a direct contracted relationship:

- the number of and geographic distribution of employees
- the dollar volume of ambulatory care claims
- the distribution of those claims across categories of service and providers of care
- the cost to the organization of developing and maintaining a provider network

The main environmental consideration for the purchaser is whether direct contracting of a PPO network represents a better option than using an existing intermediary's PPO network. Factors that are particularly important include these:

- provider distribution and representation in existing PPOs
- the "fit" between PPO provider networks and those providers frequently used by employees
- the anticipated level of savings generated by using an intermediary's PPO network versus a directly contracted PPO network
- the administrative costs of implementing and maintaining a directly contracted PPO network compared to the cost of using an intermediary's PPO network

The purchaser should select a direct contracting strategy when it is determined that the following are true:

- There are sufficient numbers of geographically concentrated employees to pique the interest of providers.
- There are appropriate internal management systems to support directly contracted provider networks.
- It makes economic sense to pursue direct contracting rather than engaging an intermediary PPO network.

IMPLEMENTING THE DIRECT CONTRACTING PROCESS

Provider. When considering the benefits of a specific direct contract, the provider must determine whether that contract represents a growth opportunity, protects the existing patient base, or simply discounts current business. The key factors in making this determination are

- the size of the purchaser and current volume of health care visits
- the benefit plan incentives to use contracted providers
- the benefit plan limitations on specialty referrals

The overriding consideration will be the size of the purchases and the proportion of the provider's business that the purchaser's employees represent. A Fortune 500 employer may be knocking at the door but have only a handful of employees located in the community. At the same time, the largest employer in town may have thousands of employees but more than half of them may be enrolled in HMOs.

The potential for growth from participating in a contracted network is directly related to the structure of the health care benefits offered to the purchaser's employees. Thus, an attempt must be made to realistically evaluate the cost of losing the purchaser's existing business compared with the cost of discounting that existing business plus the value of the estimated growth.

Benefit plan designs that make the out-of-pocket expense greater for patients who see noncontracted providers help to channel employees toward contracted providers. A significant difference in out-of-pocket expense is particularly important to primary care and other providers to whom patients can self-refer, since individuals are unlikely to change to an unknown physician in the absence of financial incentives. Providers should be wary of benefit plans that offer employees little or no financial incentive to use contracting providers.

For specialty providers to whom employees are referred, the benefit plan requirements to use "gatekeepers" or to obtain referral authorization from utilization review organizations are important. If the purchaser incorporates such control mechanisms into the benefit plan design, there should be a clear description of these requirements and a clear delineation of the contracting physicians' obligations to refer patients to other contracted providers. The degree of limitation on specialty referral is also an important factor for primary care providers to consider before entering into directly contracted arrangements.

Also, the ambulatory care provider should request a roster of other providers with whom the employer intends to contract. Ambulatory care providers who are heavily dependent on patient referrals might make participation conditional on being able to market their services to the physicians and hospitals from which they will receive referrals.

Finally, the ambulatory care provider must evaluate both the proposed financial arrangements and the purchaser's ability to pay promptly in exchange for financial concessions. As mentioned previously, these arrangements generally reimburse providers on a fee-for-service basis. Specific reimbursement mechanisms may include fee schedules, case rates, or discounted charges. Some contracts may stipulate the withholding of a portion of payment that will be redistributed back to the providers based on performance.

Although virtually all of these contracts are likely to reduce income, they represent payment rates established by agreement rather than unilaterally, as currently done. Providers are willing to make such concessions, because they believe that increased volume will offset decreases in unit price and that the purchaser will pay promptly, usually within 30 days. The potential contract must be evaluated on the basis of the provider's prior experience with the purchaser with respect to speed and accuracy of claim administration. Obviously, the purchaser's financial status will also affect its ability to honor the contract. The provider should request financial statements if there are any concerns about the purchaser's long-term viability.

Purchaser. Once the purchaser decides to engage in direct contracting, the desirable participating providers should be identified. Criteria for provider selection include

- the scope of services provided
- the ease of access for users
- the organizational structure of the provider and the consequent ease of initiating and managing a contractual relationship
- the quality assurance programs that the provider maintains
- the provider's ability to manage increased patient volume

In addition to targeting providers for participation in the network, a critical component for success is communication with the employees as to how the network should be used, which providers will be in the network, and what the difference in benefits will be between staying in the network and going outside of it. Although comprehensive information cannot be supplied until after completion of the contracting process, the commitment of the purchaser to an effective communication process and the willingness of the providers to cooperate in that effort should be included as part of the contracting process.

CONTRACT NEGOTIATION AND MANAGEMENT

Once an ambulatory care provider and a purchaser agree to enter into a direct contractual relationship, it is important that the contract terms be as favorable as possible for both parties.

Provider. The provider should be especially attentive to the following provisions:

- Payment arrangements should be clearly delineated, including the payment time frame and penalties, such as loss of discounts, for not meeting payment deadlines.
- An exclusive service area should be designated for the provider whenever possible.

- The provider should be able to collect fees from patients in the event the purchaser does not pay.
- Performance criteria and incentive arrangements should be clearly delineated, with examples if necessary.

After the contract is negotiated and signed, the provider should establish tracking mechanisms to evaluate contract performance. Areas that should be monitored include the effect on patient volume, the timeliness of payment by the purchaser, and the administrative cost of maintaining the contract and complying with its requirements.

Purchaser. The purchaser should include provisions such as the following:

- The purchaser should retain the right to terminate the contract immediately if there is reason to believe that the provider is jeopardizing employees.
- The provider should be required to notify the purchaser immediately of any criminal or malpractice actions.
- Fee increases should be linked to standard indices, such as the medical component of the consumer price index.

The purchaser should set up systems that monitor utilization, charges and payments, and patient volume for each preferred provider. The purchaser should also establish a provider relations function to follow through on claims administration, utilization review, and network management problems, as needed.

MANAGING RISKS

Provider. For providers, a major risk of direct contracting is purchaser solvency and the potential for provider exposure. However, given the size and stature of many of the employers involved in direct contracting, the degree of risk is often no greater than with some more traditional contracting partners, such as insurance companies. Also, as provider contracts are generally not risk-based, the exposure is no greater than providing service for a self-insured plan in a noncontracted environment.

However, greater financial risks to providers do result from arrangements that are not structured properly, discounts for existing business that are not offset by new business, and administrative costs that rise disproportionately to the income from the contract. Such risks are managed by conducting a thorough analysis prior to contracting and by closely monitoring contract performance once an agreement is struck.

Purchaser. As mentioned previously, some legal experts believe that employers may be liable for the professional negligence of contracted providers through the legal theory of corporate negligence. That exposure is heightened by the degree to which employee freedom of choice is limited. Employers can manage their liability by choosing providers with care and by developing a strong contract document.

Mutual Safeguards. In addition to the contract areas discussed above, certain additional contract provisions should be included to minimize the mutual risk inherent in direct contracting. These include the following:

- The contract should allow for immediate termination in case of purchaser insolvency or provider malfeasance.
- Favorable payment arrangements should be linked to incremental volume increases.
- The provider should review and approve any utilization review program that is presented as part of the contract and should have the right to review any program changes after the contract is implemented as well as the right to terminate the contract if the new program requirements are not acceptable.
- Each party to the contract should be informed of any change in the organizational status of the other party, such as acquisition or merger.
- The contract should address legal and liability concerns, including employer liability coverage and indemnification provisions whereby the parties to the contract indemnify each other for losses incurred due to errors or omissions of the other party.

CONCLUSION

Managed care systems are the latest variation of nongovernmentally sponsored and organized health care delivery. The future of the private health care delivery system lies in the voluntary alliances that are being forged today. In order to be positioned for the next decade, health care providers should consider contracting strategies that are both compatible with the health care environment and advance their own organizational goals. Direct contracting is only one option in the continuum of managed care, but careful selection of direct contracting partners may be beneficial to both ambulatory care providers and health care purchasers in achieving their organizational goals and meeting their financial needs.

11

Organization of Outpatient Practice Associations

Noah D. Rosenberg

During recent years, many independent practicing physicians have begun to recognize the importance of developing a physician contracting capability in the ambulatory care arena. Some of these independent practicing physicians have begun to form contracting vehicles, which the author will refer to as outpatient practice associations (OPAs). Several of these OPAs have evolved into organizations that are capable of representing independent physician interests in negotiations with a diversity of prepaid, indemnity, and self-insured purchasers of physician services for both professional medical services and, for the first time, institutional medical services.

Independent practicing physicians participating in OPA development projects have begun to examine seriously the economic and service advantages of integrating their medical practices around the OPAs. These physicians have begun to think of the OPAs as all-inclusive business entities. These same OPAs have begun to design, develop, and implement mechanisms for centralizing, among other things, billing and claims administration, data collection and evaluation, equipment and supply purchasing, ancillary service purchasing, capital financing, marketing, product development, and a diversity of office management functions. Physicians participating in an OPA are rapidly recognizing that the OPA can be used as a vehicle for reducing office overhead while simultaneously improving office administration, thereby enabling them to concentrate their efforts and financial resources on providing quality and cost-effective medical and institutional services in an effectively managed network of office locations and ambulatory care settings.

Several OPAs that have chosen to aggressively expand their OPA capabilities have begun by following a series of well-planned phases of business development. These phases have included, but are not limited to, drafting an OPA business plan and detailed pro forma budget, establishing physician selection and credentialing criteria, structuring an OPA–individual physician agreement, structuring an OPA–ancillary provider agreement, structuring an OPA–hospital agreement, and developing a sophisticated OPA management infrastructure.

It is important in trying to decide whether to develop an OPA that criteria are selected for the purpose of measuring the prospective OPA's administrative, financial, and medical viability. Appendix 11-A contains, in outline form, a set of criteria that may be used for this purpose. These criteria can also be used in determining whether to expand an existing OPA.

PHYSICIAN SELECTION AND CREDENTIALING

During the earlier years of independent practice association (IPA) development in acute care hospital settings, an individual physician's medical staff credential was often used by the leadership of an IPA as the only basis for credentialing the physician as an IPA participant. This "credentialing" process commonly led to the formation of large organizations that lacked a common direction among participating physicians, an appropriate mixture of primary care and specialty physicians, and an adequate number of physician participants who were proponents of providing medical services in a quality and cost-effective manner. Many of the participating IPA physicians were antagonistic toward the IPA and worked to its detriment.

More recently, independent practicing physicians developing OPAs have realized the importance—from a professional malpractice, restraint-of-trade, and business standpoint—of carefully screening and credentialing the physicians who will participate as members. OPAs now realize that participating OPA physicians and OPA directors and officers may be held legally accountable for the quality of professional services and ancillary services provided to enrollees by participating OPA physicians. These same OPAs have been confronted with numerous requests by individual physicians to be given the opportunity to become participating OPA physicians. Although state laws typically do not require a physician group to grant an applicant participating physician status, as the market power of an OPA increases in a geographic area, the OPA and its participating OPA physicians may be subjected to enhanced restraint-of-trade exposure from the individual physician who loses many of his or her patients to the OPA and who is not granted participating OPA physician status by the OPA. Many of OPAs have, therefore, begun to design and develop more sophisticated credentialing procedures, which are usually implemented through the auspices of an OPA quality assurance committee and the OPA board of directors.

OPAs have begun to establish rigorous credentialing procedures separate from those of acute care hospitals. Defined criteria for participant selection used by OPAs have included, but are not limited to: current licensure, appropriate training and experience, board eligibility or certification, peer review recommendations, challenges to membership, medical staff privileges, reprimands and suspension, professional liability insurance, malpractice claims status, practice patterns, patient cases, economic profile, results of quality assurance and risk management studies, need for specific specialties (internal needs of OPA, external needs of purchasers), use of particular ambulatory care facilities, state and federal reports, commitment to the OPA organization, patient discrimination history, and investment in particular ambulatory care facilities. Credentialing procedures used by OPAs have included, but are not limited to, discreet distribution of OPA applications to selected providers in a geographic area, uniform application of standard selection criteria, establishment of the complete confidentiality of peer review proceedings and minutes of said proceedings, and compliance with federal and state peer review reporting requirements.

STRUCTURING AN OPA–INDIVIDUAL PHYSICIAN AGREEMENT

OPAs are beginning to understand the importance of protecting themselves as business entities. They have thus begun to structure written agreements with physician participants that are designed to make these physicians aware of the importance of thinking like members of an organization that has substantial medical service and economic responsibilities. These new OPA–individual physician agreements include provisions specific to, among other things, stringent physician qualification requirements (e.g., board certification), *locum tenens* responsibilities, certification and referral authorization procedures, well-defined reimbursement mechanisms (e.g., capitation of the primary care physician in a prepaid setting, payment of the specialty physician in some instances on a capitation basis), stringent professional liability and comprehensive liability insurance requirements, diverse termination provisions (e.g., 90 days with or without cause, material breach), medical record documentation requirements, penalties for discrimination against prepaid plan patients, compliance with state and federal statutes, and required participation in OPA utilization review and quality assurance activities.

OPAs are also now requiring participating OPA physicians to authorize the OPAs on a nonexclusive basis to represent the physicians' interests in negotiations with a diversity of purchasers.

STRUCTURING AN OPA–ANCILLARY SERVICES AGREEMENT

Participating OPA physicians have begun to realize the importance of using the OPA as a vehicle for developing favorable relationships with a diversity of ancillary service providers. OPAs have thus begun to contract for outpatient laboratory services, outpatient surgery services, occupational therapy, physical therapy, home health services, durable medical equipment, prosthetics, and myriad other ancillary services. In many instances, the individual participating OPA physician may take advantage of OPA service discounts through his or her individual office.

STRUCTURING AN OPA–HOSPITAL AGREEMENT

Many independent physicians were previously concerned, and to a certain extent are currently concerned, about the amount of control that a hospital or hospital system may exert over an IPA. Although the participating OPA physicians' ownership in the ambulatory care setting has reduced the importance of the physician-hospital relationship, the physicians realize the importance of working together with a hospital or hospital system for the purpose of approaching a very complex purchasing community. OPAs have thus begun to structure affiliations with hospitals, including the negotiation and execution of agreements, to provide the OPAs with, among other things, technical support services (e.g., office space, equipment and supplies, secretarial staff, marketing services, computer services), ancillary support services (e.g., laboratory and radiology services, social services, dialysis), financial support services (e.g., development costs, lines of credit, low interest loans, and financial grants), and management support services.

Several OPAs have begun to explore more seriously integrating their contracting and management functions with those of an affiliated hospital or hospital system. These OPAs have begun evaluating the feasibility of establishing and supporting an investment or management vehicle (joint venture) with an affiliated hospital or hospital system. The joint venture would provide the OPA with, among other things, medical management (e.g., assistance in the hiring of office staff, the performance of billing and eligibility verification tasks, and the purchase of professional and general comprehensive liability insurance), equipment (through lease arrangements), access to capital (through debt financing), contract management (e.g., negotiating contracts with purchasers and maintaining positive relationships with purchasers), and strategic planning and marketing services.

DEVELOPING A MANAGEMENT INFRASTRUCTURE

Probably the single most important realization that many participating OPA physicians have recently come to has been the importance of identifying an experienced and well-organized management team to administer the OPA and the related administrative, operational, and economic activities of the affiliated ambulatory care setting. These physicians have thus begun to search for, identify, and hire experienced medical group managers to manage their OPAs. These managers have facilitated, among other things, the negotiation and execution of significantly better agreements with purchasers of physician services and vendors of equipment and supplies, open communication among participating OPA physician offices and the administrative offices of those entities who purchase physician services (e.g., physician roster changes, coordination of new office locations), resolution of grievances between physicians and those who purchase physician services, and the identification and purchase of appropriate software and hardware systems. These OPA managers have further been better able to advise OPAs in the selection of systems for the centralization of claims administration and eligibility determination, the performance of utilization review and quality assurance activities, and the development of the data collection and evaluation procedures that are becoming so important to those entities who purchase physician services.

PRODUCT DEVELOPMENT

Many participating OPA physicians have begun to realize the advantages of using OPAs for purposes of developing new medical service products that can best be implemented through an organized group of physicians who have ownership of the ambulatory care setting. These products include, but are not limited to, hardware and software systems, marketing and contracting mechanisms, financial investment strategies, reciprocal physician agreements, shared purchasing capabilities, at-risk self-insured products, and specialty-focused products.

CONCLUSION

Clearly, many independent physicians are beginning to realize the benefits of affiliating with a well-managed and integrated physician organization in the ambulatory care setting. It is quite likely that many of their peers will concur with these physicians in the near future and develop their own OPAs. Furthermore, these more fully integrated OPAs seem likely to evolve into organizations that look and act much like existing medical group practices.

Appendix 11-A

Guidelines for the Evaluation of a Prospective OPA

I. Administrative Viability

A. Experience of physician leadership

B. Experience of administrative staff

C. Experience of ancillary administrative staff

D. Experience of operational, financial, and legal advisors

E. Experience working with sophisticated eligibility and claims administration systems

F. Experience working with sophisticated data collection and evaluation systems

G. Experience working with insureds or employees of purchasers

H. Experience working with underwritten and administrative services–only products

   1. Risk-based

   2. Indemnity-based

I. Experience working with open-access versus closed-access systems

J. Experience working with integrated physician, institution, and ancillary health care provider network

II. Management Viability

A. Establish and maintain participating provider network.

   1. Establish physician and health care professional network through provider contracting.

   2. Negotiate agreement between hospital and OPA for the provision of ancillary and administrative services and for the establishment and monitoring of a hospital-OPA shared-risk pool.

   3. Negotiate agreements with nonhospital ancillary service providers.

   4. Negotiate reduced rate structures with out-of-area hospitals and physician providers.

   5. Negotiate agreements pertinent to ongoing management of OPA.
B. Establish and maintain participating plan-OPA liaison.
   1. Coordinate OPA-participating plan communications.
   2. Inform participating plans of participating provider roster.
   3. Provide participating plans with participating provider roster.
   4. Establish communication channels between participating provider offices and participating plans.
   5. Coordinate participating provider network and OPA office expansion to meet requirements of participating plans.
   6. Assist in resolving any grievances between OPA and participating plans.
   7. Resolve participating provider and participating plan member grievances.
C. Administer plan member eligibility process.
   1. Assist participating provider offices with determination of eligibility of participating plan members prior to provision of medical services by participating providers.
   2. Reconcile retroactive denial of eligibility against provision of medical services and authorization process by OPA in accordance with participating plan–OPA agreement.
   3. Administer system for retroactive eligibility determination and assist in collection of outstanding accounts receivable from ineligible patients.
D. Administer OPA distribution of capitation revenue.
   1. Receive and deposit capitation payment from participating plans.
   2. Reconcile capitation payments with participating plan–OPA agreement requirements, benefit plan components, and membership roster.
   3. Prepare budgets for internal OPA management.
   4. Distribute primary care physician capitation payments.
   5. Distribute specialty physician payment based upon authorized referrals and matching claims.
   6. Maintain operational bank accounts and trust bank accounts for OPA.
   7. Provide third-party payer information for coordination of benefits to all participating providers.
   8. Distribute payments to all ancillary and administrative providers.
   9. Prepare monthly, quarterly, and yearly financial statements and accounting protocols for all participating providers and for OPA.

10. Provide for yearly audit by outside firm or public accountant selected by OPA.

E. Administer OPA distribution of institutional revenue.

   1. Receive and deposit revenue from participating plans.

   2. Reconcile payments with participating plan–OPA agreement requirements.

   3. Maintain operational bank account and trust bank account for ambulatory care setting.

   4. Distribute payments to all ancillary and acute care hospital providers.

   5. Prepare monthly, quarterly, and yearly financial statements and accounting protocols for ambulatory care setting.

   6. Provide for yearly audit by outside firm or public accountant selected by OPA.

   7. Distribute institutional risk pool bonus.

F. Administer utilization review, quality assurance, and medical policy committee functions.

   1. Provide the necessary personnel to administer medical and hospital referral authorization procedures.

   2. Interface with each participating provider's office staff to monitor the referral authorization procedures.

   3. Provide administrative assistance prior to and at all utilization review, quality assurance, and medical policy committee meetings (e.g., meeting schedules, setup, agenda, minutes).

   4. Provide administrative support at utilization review committee meetings, including the discussion of information on participating plan benefits, billing, the referral authorization process, referral and practice patterns, compliance with referral authorization process by participating providers, referral limitations, monitoring of coding procedures, and participating plan utilization guidelines.

   5. Provide administrative support for all quality assurance activities, including policy and procedure development, data collection, meeting administration, documentation of findings, monitoring of OPA-developed requirements for medical record documentation, and making arrangements with participating plans for office or site visits.

   6. Provide administrative support for medical policy committee, including policy and procedure development, meeting adminis-

tration, documentation of findings, and consistent application of adopted policies.

G. Provide general administrative assistance.

1. Provide all administrative support for hiring and (if necessary) training of staff in each participating provider's office.

2. Provide all support for daily interface with participating providers and their office staffs.

3. Provide support for OPA-hospital interface pertinent to the coordinated delivery of medical services to plan members.

4. Assist with the resolution of all nonmedical problems relating to the operation of the OPA and the provision of medical services to plan members.

H. Manage payment structure.

1. Pay percentage of OPA revenues.

2. Pay for management services as provided.

3. Pay fixed monthly fee for management services.

III. **Financial Viability**

A. Experience working with multiple types of purchaser reimbursement

1. Risk reimbursement

a) Professional risk

b) Hospital risk

c) Ancillary risk

2. Indemnity reimbursement

B. Historical financial experience

C. Current financial experience

D. Claims payment experience

1. Incurred but not reported claims

E. Allocation of financial resources

1. Amount allocated to administration

2. Amount allocated to professional services

a) Primary care

b) Specialty care

3. Amount allocated to hospital services

4. Amount allocated to ancillary services

5. Amount allocated to financial reserves

F. Relationships with sources of capital

1. Hospitals and hospital systems

2. Physician investors
3. Third-party investors

IV. Sophistication of OPA Credentialing Program

A. Criteria used for credentialing and recredentialing of providers

1. Current licensure
2. Appropriate training and experience
3. Board eligibility and certification
4. Medical staff privileges
5. Peer recommendations
6. Challenges to membership, medical staff privileges, reprimands, suspensions
7. Professional liability insurance
8. Malpractice claims status
9. Practice patterns
10. Patient case mix
11. Economic profile
12. Results of quality assurance and risk management studies
13. Need for specific specialties
    a) Internal needs of OPA
    b) External needs of purchaser
14. Use of ambulatory care facilities

B. Procedures used for credentialing

V. Sophistication of OPA Utilization Review Mechanisms

A. Experience of professional staff

1. Nursing staff performance review
2. Physician staff performance review

B. Liability insurance procured and maintained by OPA

C. Purchaser role relative to deciding coverage issues for specific medical services

1. Informing the patient and provider system regarding coverage

D. Nature of utilization review process

1. Inpatient
   a) Nurse reviewers should be licensed and should have received demonstrated training in performing utilization review.
   b) Physician reviewers should be practitioners specializing in the medical subject area for which a patient is to be hospitalized.

c) Before issuing a denial, each patient's attending physician must be consulted by the physician reviewer and the case must be thoroughly discussed with the attending physician.

d) Before issuing a denial, physician reviewers should be required to have reviewed applicable portions of the patient's charts and records and not to have relied exclusively on summaries of these records prepared by a nurse reviewer or other health professional. In addition, physician reviewers should actually examine the patient if he or she has any doubt regarding the appropriateness of a denial.

e) Emergency admissions and procedures should always be exempted from the requirement of preauthorization review.

f) Nurse and physician reviewers should keep concurrent notes of all their review activities and of the basis for each decision. If such records are maintained, it will be easier for purchasers and the health professionals themselves to defend against any future malpractice claims arising out of such review activities.

g) Time frames should be specified for when review by a nurse coordinator and review by a backup physician must routinely be completed. If such reviews are not performed within a specified time period, authorization for an admission or procedure should be deemed given.

h) When a denial for an admission or procedure is issued, the patient and physician should be entitled to appeal the denial. This type of appeal should be in addition to patient rights pertaining to the utilization review program.

i) Medical criteria, including those related to determining appropriateness of an admission or procedure and the length of stay, should be based upon local practice standards and be subject to prior review and approval by the purchaser before they are used.

2. Outpatient (same as inpatient)

E. Adequacy of computer system

VI. Adequacy of OPA Physician Delivery System

A. Service access (professional, hospital, and ancillary)

1. Specific to purchaser employee population

a) Age

b) Sex

c) Illness exposure

B. Geographic access

C. Scheduling access

D. Sophistication of OPA, hospital, and ancillary provider relationships

    1. Integration of OPA, hospital, and ancillary provider utilization review and quality assurance systems

    2. Integration of OPA, hospital, and ancillary provider utilization data collection and evaluation systems

    3. Sophistication of OPA, hospital, and ancillary provider financial relationship (e.g., hospital risk pools)

        a) Outpatient laboratory

        b) Outpatient surgery

        c) Outpatient mental health

        d) Outpatient alcohol and drug abuse

        e) Occupational therapy

        f) Physical therapy

        g) Home health

        h) Durable medical equipment

        i) Prostheses

        j) Implantable devices

        k) Out-of-area reciprocity agreements

        l) Subacute care

    4. Sophistication of OPA, hospital, and ancillary provider medical management systems

VII. Sophistication of OPA–Individual Professional Relationship

A. Qualification of providers

B. Compensation of providers

    1. Risk reimbursement

        a) Primary care versus specialty care

        b) Hospital inpatient incentives

        c) Hospital outpatient incentives

        d) Ancillary service incentives

    2. Compensation models

        a) Model 1

            (1) Capitation of primary care physicians and payment of specialty care physicians on a modified fee-for-service basis

            (2) Distribution of OPA incentive pools to primary care and specialty care physicians

        (3) Distribution of hospital–OPA incentive funds and/or participating plan–OPA incentive funds

    b) Model 2

        (1) Payment of primary care and specialty care physicians on a modified fee-for-service basis

        (2) Distribution of OPA incentive pools to primary care and specialty care physicians

        (3) Distribution of hospital-OPA incentive funds and/or participating plan–OPA incentive funds

    b) Model 3

        (1) Capitation of primary care and specialty care physicians

        (2) Distribution of OPA incentive pools to primary care and specialty care physicians

        (3) Distribution of hospital–OPA incentive funds and/or participating plan–OPA incentive funds

  3. Fee-for-service reimbursement

C. Insurance required

  1. Type of insurance

  2. Level of insurance

  3. Quality of insurance

D. Hours of service

E. Scheduling requirements

F. Referral requirements (e.g., prior authorization)

G. Billing of patients

H. Coordination of benefits

I. Access to financial records of providers

J. Access to medical records of patients

K. Administrative responsibilities of physician office (e.g., eligibility procedures)

L. Grievance procedures

M. Nondiscrimination requirements

N. Termination provisions

  1. Termination for material breach

  2. Termination for provision of poor quality care

  3. Termination for expiration of health plan–OPA agreements

  4. Termination without cause

  5. Continuing care responsibilities in the event of termination

      6. Due process rights in the event of termination

  O. Compliance with pharmaceutical formulary

  P. Ability of OPA to charge administrative or operational fees

  Q. Claims submission requirements (e.g., deadline for claims submission)

  R. Stop-loss capability

VIII. Sophistication of OPA Utilization Data Collection and Assessment Systems

  A. Adequacy of computer system

  B. Experience of MIS staff

  C. Compatibility of computer systems of OPA and purchaser

  D. Compatibility of utilization data requirements of OPA and purchaser

  E. Ability of OPA to collect data required by purchaser

  F. Ability of OPA to generate machine-readable format for data referenced above

  G. Timing of data distribution

  H. Ownership of data

  I. Use of data

  J. Compensation for data

12

Risk Management

Annie Stoeckmann

In order to develop a risk management program, a system that identifies, analyzes, resolves, and monitors areas of risk within the organization or practice must be established. Such a system is an essential tool for an effective loss prevention program. The potential for a loss must be identified and analyzed before the loss can be prevented, minimized, or resolved.

Identifying and analyzing risk within the ambulatory care setting requires a focused approach directed toward areas with actual or potential loss exposure. Several sources for retrieving the necessary data are claim histories, the quality improvement program, utilization management findings, credentialing and peer review activities, patient complaints, direct inspections, and consultation with experts (if needed). Claim histories are retrievable from current and previous professional liability carriers or from the entity's own records if self-insured. Unusual occurrence reports, whether through incident reporting systems or quality assurance programs, are a current source of data concerning potential losses. Peer review activities will help define problem-prone practitioners or clinical areas at risk, while patient complaints and direct observation from walking rounds provide first-hand information. Utilizing the expertise of inside or outside consultants for highly technical areas such as hazardous waste, plant safety, and current legislative health care issues is another valuable method for identifying risk exposure. Once the data are collected, careful review and trending for specific patterns can be done to assist in managing any potential loss.

One question that occurs in managing risk in ambulatory care is where to affix liability. Are practitioners or system breakdowns at fault? In a review of five years of data reported by HMOs and managed care plan providers, it was discovered that the highest percentage of alleged events were due to failure to diagnose, delayed diagnosis, or delayed treatment. Analysis of these claims revealed, for example, that delayed diagnosis or misdiagnosis of cancer of the breast, colon, and cervix frequently occurred when laboratory and radiology reports, although properly obtained, were not even reviewed by the primary physician. Wrongful death due to misdiagnosis or delay in treatment showed patient noncompliance with follow-up appointments with primary care providers and referral physicians. In these cases, there were often no procedures in place to assess whether patients actually followed through with referrals, consultations, and recommended recheck visits.

Whether analysis reveals a tendency toward system breakdown, inappropriate medical judgment, or practitioner error, the following are well recognized as areas that most frequently give rise to potential compensatory events: medical records, medication administration, communication, informed consent, quality of care, and credentialing.

THE MEDICAL RECORD

The medical record is often referred to as the determining factor in the validity and viability of a medical malpractice lawsuit. It has been amply shown that if health care professionals recorded all care and treatment in the records, most lawsuits could be discouraged, defended against, or settled reasonably. Terms such as *timely, accurate, consistent, objective, complete,* and *legible* are not new. They describe the very elements of good recordkeeping that may protect the patient from a misdiagnosis, delay in treatment, negligent prescribing or medication and prescription errors.

All entries into the medical record should be timely, and yet lack of timeliness is one of the most common problems. Many patients new to a practice receive a history and physical at the initial visit, yet evidence of subsequent or updated histories and physicals vary considerably from one practice to the next. Allegations of negligence surface when cancer of the colon or breast is diagnosed in patients whose last recorded physical was five years earlier. Entries in progress notes or reports, if dictated weeks after office visits, are of little value to the patient or practitioner in diagnosis or treatment. In fact, late entries will more likely discredit the record in a court case if the plaintiff claims there was altering of records or tampering with evidence. In some limited situations, late entries may be appropriate if the record clearly identifies the date and time of the entries as well as the date and time of the examinations. But more often than not, late entries are perceived as self-serving by a jury.

The section of the medical record that is most important and helpful as a risk management tool is the active problem list. The purpose of this page is to provide the health care practitioner with a current summary of the patient's problems, the clinical management, and the prescribed medications. A complete and current problem list may decrease the potential for delayed or failed treatment or misdiagnosis. Being able to quickly note that the patient has not had a mammogram in two years or that the previous pregnancy revealed gestational diabetes may affect the current plan of care and enhance the practice of good medicine.

Inconsistencies in the medical record attack the credibility of the health care practitioner. Frequently, the recorder or nurse will document a patient complaint or the reason for an office visit but the physician will fail to address it in the chart. Too often a practitioner will not document thought processes or conversations with the patient. Complaints of numbness or tingling in lower extremities, for example, if recorded by the nurse but not addressed by the health care practitioner, can make defense difficult when litigation arises due to the amputation of a diabetic patient's leg.

Objective and accurate reporting makes everyone's job easier. Subjective, patronizing, or critical remarks should never appear in a medical record, since they can be misinterpreted by cotreating practitioners or provide a prospective plaintiff with an incentive to pursue a lawsuit. Likewise, omitting medically relevant information regarding chemical dependency, altered life style, or mental health problems may interfere with a subsequent treating physician's diagnosis and plan of care. Developing criteria that screen for objectivity in the record will assist in identifying the existence or nonexistence of such problem records. Using these criteria for both random and focused chart reviews will help identify such omissions and misstatements. Formulating a procedure for controlling the release of sensitive medical information will encourage complete and accurate charting while protecting patient confidentiality.

Legibility is always an issue in documenting the care and treatment of patients. It is understood that treating and cotreating health care practitioners must be able to read the medical record in order to render appropriate and safe care. Miscommunications and medication errors frequently arise from illegible charting. If a lawsuit should arise, the only evidence of the quality of care rendered is the written record plus the patient care outcome. Risk management efforts that encourage legible records include recommending dictation in lieu of handwritten narrative notes, providing forms that allow for check boxes to be filled in when appropriate, and instituting an active quality improvement program that identifies practitioners with illegible handwriting.

PRESCRIPTION AND MEDICATION ERRORS

Prescription and medication errors occur often, yet most are preventable. Medication errors occur because the basic common-sense rules of administering and prescribing drugs are ignored. Improper dosages, inappropriate medications, failures to note drug allergies, multiple prescriptions leading to overdose, and failures to warn of side effects are the most common mistakes in drug management.

Proper dosages and routes can be assured by checking manufacturer recommendations prior to prescribing or giving patients take-home samples. Too often physicians rely on medical assistants to double-check medications.

Illegible physician handwriting is also a well-known contributor to medication errors that result in patient injury. Prescribing the right drug requires a continued awareness of new and improved drugs as well as an awareness of drugs with similar chemical compositions but different trade names. Drug reactions and interactions place an added burden on physicians and staff to continually update their knowledge.

A history of allergies can easily get buried in the medical record. A patient's allergy to one drug is often indicative of other sensitivities and should be recorded in the active problem list. When in doubt, a practitioner should clarify with the patient whether a previous reaction was a true allergy or sensitivity.

Overdoses and underdoses of medications often cause problems in risk management. All too often a patient will be seeing several different practitioners at the same time. Each may be treating the same or different conditions and each may be prescribing a drug therapy. In this situation, the probability of overdose or of a drug interaction rendering a medication less effective is great. The chart should be reviewed prior to prescribing. The patient's current active medication list should be displayed in the front of the chart so all practitioners will be aware of the patient's drug therapy plan. Prescription refills should be tracked and documented (together with any history of drug intolerance). All refills should be authorized by a licensed practitioner. Too often litigation reveals that a patient received regular refills for months with no intervening interview or exam.

Failure to warn patients of drug actions, side effects, and interactions has recently earned much attention from juries. The obligation to warn has been placed on the practitioner, who acts in the legal role of intermediary between the drug companies and the patient. Discussing proper use and potential adverse effects of the prescribed drug, as well as the consequences of not taking the drug or not taking it as prescribed, should become an automatic step in drug therapy.

Sample drugs, made available to office practices, clinics, and urgent care centers, present several additional risk management challenges. The generous intent to provide the patient with free drugs or as a starter to test tolerance holds the potential for serious risks. Often neither the drug nor the dosage prescribed is documented in the medical record. There may be no labeling on the medication as to how often it should be taken. And there is seldom any system for monitoring of outdated or recalled drugs in this mini-pharmacy in the hallway or desk drawer. Strengthening staff education and orientation regarding drug therapy, developing specific quality assurance and utilization review criteria for monitoring prescription practices, and minimizing or eliminating the dispensing of sample drugs may help reduce risk exposure due to prescription and medication errors.

COMMUNICATION

Lack of communication can be the single major factor that turns a patient into a plaintiff. Effective communication—which includes active listening—builds trust, demonstrates caring, and is tantamount to the development of a positive relationship between the patient and the health care team. It is a well-known fact that patients are more likely to overlook an unfavorable medical outcome if they trust and believe in their health care providers.

The first impression, frequently a lasting one, occurs when the patient first makes contact. The initial exchange may be face to face or by telephone. A professional but caring manner will go a long way toward mollifying an anxious patient who has experienced a lengthy wait to see his or her physician. Patient surveys as well as direct observation can be used to assess the courtesy, professional demeanor, and efficiency of the practice staff.

Telephone encounters and advice can be a sensitive area of risk exposure. Claims of delayed diagnosis, delayed treatment, and practicing outside the scope of licensure are frequently made. Patient information obtained by staff that is not properly relayed to the practitioner may result in a ruptured appendix or irreversible drug reaction. Telephone call protocols that include directions for gathering patient information, recording it, and transmitting it to the appropriate health care provider can minimize the risk of patient injury. Staff education regarding the exact responsibilities of each staff member, as well as a quality improvement program that monitors compliance with protocols and appropriateness of advice, is a necessity.

Breakdown in communication occurs not only between physicians and patients and their families. It is prevalent among providers themselves and can be a source of potential compensatory events. The failure to follow-up with referral physicians, for example, can result in a delayed diagnosis of cancer. Setting up tickler files or follow-up logs to ensure that return visits are made and consultant referrals and ancillary services are obtained guarantees improved communications and reduces the risk of patient harm. Whether it is practitioner to patient or primary care provider to consultant, effective communication builds bridges of trust between the health care team and their patients and reduces the risk of malpractice lawsuits.

INFORMED CONSENT

"Every human being, being of adult years and sound mind has a right to determine what shall be done with his own body and cannot be subjected to medical treatment without his consent" (*Schloendorf vs. Society of New York*, 211 NY 125, 105 NE Rptr 92, 1914).

This famous statement was made by a well-respected New York judge, Benjamin Cardozo. Consent law is premised on the patient's right to make a knowing and informed decision when a medical procedure presents significant risks. The most qualified and appropriate person to provide the patient with the necessary information regarding his or her medical condition and the proposed procedure or treatment is the health care practitioner.

The patient or an appropriate representative needs to be told about the nature of the medical condition, the procedure or treatment proposed, the practitioner who will perform the procedure, the risks and benefits of the procedure, the alternatives, and the consequences of refusing. The informed consent process is really a dialogue between the patient and the health care practitioner. It affords the patient the opportunity to ask questions and to have explained, in easily understood language, what procedures are planned or anticipated. Should litigation arise, the practitioner who performed the procedure must convince a jury that the patient made an informed decision. When determining which procedures or treatments require informed discussion and the extent of disclosure needed, some states use the "reasonable physician" standard—what would a reasonable physician in the medical community disclose under the same or similar circumstances? The recent trend is to use the "reasonable patient" standard—what would a reasonable person in the patient's position want to know in similar circumstances?

The best evidence that informed consent was given is documentation. This can be accomplished by narrative notes in the chart, by a preprinted consent form personalized to the patient and procedure, copies of diagrams, patient information sheets, and references to videos and pamphlets used during discussion. The written word will frequently lend more credibility in a dispute before a jury. It is imperative to remember that informed consent is a communication process and not a piece of paper. An interpreter should be used if the practitioner speaks a language other than the patient's. It is also wise to remember that the patient has the right to refuse treatment or withdraw consent at any time. It would then be the practitioner's responsibility to inform the patient of the risks and complications of such refusal or withdrawal. A patient who is prepared in advance for a possible unfavorable outcome of therapy will better accept that outcome and is less likely, therefore, to sue the health care practitioner.

UTILIZATION AND QUALITY OF CARE

Whenever there is any possibility of inferring that a medical decision may have been based on economic incentives, there exists potential risk exposure. This includes the sometimes time-consuming and complex procedures required to obtain authorization for treatment in a capitated payment system, which can be interpreted as incentives not to pursue care. Representations that high-quality care and low utilization are synonymous must be closely examined by risk managers. Courts have warned that "it is essential that cost limitation programs not be permitted to corrupt medical judgement" (*Wickline vs. State of California,* 228 Cal. Rptr 661 1986). A more recent case, *Wilson vs. Blue Cross of Southern California, et al.* (271 Cal. Rptr 876 [1990]), shows that third-party payers and utilization review entities may also be subject to legal consequences if a patient is harmed by an improper decision. Working closely with managed care plan providers to ensure the patients' well-being, as well as an understanding of the benefits offered under their plan, is crucial to avoid conflicts. A team approach is the only sure way to provide the most cost-effective and safest care.

CREDENTIALING

Liability theories such as "corporate liability and ostensible agency" are well known in the malpractice litigation arena. Extending legal responsibility to a hospital for failing to ensure the competence of its medical staff through careful selection and review, as prescribed in *Elam vs. College Park Hospital* (132 Cal. App. 3rd 332 [1982]), is now being extended to medical groups and contracted providers for managed care plans. Recent case law suggests that there is an emerging trend to hold HMOs and their provider medical groups liable for the negligence of their independent contractors or referral physicians. In a Missouri appellate court decision, *Harrell vs. Total Health Care, Inc.* (1989 Mo. App. Lexis 377), though not released for publication and subject to modification, the judge stressed the similarity in the duty to protect patients from foreseeable risk of harm for both hospitals and health care plans. Although this case was eventually dismissed due to a statutory immunity, the court recognized a duty owed by the HMO to "conduct a reasonable investigation of the physicians to ascertain their reputation in the medical community for competence." The court in *Harrell* did not specify what constitutes a reasonable investigation, but it did point out that if no investigation is made regarding the competence of referral physicians, the duty to prevent foreseeable harm has not been met.

In *Schleier vs. Kaiser Foundation Health Plan* (876 Fed. Reptr. 2nd 174 D.C. Cir. 1989), the court found Kaiser liable for consultant's negligence based on agency and master-servant theories. The court said that because the consultant answered to the primary care Kaiser physician, enough control existed to hold the employer liable for the negligence of an independent contractor. Furthermore, when the consultant was brought in to examine the patient, the patient had every reason to believe that the consultant was Kaiser's agent.

In a recent Missouri case, *Ashley Stalmach vs. Physicians Multispecialty Group* (No. 53906, Court of Appeals of Missouri, June 13, 1989 Mo. App.

Lexis 852), which was settled prior to Supreme Court review, it was held that an enrollee in a health plan may sue the medical group under a breach of contract theory as a third-party beneficiary. Here the contract between the medical group and the health plan was entered into in order to provide benefits (services) to the enrollee, the third party. The plaintiff sued the medical group for substandard care by the subcontracting physician. This was not done under an agency theory, as in *Schleier,* but under contract law. Although the case holds no precedence due to the fact it was never published, it may point a finger to future trends. Now, along with the theories of corporate liability and ostensible agency, there exists another possible theory for litigation, breach of contract, for extending liability to managed care plan providers.

The consensus of these cases dictates the importance of implementing a strong credentialing program for all physicians and allied health care professionals, whether they are employees, independent contractors, or noncontracting referral practitioners. The credentialing should at the very minimum include verification of the following: licensure, education and training, hospital affiliations, listed references, disciplinary actions, malpractice claims history, and professional liability coverage. Frequently this process can be facilitated through the cooperation of the physician's affiliated hospital or by using a centralized credentialing service. The duty to prevent a foreseeable risk of harm to a patient who sees a primary care provider or referral specialist as contracted under the plan places a recognized responsibility for credentialing all providers of care.

CONCLUSION

Early assessment of the potential for compensatory events, by reviewing incident or quality improvement reports as well as patient complaints on a daily basis, can greatly reduce risk and minimize patient injury. To adequately protect the patients and the health care team, ongoing monitoring by means of claim reviews, quality improvement and utilization management programs, and peer review activities is essential. A strong risk management system can assist practitioners in delivering and documenting safe, high-quality care, which is the best way to prevent or minimize patient injury and subsequent loss.

13

Measuring Productivity

Gloria Gilbert Mayer

The concept of productivity is well developed in manufacturing industries but has been applied to service industries only recently. Although there are many complicated methods of defining productivity, in general, productivity is a ratio that describes the relationship between units of input and units of output. However, productivity measurements are difficult to apply to health care because of the great variability of the inputs and outputs and the consequent lack of reliable data. The ratio that determines productivity can be expressed either as inputs (resources used) divided by outputs (services produced) or outputs divided by inputs. However, no matter how productivity is measured, there must be an agreed unit of measure to quantify productivity.

In hospitals, the basic units of measure are well established. Table 13-1 lists some typical hospital departments with associated units of measure. In ambulatory care settings, the basic units of measure are not well established. In addition, if an ambulatory care setting is predominantly reimbursed through capitation, the units of measure are even more complicated. Table 13-2 lists ambulatory care areas with associated units of measure in a large multispecialty medical group reimbursed through capitation.

EXAMPLE OF PRODUCTIVITY MEASUREMENT

Since the ambulatory care medical records department is a complex area, it can be used to demonstrate several methods of measuring productivity. The most simple method of measuring productivity is to divide the number of charts required by physicians by the number of charts actually received by physicians. If 1,000 charts were requested in a week and 1,000 charts were delivered, then the department could claim it achieved high productivity (100 percent). If, on the other hand, only 900 charts of the 1,000 requested were received by physicians, then it would have achieved 90 percent productivity. This is an example of a very crude way of measuring the productivity of the medical records department.

Table 13-1 Sample Units of Measurement in Selected Hospital Departments

Department	*Unit of Measurement*
Individual patient unit	Unit patient days
EKG	Procedures
Labor and delivery	Deliveries
In-service education	Number of hours
Emergency room	Visits
Radiology	Relative value units/100
Social services	Contacts
Dietary	Meals served
Admitting	Admissions
Central supply	Line items
Quality assurance	Discharges
Medical records	Admissions
Transcription	Lines transcribed
Medical library	Number of active physicians
Housekeeping	Square feet serviced
Printing and duplication	Reams of paper used

Another method of measuring productivity is to examine the full-time equivalents (FTEs) needed to pull the 1,000 records. If one FTE can pull 50 charts an hour, then it should only require 20 hours of personnel time, or 2.5 FTEs, to pull the 1,000 charts (assuming one FTE works 8 hours a day). If the number of charts pulled by each person per hour is increased by 5, then productivity would

Table 13-2 Sample Units of Measurement for Selected Ambulatory Care Departments in a Capitated Multispecialty Medical Group

Department	*Unit of Measurement*
Medical records	Charts pulled monthly
Patient education	Participants
Managed care	Claims adjudicated
Management information systems	Enrollees
Accounting	Enrollees
Quality assurance	Patient visits
Appointments	Calls
Human resources	Employees
In-service education	Participants
Marketing	Enrollees
Medical staff recruitment	New physician hires
Patient relations	Enrollees
Risk management	Patient visits
Housekeeping	Square footage serviced

be increased by 10 percent and approximately 18 hours of work would be needed to pull the same 1,000 charts. If 50 per hour is the standard in the department, then the productivity can be calculated thus:

$$\frac{55}{50} = 110\% \text{ productivity}$$

On the other hand, if the staff only pull 45 charts per hour, then productivity falls:

$$\frac{45}{50} = 90\% \text{ productivity}$$

Most productivity standards are based on hours worked and the unit of service. Roey Kirk (1986) developed a simple chart that describes the four situations that increases productivity:

Productivity increases

when the hours worked	*and the units of service*
decrease	stay the same
decrease faster	decrease
stay the same	increase
increase	increase faster

Again, using the medical records department example, if one of the medical records clerks worked less hours but was still able to pull the required number of charts, then productivity would have increased. If one medical records clerk resigned but the decline in required charts pulled was only 30 percent, productivity again would have increased. If the hours of work by the medical records department stayed the same but the charts pulled increased to 60 charts per hour, this also would be an improvement. Finally, if two additional medical records clerks were hired, and now everyone could pull 60 charts per hour, productivity would also have improved.

Although this is an example from one small segment of an ambulatory care clinic, the same productivity principles can be applied to any area. Exhibit 13-1 provides some other ratios that can be used to calculate productivity.

Productivity should be measured on a routine basis in all departments. Most productivity calculations are performed on a monthly basis. The calculations are typically computerized by the MIS department and the results are given to department managers soon after the close of each month. It is very important to let managers review their own department's productivity and share the results with their staff. Goals can then be established by the entire department, and accomplishments, praise, and rewards can also be shared.

If, on the other hand, productivity goals are not met, reasons for the variances can be discussed and methods of improvement instituted. The variances should be shared with senior management, who can institute systems to help the

Exhibit 13-1 Productivity Ratios for a Medical Group Practice

LABOR PRODUCTIVITY RATIOS

$$\frac{\text{Total patient visits}}{\text{Total labor hours*}}$$

$$\frac{\text{Total patient visits}}{\text{Total hours worked per physician}}$$

$$\frac{\text{Total patient visits}}{\text{Total nursing hours}}$$

$$\frac{\text{Hours of staff absenteeism}}{\text{Total staff labor hours}}$$

$$\frac{\text{Tests performed}}{\text{Labor hours of technicians}}$$

FEE-FOR-SERVICE PRODUCTIVITY RATIOS

$$\frac{\text{Total charges}}{\text{Full-time equivalent support staff}}$$

$$\frac{\text{Total charges}}{\text{Full-time equivalent physicians}}$$

$$\frac{\text{Total collections}}{\text{Total charges}}$$

$$\frac{\text{Total collections}}{\text{Total support staff}}$$

MANAGED CARE PRODUCTIVITY RATIOS

$$\frac{\text{Total tests}}{\text{Total enrolled patients}}$$

$$\frac{\text{Total visits}}{\text{Total enrolled patients}}$$

$$\frac{\text{Costs per visit}}{\text{Expense per visit}}$$

* Includes physicians, nurses, and support personnel.
Source: Based on *The Productivity Prescription: The Manager's Guide to Improving Productivity and Profits* by D. Bain, p. 62, McGraw-Hill, 1982, and "Productivity Enhancement: Implications for Medical Group Management" by T.D. Holts, p. 35, *College Review,* Fall 1990.

department meet its productivity goals, evaluate why the goals are not being met, or adjust the current goals if they are felt to be too high. This productivity analysis must be done within two or three weeks after the close of the previous month to have a meaningful impact. A longer reporting interval loses effectiveness, since people may then forget what happened, making a proper analysis impossible. Therefore, a predetermined monthly schedule should be established for the completion of reports and analyses.

PRODUCTIVITY IN PREPAID SETTINGS

Although in the global sense total enrolled patients is the most meaningful measure for prepaid practices, individual departments must often use other statistics for inputs and outputs. In the case of medical records, it might be unfair to measure productivity against total enrolled patients, since the record clerks might have to respond to unnecessary requests for records due to sometimes inefficient systems or processes over which they have no control. For example, if a physician requests the same record on three successive days because she has been unable to contact a patient, the added time needed to service the report requests should not show up as a reduction in the productivity of the medical records department.

However, it is probably appropriate for physicians to use total enrolled patients in their formulae, since they and their clinical departments together must service the entire population of enrollees. In their efforts to demonstrate productivity, physicians may fill all their time slots with unnecessary rechecks and extended visits, but if they are not able to care for the needs of all enrollees, the "increased" productivity is a false measure.

The statistics used in other areas are again based on total enrolled patients, such as bed days per thousand (for hospital utilization), visits per thousand, x-rays per thousand, and so on. In using this type of information, a comparison of the projected and actual usage or costs yields useful information. Essentially, a budget is formulated or a standard established, and this preestablished figure is compared with the actual figure. If there is no preestablished figure, current statistics should be documented and attempts should be made to improve them. Trending is useful in the analysis of current practice and in documenting improvements.

AMBULATORY CARE STAFFING PRODUCTIVITY

In ambulatory care organizations, one of the biggest but least defined cost items is the staffing ratio. Staffing in the hospital has been studied and developed into a fine art, with variable staffing and the matching of patient needs with staff abilities. Nurses are called off if the patient count is below certain budgeted numbers. Likewise, nurses are added to the staff if the census increases beyond predicted statistics. Yet in most ambulatory care settings, nurses, receptionists, medical record personnel, and so on, are guaranteed 40 hours per week whether needed or not.

The staffing variables that must be considered in the ambulatory care setting are as follows:

1. volume of patients
2. complexity of patients

3. physical design
4. ability and skill level of staff
5. unit-related and other activities not associated with patient care
6. system sophistication

Volume of Patients

The total volume of patients seen in the ambulatory care setting has a direct effect on staffing patterns. In a large clinic, the total number of patients seen in the clinic and the number of patients seen by individual practitioners affect staffing. For example, if a practitioner sees five or more patients an hour, two assistants may be required. One assistant may just call patients in, obtain basic data, assist in basic care, and clean rooms. The other may be kept busy on the phone, charting, arranging follow-up care, calling consultants, and so on. If a provider sees less than four patients an hour, one support person may be sufficient.

The volume of patients also affects the number of business people needed in a clinic. Receptionists, medical records personnel, business staff, and so on, are needed if larger numbers of patients warrant them.

Complexity of Patients

The type and complexity of patients seen also affect the staffing in ambulatory care settings. Complex patients may require a higher level of personnel—for example, RNs or LPNs, who are able to perform such functions as patient education and assessment. If patients' conditions are routine and do not have comorbidities, unlicensed medical assistants may suffice. However, if patient illnesses become increasingly complex, assistants with more knowledge and capabilities may be necessary.

Physical Design

The physical design of the practice can affect staff efficiency. If the reception area is next to the back office, then staff can cover for each other in busy times. If two nursing units are in close proximity, again nursing staff can be shared. There are some physical designs that do not allow for any sharing of staff, in which case double staffing is needed. The physical design of the practice should create efficiency and ease of movement for staff and patients and allow staff to visualize areas other than their immediate work area (see Chapter 35).

Ability and Skill Level of Staff

The higher the level of staff expertise, the easier it is to establish more efficient, more flexible staffing patterns. Cross-training all staff helps to keep staff costs down. If an office medical assistant can make appointments, take cash, find charts, and answer the telephone, then the number of staff or the amount of overtime may be reduced. However, those tasks that require a license must not be delegated to a nonlicensed employee (of course, licensed staff members can undertake any task unlicensed staff members perform).

Unit-Related Activity

If licensed staff have a lot of tasks that are not patient-related, then more unlicensed staff may be needed. Activities such as stocking rooms, taking inventory, ordering supplies, and cleaning should be delegated to the lowest-salaried workers. If licensed personnel have to participate in routine tasks, they have less time to provide patient care.

System Sophistication

The most efficient practice has systems that have kept up with the growth in the volume of patients. Computerized appointment, billing, and scheduling systems provide accuracy and speed. Workflow analysis and work redesign may correct inefficient procedures. Each procedure should be examined to determine who performs it, when and where it occurs, how it could be performed more efficiently, and whether it is necessary. This analysis of current systems and procedures could significantly increase productivity.

MEASURING STAFFING PRODUCTIVITY

There are various methods of measuring nursing and other staff productivity in the ambulatory care setting. The ratio most commonly used to measure productivity is staff hours per patient visit. The formula is fairly easy to calculate:

$$\frac{\text{Number of hours worked}}{\text{Total number of visits}} = \text{Staff hours per patient visit}$$

If an internal medicine unit has three nurses working for a total of 24 hours and there are 50 patient visits during that period, the formula would read:

$$\frac{24 \text{ hours}}{50 \text{ patients}} = .48 \text{ hours per patient visit}$$

This measure indicates that almost 30 minutes of nursing time are devoted on average to each patient.

The difficulty in obtaining this statistic is in securing accurate data on the actual number of patients seen and the actual paid hours of nursing. Does a nurse receive compensation for lunch? Do nurses clock out early? Are patients who cancel their appointments captured? This system must be based on a completely accurate set of data. Figure 13-1 demonstrates a comparison of hours per visit for three different clinic departments for ten periods. As can be seen, units D-1 an D-2 require around 1 hour of nursing time. In periods 7 and 8, staffing time dropped to about .6 hours. Unit D-3 staffed at much higher levels, around 1.5 hours of nursing time per visit. This is a significant difference and could be extremely costly to the group if it represents overstaffing. However, if this variance is due to real patient needs, then the staffing may be at appropriate levels.

Productivity data are collected on a daily basis and summaries are presented to the clinic managers. The managers then analyze trends and variances. Since there is little national data on appropriate hours per visit, the clinic must compare its current performance with its performance in the past. Each manager attempts to "do better" with staffing patterns by utilizing part-time help for busy periods, cross-training employees, and using other methods. The same productivity measurement technique can be used for other staff, including nurses, receptionists, business office staff, and medical record clerks.

Another ratio for measuring productivity is staff hours per physician hour. Although this is easily calculated, it is of little use unless the number and type of patients is included in the formula.

A patient classification system categorizes patients according to their need for care. Some specialties are known to require more staffing, such as surgery, because of the large number of office surgical procedures. If a clinic can accurately classify patients according to their complexity and need for nursing care, staffing will become much more precise. However, patient classification systems are difficult to install and maintain, and reliability and validity studies must be performed routinely, which takes significant time (see Chapter 26).

POSITION CONTROL

Position control is the process of predetermining personnel requirements based on defined business needs rather than individual variations and idiosyncrasies. In ambulatory care settings, position control is often extremely unstructured. Staff are hired according to physician preference, and there is no formal

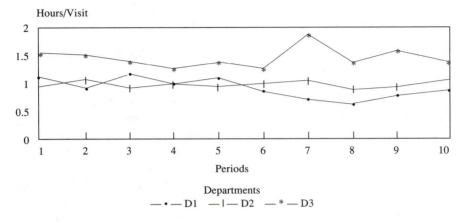

Figure 13-1 Internal Medicine and Surgery Staffing Statistics

---

method of controlling the number of full-time equivalents (FTEs). Sometimes, no one even knows the total number of FTEs, and there is no process for requesting additional staff and getting them approved. Exhibit 13-2 is an example of a position control form that may be useful in the ambulatory care setting. The form should be kept up to date and be completed in pencil so names can be erased. The most important item in this form is the position title—jobs are not created for people but people fit into predetermined positions.

Reallocation of staff is necessary if the workload is variable. When physicians are off or the patient count drops, support staff must be used by different departments, given special projects to do, or encouraged to take a vacation day.

Exhibit 13-3 provides definitions of terms needed to enforce position control and Exhibit 13-4 lists the equivalent days and hours for certain partial FTEs. It is quite critical that all managers understand these concepts and provide productivity reports utilizing appropriate terminology.

Typically there are some managers and supervisors who do not understand position control and related concepts. A staffing educational workshop may prove useful for many organizations. At the completion of such a workshop, participants should be able to

1. describe the staffing system used in their current setting
2. develop a position control form identifying the total number of FTEs
3. develop a scheduling system utilizing part-time and full-time staff that yields the greatest productivity for a hypothetical patient volume

Exhibit 13-2 Position Control Form

List by Category (Supervisors, RNs, LVNs, MAIIIs, MAIIs)

Grade	Position Title	Hours	FTE	Name	Hire Date	Pay Rate

Exhibit 13-3 Definitions of Full-Time Equivalent (FTE) Terminology

Total Annual FTEs: Includes all positions: flexible (direct), fixed, and nonproductive.

Fixed FTEs: All indirect care positions: managers, clerks, clinicians, etc.

Flexible FTEs: Volume-based budgeted positions. Includes productive and nonproductive time.

Nonproductive FTEs: Positions/hours budgeted to cover hours that will be paid but not worked. Will vary depending on the benefits given by the institution. In the example below, it is anticipated that each flexible FTE will take an average of 272 hours of benefit time.

14 vacation days + 8 holidays + 12 sick days × 8 hrs./work day = 272 hrs.

Thus,

$$\frac{272 \times 10.0 \text{ (FTEs)}}{2080} = 1.3 \text{ FTEs required to cover for vacations and other unproductive hours}$$

Position Control: Predetermined personnel requirements based on defined needs and not individual staff.

Projected Annual Visits/Year/Day: Decided/targeted by finance, administrative, and nursing management based on plan contracts, historical data, and prevailing external and internal variables.

2080: Hours a FTE is paid annually (52 weeks × 40 hrs./wk.).

Source: Based on *Nursing Quality and Productivity: Practical Management Tools* by Roey Kirk, p. 79, Aspen Publishers, Inc., 1986.

Maintaining an appropriate number of staff working at maximum capacity is essential for stability and profitability. Although many of these staffing principles are quite basic, reviewing them periodically and keeping up to date on new developments will enhance effective operations and increase productivity.

Exhibit 13-4 Day and Hour Equivalents of Partial FTEs

1.0 FTE = 5.0 days or 40 hours per week
.9 FTE = 4.5 days or 36 hours per week
.8 FTE = 4.0 days or 32 hours per week
.7 FTE = 3.5 days or 28 hours per week
.6 FTE = 3.0 days or 24 hours per week
.5 FTE = 2.5 days or 20 hours per week
.4 FTE = 2.0 days or 16 hours per week
.3 FTE = 1.5 days or 12 hours per week
.2 FTE = 1.0 day or 8 hours per week

CONCLUSION

This chapter reviewed some basic principles of productivity and its measurement. Productivity is a complicated concept and its principles can vary depending on reimbursement methods. However, no matter how it is done, productivity must be tracked, evaluated, and improved routinely in order to maintain viability in a competitive health care market.

BIBLIOGRAPHY

Bain, David. 1982. *The Productivity Prescription: The Manager's Guide To Improving Productivity and Profits.* New York: McGraw-Hill.

Budd, Geta B. 1988. "Productivity: The Challenge for Ambulatory Service." *Journal of Ambulatory Care Management,* February.

Greenfield, Alan R. 1989. "Physician Productivity: A Managerial Challenge." *Journal of Ambulatory Care Management,* February 12.

Holts, Thomas D. 1990. "Productivity Enhancement: Implications for Medical Group Management." *College Review,* Fall.

Kirk, Roey. 1986. *Nursing Quality and Productivity: Practical Management Tools.* Gaithersburg, Md.: Aspen Publishers.

14

Meaningful Information for Decision Making

Roger A. Krissman

THE NEED FOR INFORMATION

In the days when medical groups operated under the umbrella of laissez faire and insurance companies and third-party payers reimbursed charges at virtually 100 percent, there wasn't a great need for financial or statistical information. Physician offices had no problem attracting patients and at the same time increasing their profit margins. Controlling expenses, analyzing sources of revenue, researching the market, and applying business concepts within the health care industry were not priorities. As the industry started to evolve as a result of the passage and implementation of Medicare, the need for more information was spawned. When employers began to examine benefit packages for their employees, it became abundantly clear that the cost of health care was increasing at a rate faster than that of other segments of the economy both in terms of whole dollars and percentages of gross national product. The federal government, being the single largest purchaser of health care, attempted to dramatically reduce its expenditure in the market through the strict enforcement of regulations and the application of the prospective payment system. Medical groups, hospitals, and other health care providers found that there was a finite pool of dollars available and that this pool of dollars was being judiciously administered by third-party payers, especially state and federal governments.

Today, faced with possible revenue deductions or a minimal growth of revenue through enhancement of services, providers are forced to seek alternatives to maintain their profitability. Prepaid managed care is an alternative that many providers are currently examining as a way to enhance their financial viability. The rationale for switching to prepaid managed care is that it controls expenses and reduces unnecessary studies and procedures while still providing high-quality health care. Unlike fee-for-service systems, where operating units are separated into two financial categories, revenue generating and nonrevenue generating (overhead), a managed care system consists only of cost centers.

Revenue is not directly produced by volume of patient visits or by a particular department but is generated through the number of enrollees assigned to the group through its contracts with various HMOs. As a result, the expense of providing care must be closely monitored.

In order for an organization to find its way through the treacherous waters of managed care, it must gather and analyze information with the overall goal of maintaining the balance between cost control and appropriate but not excessive medical care. If the pendulum is allowed to swing to either pole for a prolonged period of time without decisive, corrective action, the organization will suffer adverse financial effects. On one hand, if cost increases are allowed to go unchecked, then costs per visit will increase at a rate in excess of revenues being generated on a per member/per month basis. If quality of care is not adequately monitored, then patients will require more care or become dissatisfied with their care and opt out of the plan. This will cause a chain of events that will eventually lead to a reduction in the enrollees assigned to the medical group and thus to a decrease of revenue.

With medical costs continuing to rise faster than the cost of living index because of technological advances, the aging of the population, and other factors, cost containment has been and will remain the linchpin that equates to financial viability. Cost containment in a prepaid practice is essential for the achievement of financial goals and objectives. Furthermore, the kind of cost containment needed extends well beyond the traditional idea of "reducing expenses by arbitrary means." It requires an analysis of utilization review, individual physician practice patterns, and overall trends in the industry as well as a complete and ongoing review of all operations.

Providers must also consider many issues. When is the proper time to contract and at what price? What impact does the competition have on the business? Within the organization, what expenses can be controlled? What expenses should decrease, increase, or be shifted to outside contractors? What is the average cost per patient visit? These are just a few of the questions that all providers must answer. Unfortunately, many times a plan of action is initiated without the necessary statistical data. Without an adequate management information system, an informed decision is not possible. Making decisions without good management information systems in place is similar to driving an automobile from Los Angeles to New York City without a road map.

MANAGEMENT INFORMATION SYSTEMS

Selecting and implementing a management information system is one of the most significant steps toward establishing a foundation upon which to make informed decisions.

It is necessary for providers to analyze their needs from a business standpoint, not only considering their current situation but also where they desire to be in the future. This is the theory that is often used in developing the financial road map for an organization. There must be an accurate tracking mechanism in place both to gauge the progress toward, or deviations from, stated organizational goals.

Unfortunately, the development of tracking mechanisms is a long, arduous process. Current accounting practices, statistical information-gathering procedures, and all information systems, whether manual or computerized, must be reviewed for accuracy and timeliness of reporting. Information that is inaccurate or stale has very little value. The old adage often heard in the era of computerization—garbage in, garbage out—is still valid.

Additionally, the review of operations may reveal that some vital information is not being gathered or reported at all. For example, suppose administration desires a report on revenues and visits being generated by fee-for-service patients according to type of payer (e.g., Medicare, insurance, employers, etc.). The reports summarizing all visits have the required categories delineated, but the accounting financial package only reports fee-for-service revenues on a consolidated basis. If the financial system and the statistical system are not synchronized, the report cannot be easily produced. It is imperative that the systems in place gather the required data elements and, if more than one system is computerized, that the software packages are compatible. A management information system must have the capability to combine statistical and financial data and compare them to the budgeted baseline projections. In addition, the overall system will need to have the flexibility to gather data from many different sources, indicated in Figure 14-1.

An organization might have several computerized systems in place. The budgeting and financial systems might use one type of software, patient scheduling might use another, and physician practice profiles might use still a third software package. Compatibility among the software packages is necessary for executive summary report generation or report writing. Report writing allows the user to access the data elements from several different systems and present them in a format that is accurate, concise, logical, and easy to understand. It also gives the user the ability to generate special reports for departments or specialties where a problem has been identified and additional detailed information is required for further analysis.

BUDGETS

A budget, by definition, is a plan or schedule adjusting expenses during a certain period to the estimated or fixed income for that period. The primary

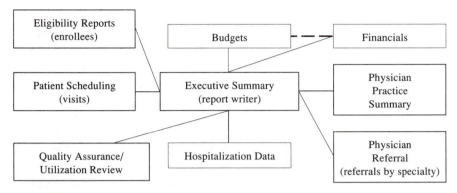

Figure 14-1 Medical Organization Management Information Systems

---

goal of any budget system is to establish a baseline so that operational activity can be formalized (written down or stored in a computer system) and of course quantified (expressed in numbers or dollars). Budgets also function as a planning tool for department managers.

When plans, instead of being devised in a crisis, are made well in advance, various alternatives can be more fully explored and the decision-making process can be more effective. Once decisions are made, they must be acted upon by the organization. Budgets can be used as an effective method for communication and coordination. Administration may labor and agonize over assembling business plans. However, these plans can only be put into operation if they are communicated to the appropriate individuals in the organization in budgetary terms.

The budget is a projection of key financial statements: The balance sheet, the income statement, and the statement of changes in financial position. In addition, there are supporting schedules listing assumptions and calculations used as components for each statement. Budgets are generally prepared annually. But besides the annual budget, there are usually monthly projections. These allow administration to make evaluations after each month and to make necessary adjustments throughout the year.

Before budget forecasting by departments can begin, there are four tasks that administration should perform:

1. It should review the operating environment. A provider cannot effectively plan for the coming year without a review of health care trends, changes in the patient population, and other factors.
2. It should define the organization's goals and provide a statement that describes these goals. Is the main goal for the coming year to hold the line

against competitors? Will additional HMOs be contracted? What will be the goals for fee-for-service business? What new services can be offered? If top management communicates the desired direction, management can then set out to move in that direction.

3. It should list a set of assumptions to be used in the budget process. What will inflation be in the coming year? What is the enrollment growth projections from the HMOs? Will fee-for-service activity increase, decrease, or remain the same? Many more questions will need to be addressed by administration and communicated to those directly involved in the budget preparation process.

4. It should establish measurable objectives. For example, capitation revenue growth may be projected at 10 percent, with expenses increasing by 6 percent. By establishing measurable objectives, the organization can more accurately measure its progress toward its goals.

After accomplishing these four tasks, the actual budget preparation and forecasting can begin. A specific plan should be set up to meet the established goals. The specific plan requires a forecast of what might occur under a variety of alternatives. These might include opening new services, changing the dates of salary increases, and purchasing additional office space. Forecasting can be very elementary, such as projecting that the coming year will be a repeat of the prior year. But it can also be based upon more complex formulas that measure trends and patient referral patterns. The vast majority of forecasting is based upon historical patterns. Forecasting, in order to be accurate, must also take into account any changes that may impact the organization. These changes can be due to improved medical technology, changes in patient mix, changes in disease prevention or treatment, and so on.

Everyone involved with the forecast must remember that it is but a guess about the future. Although these guesses are based upon historical data, there are variables that only administrators and department managers can address. Administrators should allow themselves to make modifications to the forecast based upon their experience and intuition.

In an ambulatory health care practice, there are generally three different areas to be budgeted: service demand, operations, and capital equipment.

The service demand budget projects expected patient volumes and facility utilization. It is a projection of overall expected activity and statistics for the organization. An example of a service demand budget is presented in Table 14-1.

In this example, the projected number of enrollees increases over the 12-month period for both commercial and senior HMO plans. The number increases at a higher rate in the first and fourth quarters of the year to take account of the HMO's open enrollment and the expected su:ge of new patients entering the system. Since an increase in enrollment correlates directly with revenue

Table 14-1 Service Demand Budget

	Jan	Feb	Mar	Apr	May	Jun	Jul	Aug	Sep	Oct	Nov	Dec	Total
Enrollees													
Commercial	25000	25420	25840	25980	26120	26260	26400	26540	26680	26900	27200	27500	315840
Senior	3000	3040	3080	3100	3110	3125	3140	3155	3170	3200	3225	3250	37595
Total	28000	28460	28920	29080	29230	29385	29540	29695	29850	30100	30425	30750	353435
Patient Visits													
Family Practice	6720	6825	6940	6975	7015	7050	7085	7125	7170	7230	7300	7380	84815
Internal Medicine	2800	2845	2890	2900	2920	2935	2950	2970	2985	3010	3040	3075	35320
Surgery	1120	1140	1160	1160	1170	1180	1180	1190	1190	1200	1220	1230	14140
Orthopedics	560	570	580	595	585	585	595	595	605	610	610	615	7105
Total	11200	11380	11570	11630	11690	11750	11810	11880	11950	12050	12170	12300	141380
Lab Determinations	4480	4552	4625	4650	4675	4700	4725	4750	4780	4820	4865	4925	56547
X-ray Procedures	1680	1700	1735	1745	1750	1760	1770	1785	1790	1800	1825	1850	21190
Hospital Utilization													
Commercial													
Days	638	567	644	602	553	546	546	552	552	598	638	698	7134
Admits	145	135	140	140	135	130	130	120	115	130	145	155	1620
ALOS	4.4	4.2	4.6	4.3	4.1	4.2	4.2	4.6	4.8	4.6	4.4	4.5	4.4
Charges	478500	425250	483000	451500	414750	409500	409500	414000	414000	448500	478500	523500	5350500
Charges/Admits	3300	3150	3450	3225	3072	3150	3150	3450	3600	3450	3300	3377	3303
Senior													
Days	403	354	403	378	341	285	248	261	295	354	360	448	4130
Admits	65	60	65	60	55	50	45	45	50	60	60	70	685
ALOS	6.2	5.9	6.2	6.3	6.2	5.7	5.5	5.8	5.9	5.9	6.0	6.4	6.0
Charges	382850	336300	382850	359100	323950	270750	235600	247950	280250	336300	342000	425600	3923500
Charges/Admit	5890	5605	5890	5985	5890	5415	5222	5510	5605	5605	5700	6080	5728

growth, it is vitally important to be as accurate as possible in projecting both the number of enrollees and the capitation rate to be paid on a per member per month basis.

Patient visits (by specialty) and laboratory and x-ray procedures are used as the productivity statistics for each specialty or department. These data will be utilized in estimating the direct expenses for these cost centers. By establishing the departmental workload, staffing requirements for the operational budget, in terms of FTEs and manhours, can be finalized. After deciding staffing requirements, salary and wages and other direct costs such as benefits and repairs can be estimated. Hospital utilization is projected to measure the effectiveness of the organization's utilization review program. By tracking hospital days, an estimate of the total number of days per 1,000 enrollees can be derived. This unit of measurement is standard throughout the managed care–HMO industry, as is the average length of stay (ALOS).

The operating budget provides all the information necessary to prepare a budgeted income statement. It includes revenue projections, salary expenses, employee benefits expenses, supply expenses, repair and maintenance expenses, administrative expenses, and, finally, financing (depreciation interest cost) expenses. These separate elements are combined into a projected income statement. Each department, or cost center, should be budgeted separately, and then the data from all departments should be consolidated in the organization's income statement.

Table 14-2 is an example of a completed budget for a family practice department. Note how the forecast includes both financial and statistical data. Payroll hours include both productive and nonproductive hours. The financial portion of the departmental budget shows the estimated costs that will be incurred at the given patient volumes. Variable costs such as salaries, benefits, and supplies are budgeted based upon expected patient volumes. Nonvariable costs such as maintenance contracts, rental payments, and utility bills are based upon historical data. By budgeting in this fashion (combining statistical and financial information), a budget or baseline for the family practice department can be established against which operations and productivity for the budget year can be measured.

The capital equipment budget is simply a forecast, usually by department, of the capital needs for the coming year translated into dollars.

DEPARTMENTAL FINANCIAL REPORTS

The department financial report is a vital link in information feedback. It is necessary to inform department managers how resources are being expensed in their departments. This report compares budgeted data to actual data on a

Table 14-2 Family Practice Department Operating Budget

	Jan	Feb	Mar	Apr	May	Jun	Jul	Aug	Sep	Oct	Nov	Dec	Total
Patient Visits	6720	6825	6940	6975	7015	7050	7085	7125	7170	7230	7300	7380	84815
Revenue													
HMO Allocation	280000	284600	289200	290800	293200	293850	295400	296950	298500	301000	304250	307500	3535250
Fee-for-Service	50000	48000	49000	49500	50000	50000	51000	52000	48000	52000	51000	50000	600500
Total Revenue	330000	332600	338200	340300	343200	343850	346400	348950	346500	353000	355250	357500	4135750
Expenses													
Salaries	74600	75750	77030	77400	77850	78250	79700	80150	80650	80950	81750	82650	946730
Benefits	14920	15150	15400	15480	15570	15650	15940	16030	16130	16190	16350	16530	189340
Supplies	30240	30710	31230	31385	31565	31725	31880	32060	32265	32535	32850	33210	381655
Repairs	1000		1250	1500			1800		1200		900		7650
Rentals/Leases	20000	20000	20000	20000	20000	25000	25000	25000	25000	25000	25000	25000	275000
Utilities	1000	1000	1100	1100	1100	1200	1200	1200	1100	1100	1200	1200	13500
Education	500	500	750	2000	500		750		800		3500	2000	11300
Other Expense	12000	11500	10400	10000	10800	10600	10000	12000	12500	10000	800	11000	121600
Total Expense	154260	154610	157160	158865	157385	162425	166270	166440	169645	165775	162350	171590	1946775
Profit/Loss	175740	177990	181040	181435	185815	181425	180130	182510	176855	187225	192900	185910	2188975
Payroll Hours	7460	7575	7703	7740	7785	7825	7970	8015	8065	8095	8175	8265	94673

monthly and year-to-date basis. Differences between budgeted and actual data are called variances. If the amount actually spent on an expense item is greater than the budgeted amount, it is considered to be an unfavorable (negative) variance. On the other hand, if less was spent than anticipated, it is a favorable (positive) variance.

The financial report for the family practice department (Table 14-3) shows both financial and statistical data. The expenses, budgeted and actual, are reported at the given volume of patient visits. This section of the departmental financial report is a "static" budget. It provides an expected cost for one particular volume (patient visits). At the end of the reporting period such as a month or a year it is highly unlikely that exactly the number of patients projected will actually have been seen. If substantially more patients are seen than were planned for, it is logical to assume that the budget will be exceeded. On the other hand, if patient visits are down, then costs should be under the budgeted amounts. In Table 14-3, budgeted patient visits exceed actual visits by 450 or 6.7 percent, while total revenue has increased by $13,000, or 3.9 percent, over the expected amount. The greater-than-expected volume of patients is reflected in the expense section, where almost every line item is a negative variance. It would be logical to assume that since more output (patient visits) occurred, expenses should be greater than expected. But what is the amount that should have been expended at the actual patient volume? Is resource usage more efficient or less efficient than expected?

The second section of the departmental financial report takes into consideration volume variance in departmental work units and gives the user the ability to analyze the effects of workload increases or decreases on a per-line-item basis. The per-statistic section presents budget and actual financial information (in this example, on a per-patient-visit basis). As noted in the "static" budget section of the report, most expense line items show a negative variance. For example, salaries were over budget by $700. However, an analysis of salary expense on a per-patient-visit basis demonstrates that $11.10 of salary expense per patient visit was budgeted but that the actual salary expense was $10.50 per patient visit. This yields a positive variance of $.60 per patient visit. There was more efficiency at allocating and expending resources than anticipated, thus fewer dollars were spent given the actual patient load.

The third section of the departmental financial report (Table 14-3) allows the department manager to review departmental productivity. Paid manhours per the budget totaled 7,460, whereas actual paid manhours totaled 7,590, which would appear to be a negative variance. However, once again, reviewing manhours on a per-statistic basis reveals a budgeted hour per statistic (visit) of 1.11 versus an actual hours per statistic of 1.06—a favorable variance of .05 hours per patient visit. This is equivalent to an increase in productivity of 4.5 percent.

Table 14-3 Family Practice Department Financial Report for January

	Budget	Actual	Variance	Percentage
Patient Visits	6,720	7,170	450	6.7
Revenue				
HMO Revenue	280,000	290,000	10,000	3.6
Fee-for-Service Revenue	50,000	53,500	3,000	6.0
Total Revenue	330,000	343,000	13,000	3.9
Expenses				
Salary	74,600	75,300	(700)	(.9)
Benefits	14,920	15,100	(180)	(1.2)
Supplies	30,240	33,400	(3,160)	(10.5)
Repairs	1,000	750	250	25.0
Rentals/Leases	20,000	20,000		
Utilities	1,000	1,075	(75)	(7.5)
Education	500	475	25	5.0
Other Expense	12,000	14,000	(2,000)	(16.7)
Total Expense	154,260	160,100	(5,840)	(3.8)
Profit/Loss	175,740	182,900	7,160	4.1

Per Statistic

	Budget	Actual	Variance	Percentage
Revenue				
HMO Revenue	41.67	40.45	(1.22)	(2.9)
Fee-for-Service Revenue	7.44	7.39	(.05)	(.7)
Total Revenue	49.11	47.84	(1.27)	(2.6)
Expenses				
Salaries	11.10	10.50	.60	5.4
Benefits	2.22	2.11	.11	5.0
Supplies	4.5	4.66	(.16)	(3.6)
Repairs	.15	.10	.05	33.3
Rentals/Leases	2.98	2.79	.19	6.4
Utilities	.15	.15		
Education	.07	.07		
Other Expense	1.79	1.95	(.16)	(8.9)
Total Expense	22.96	22.33	.63	2.7
Profit/Loss	26.15	25.51	(.64)	2.4

Productivity

	Budget	Actual	Variance	Percentage
Payroll Hours	7460	7590	(130)	(1.7)
Average Hourly Rate	10.00	9.92	.08	.8
Hours per Statistic	1.11	1.06	.05	4.5
Full-Time Equivalents	43.1	43.9	(.8)	(1.9)

The average hourly rate indicates the cost for each payroll hour. It is an indicator of the employee mix that is being utilized. Licensed personnel, such as RNs and LVNs, are more highly compensated than receptionists or medical assistants. A large variance in the average hourly rate may be a signal that more highly compensated personnel are being utilized to a greater extent than expected. The full-time equivalents (FTEs) statistic measures the total number of personnel in terms of a 40-hour workweek full-time equivalency. For example, two part-time employees working 20 hours per week equals one full-time equivalent. By analyzing this statistic, the overall staffing pattern for the department can be determined. It is most important to analyze the productivity information contained in this report, since efficiencies in employee staffing and productivity directly result in a savings in payroll costs and employee FTEs. Since payroll costs are generally the largest expense that is directly controllable, all ambulatory care practices must have a system that measures and controls productivity and payroll expenses.

A physician hospital referral report providing feedback to administration and physicians on referral patterns is also an important tool. A medical group that contracts with an HMO and has a risk-sharing program (a program in which the medical group shares in the profits and losses of a hospital funding pool with the HMO) must review its hospital usage to ensure proper utilization and thus maximize its profit from such a program. The physician hospital referral report (Table 14-4) is essential for overseeing physician hospital utilization. This report is generated on a monthly and year-to-date basis so that unfavorable trends can be noted, analyzed, and discussed with the physicians and so that subsequent follow-up can occur. It lists physicians by name, hospital admissions for all diagnostic-related groups (DRGs), the average length of stay across all admissions, the average length of stay that is normal in the industry, and percentage of variance of average length of stay between the norm and the actual. The patient billings compose the actual charges versus the targeted amounts as determined by historical experience. The admission rate per 1,000 patient visits is presented for comparison purposes. Each specialty has a separate report generated to account for differences in admission patterns according to clinical areas. In Table 14-4, Dr. Brown's numbers would indicate that a review of hospital utilization should be performed. Further analysis may reveal that one or several of Dr. Brown's patients were outliers (patients whose complications or comorbidity made the discharge of the patient within the normal length of stay not possible) or that Dr. Brown's practice utilization should be reviewed for appropriateness.

Another benefit of tracking hospital admissions, days, and charges is that it enables the medical group to reconcile its hospital utilization data with those of the HMO. In the case of a risk-sharing program, in which a hospital funding pool is controlled by the HMO, it is imperative that the medical group maintain

Table 14-4 Physician Hospital Referral Report

Physician No.	Physician Name	No. of Hospital Admits	Actual ALOS	Physician Target ALOS	Hospital ALOS Variance %	Referral Actual Hospital Chgs/Admit	Report Target Chgs/Admit	Share Variance %	No. of Patient Visits	Admits per 1000 Visits
227	Smith	18	4.3	4.0	(7.5)	3214	3115	(3.2)	2125	8.47
300	Jones	26	3.9	4.2	7.1	3022	3216	6.0	2650	9.81
151	Brown	14	8.2	4.8	(70.8)	7162	3739	(91.5)	2200	6.36
219	Evans	32	4.5	5.1	11.8	3945	3710	(6.3)	3325	9.62
Average		22.5	5.2	4.5	(15.6)	4336	3445	(25.8)	2575	8.74

a separate data base. The separate data base would enable the medical group to quickly identify errors and omissions that could have a substantial effect on the profitability of the programs.

The operating indicators report (Table 14-5) combines statistical and financial information for the entire organization. Key indicators in the areas of utilization—profit/loss statements, referral claims paid, and labor cost management—are summarized in this report. Its purpose is to supply administration with a quick synopsis of financial operations. By utilizing it, administration will be able to quickly identify trends or possible problem areas that may require additional investigation for subsequent corrective action. This report is a by-product of the management information systems that were discussed earlier in the chapter—the report writer function is used to abstract and summarize specific data from several different software packages.

Table 14-5 Operating Indicators Report

	Month to Date		
	C/Y Actual	P/Y Prior	C/Y Budget
Utilization			
Enrollees - Comm	26,500	23,000	25,000
Enrollees - SR	3,500	2,000	3,000
Enrollees - Total	30,000	25,000	28,000
Visits - Comm	7,500	7,200	7,400
Visits - SR	1,500	1,450	1,500
Visits - FFS	100	125	125
Visits - Total	9,100	8,775	9,025
Visit/Enrollee - Comm	.28	.32	.30
Visit/Enrollee - SR	.43	.73	.50
Cap/Enrollee - Comm	40.00	39.50	42.00
Cap/Enrollee - SR	75.00	76.00	78.00
Cap/Enrollee - Total	44.08	42.42	45.86
Summary P & L			
Operating Revenue	1,322,500	1,060,500	1,284,000
Other Revenue	100,000	75,000	125,000
Operating Expense	1,251,800	999,500	1,240,000
Depreciation/Interest	99,575	79,000	98,500
Earn before Partner Draw	71,125	57,000	70,500
Partner Draw w/o Dist.	35,000	25,000	35,000
Profit/(Loss)	36,125	32,000	35,500
P & L Enrollee			
Operating Revenue	44.08	42.42	45.86
Other Revenue	3.33	3.00	4.46

(continued)

Table 14-5 Continued

	Month to Date		
	C/Y Actual	P/Y Prior	C/Y Budget
Operating Expense	41.73	39.98	44.23
Depreciation/Interest	3.32	3.16	3.52
Earn before Partner Draw	2.37	2.28	2.52
Partner Draw w/o Dist.	1.17	1.00	1.25
Profit/(Loss)	1.20	1.28	1.27
P & L Per Visit			
Operating Revenue	145.33	120.85	142.27
Other Revenue	10.99	8.55	13.85
Operating Expense	137.56	113.90	137.40
Depreciation/Interest	10.94	9.00	10.91
Earn before Partner Draw	7.82	6.50	7.81
Partner Draw w/o Dist.	3.85	2.85	3.88
Profit/(Loss)	3.97	3.65	3.93
Referrals			
Prof Claims Paid (#)	500	375	450
Prof Claims Paid ($)	42,000	29,200	45,000
Expense per Claim	84.00	77.87	100.00
Hospital Claims Paid (#)	195	150	210
Hospital Claims Paid ($)	750,750	585,000	861,350
Expense per Claim	3,850	3,900	4,102
Labor Costs Mgmt			
Labor Cost per Manhour	10.50	10.35	11.00
Labor Cost per Enrollee	11.68	11.19	12.40
Labor Cost per Visit	38.52	31.89	38.47
Total Manhours/Visit	3.67	3.08	3.49
Total Manhours/Enrollee	1.11	1.08	1.13
FTE Employed	193	156	182
Payroll % of Revenue	24.60	24.60	24.90
Benefits % of Payroll	22.10	19.70	22.50
Total Personnel Cost			
% of Revenue	30.00	29.50	30.20
Overtime % of Payroll	5.00	4.30	5.50

Table 14-5 lists some of the indicators a medical group may wish to review on a monthly basis. However, this example is not intended to be a paradigm. Each medical practice should review its own systems to determine what information is most valuable for decision making. Accurate and timely production of this data is essential for practice management. No medical practice can expect to remain competitive without adequate financial information and the ability to implement decisions based on this information.

15

Creating a Successful Relationship with a Bank

Julie Yen and Martin D. Goldberg

Why should a medical organization be concerned with establishing a successful relationship with a bank? Too often, this question has a low priority as far as the new or emerging medical organization is concerned. "After all," physicians may say to themselves, "we are among the most highly trained, well-paid professionals, and since we are dealing with vital health issues, we really shouldn't have to spend time on these kinds of matters. Let the lenders think about how to best meet our needs. That's what we pay them for."

Changes in the economics and the regulatory environment of the health care industry make this attitude no longer practical. Numerous hospitals and some medical groups have had to close their doors because of their inability to keep pace with these changes. In addition, the incomes of many physicians have been negatively impacted by more strenuous control of reimbursement rates and methods. Thus, those doctors who fail to manage their practices prudently may find themselves no longer automatically viewed as infallible credit risks. If a medical organization needs more than a checking account or a place to put deposits, there is every reason it should be concerned to establish and maintain a successful banking relationship.

Fundamentally, banks regard medical organizations as businesses. From this perspective, medical organizations need to be well managed, well organized, financially sound, and legally established. They must provide products and services for which there is a clear demand. Those organizations that meet these conditions are definitely attractive to banks. They are excellent sources of deposits and have demands for loans and other banking products, such as cash management and trust services. All of these needs generate income for banks. Beyond this, large multispecialty medical groups count numerous physicians as partners (or shareholders), and as a result their diversified earning capacity is usually an excellent secondary source for the repayment of loans. Also, the individual partners or shareholders provide an additional customer tier for bank services.

MEDICAL ORGANIZATION CONCERNS

Given this attractiveness, why do medical organizations hesitate to cultivate successful banking relationships? There are, in fact, frustrations in dealing with banks. For the growing medical group, these can range from a lack of understanding by the banker of the unique nature of the group to overrestrictive paperwork and collateral requirements. Additional complaints about banks include slow responses to requests and excessive turnover of account officers. Because of these issues, selection of an appropriate bank is essential.

It is recommended, when considering a new banking relationship, that a medical organization "shop and compare." A number of issues need to be kept in mind when choosing a bank. First, does the bank have experience in dealing with health care entities? There are distinctive aspects to medical enterprises, such as accounting methodology, and therefore there is no substitute for dealing with a bank officer who understands the dynamics of the industry. Second, note should be taken of the size, range of services, financial condition, and lending capacity of the banking institution. The medical organization must keep in mind that the bank it selects should be large enough to accommodate its future growth, because the asset size and capital base of a bank generally determines its lending limits. On the other hand, the bank should not be so large that the medical group would be considered an insignificant account and thus not receive the level of service or attention it needs. Finally, to help address the issues of responsiveness, competence, and personnel stability, the medical organization should check with other related health care groups for recommendations and references.

BANKER CONCERNS

Of course, just as medical organizations have legitimate concerns about banks, bankers have certain common concerns regarding medical organizations. It should be recognized that banks, just like medical enterprises themselves, are institutions of public trust, with extensive regulatory and statutory constraints. It is often not understood that this is one of the reasons banks require so much information and need ongoing communication with medical organization officers. Some of the common complaints bankers voice about the medical industry are discussed below.

New and emerging medical organizations seldom have written business plans. Business plans communicate specific information about how the purpose and goals of the entity are to be achieved. They outline such items as organization structure, the management background of key individuals, operating budgets and projections, and other financial information. The specifics of business plans will be discussed later in this chapter. Bankers need a written business plan as a place to start in their evaluation of an organization. All too frequently, a medical organization will approach a prospective banker with inadequately organized verbal plans and expect the banker to guess its needs, rely on memory, and pull the bits of information together. This makes the banker's task much more difficult and often leads to delays and misunderstandings. By coming in well prepared, time and energy are saved for both parties, and the relationship begins on the right footing. Also, with everything laid out in writing, the banker has no excuse not to respond in a timely manner.

Physicians and privately owned medical organizations often do not see the need for submitting current financial information. Just as doctors need x-rays and blood tests to ascertain the health of their patients, bankers need current financial data to diagnose and monitor the financial health of their borrowers. It should be understood that deposit balances alone do not pay off loans (unless they specifically secure the loans) and therefore are not sufficient for the banker to use as an indicator of financial strength. Current financial statements are essential and allow the banker to develop confidence in the relationship over time. Moreover, as regulated institutions, banks are legally required to have up-to-date information on file to justify their credit decisions.

The need for regularly updated financial statements also extends to the individual physicians who serve as loan guarantors for the entity they own. Bankers must rely on strong individual financial statements to justify and maintain credit approvals when the medical entity has limited net worth of its own. This situation can often arise when owners draw out the majority of earnings from the entity to help with their individual tax and personal problems. Owners should recognize that financial obligations toward the entity go hand in hand with the benefits they receive.

Owners of a medical enterprise are reluctant to retain earnings to finance growth. Partners or stockholders in the enterprise may rely too heavily on borrowed funds to finance expenditures, whether operational or capital in nature. Low retained earnings and low capital expenditures indicate to bankers that the ownership may not be sufficiently committed to the entity as an organization. For this reason, bankers find it difficult to accept the usual practice according to which all income is distributed to physician-owners. In general, highly leveraged businesses have difficulty weathering problems and are candidates for failure. As such, they are not good credit risks. Bankers need to see health care enterprises exhibit discipline in establishing and maintaining sufficient levels of net worth.

Medical organizations enter into banking arrangements without fully understanding the terms and conditions of the agreements. Loans extended to any enterprise always have specific terms and conditions, sometimes called "covenants," to ensure repayment and to maintain the fiscal health of the enterprise.

(See Appendix 15-A for definitions of banking terms commonly used in loan agreement covenants.) These conditions may include such items as a minimum working capital requirement, a maximum leverage of debt to net worth requirement, cash flow coverage requirements, and a requirement to build up net equity through earnings. Unfortunately, medical organizations frequently fail to adequately appreciate these requirements and the obligations they entail.

For example, short-term working funds, such as those needed to meet daily operating expenses, are sometimes drawn upon to finance long-term capital expenditures. This drains the cash position of the entity and can lead to a violation of the covenants that govern the loan. What is more, when the banker brings such a violation to the attention of the medical borrower, it is often ignored. This not only is frustrating to the banker, but it also adversely affects the group's credibility and can undermine future loan approvals. Medical groups should be sure they comprehend and can comply with the agreements they enter into prior to the execution of the loan documents. In the event of noncompliance due to unforeseen circumstances, the medical group can help matters by keeping its banker informed and working collaboratively toward a mutually acceptable solution.

Medical groups very often lack clarity in decision making, management, and governance. Bankers like to have clearly designated individuals who can sign for and commit the medical group, preferably owner-members of the executive committee. However, bankers typically find that their contacts in medical organizations are uncertain how far their authority extends in negotiations and agreements. One of the reasons for this is that even when authority is delegated to the contact, it frequently is withdrawn. A genuine source of frustration for the banker is trying to reach decisions with representatives who may not be empowered to commit the organization. This kind of ineffective decision making is particularly evident in group practices and large executive committees that require notes on all financial matters.

A medical organization's difficulty in arriving at decisions not only causes delays in the banking relationship but, more importantly, is symptomatic of the organization's confusion about its direction, goals, and management processes. This leads the banker to question the effectiveness of the organization's management, and, as a result, the banker can become hesitant to enter into transactions. For example, decisions made through representatives of large medical groups are frequently reversed because a minority of the organization's partners or shareholders refuse to abide by the decisions. What is disturbing about this for the banker is that the medical group tolerates going back on previously established agreements and abandoning its own governance principles. This behavior cripples effective action.

Since bankers view a medical enterprise as a business, they expect it not to be managed in an arbitrary or haphazard fashion. Bankers like to see continuity in leadership and relative stability in the executive function for the same reason that physicians like to see low turnover among their bankers: It is frustrating to have to repeatedly explain a business situation and continually revisit past decisions. Developing and building upon relationships become very difficult under these circumstances. For this reason, frequently rotating individuals into the executive function for political purposes is unwise. The development of an executive takes time. Executives need to be able to learn from their experiences, and they should not automatically be replaced because of one or two mistakes. The medical entity needs to evaluate executive performance with perspective. Seasoned bankers are able to understand certain mistakes and are more interested in strategies for attacking problems than in replacing personnel. Of course, if the executives prove to have no business capacity or potential, bankers will not want to proceed without a change in leadership.

Managing a business is a full-time job and requires adherence to the policies of the organization. It requires an effective executive who can devote full attention to the running of the business. In the case of a large medical group, a full-time administrator and support staff are needed. Physician executives who think they can divide their time between carrying a heavy patient load and managing the enterprise are unrealistic. Unfortunately, having full-time physician executives may collide with the common belief that administrative work is somehow inferior or unproductive compared to clinical practice. This belief is unfounded. Effective medical practice carried out by the entity can only be sustained through an organizational environment supported by clear and committed leadership. It requires talent, experience, and skill in business operations, strategic management, and group interaction to develop an organization that can reach its potential. Clinical credentials alone are not enough. The value of executive ability needs to be recognized and appropriately compensated.

Medical organizations often do not communicate well with their bankers. Bankers actually do understand that administrators have busy schedules and numerous demands on their time. That is why alert bankers try to keep calls to a minimum. However, when a banker does call, the administrator should realize that the matter needs prompt attention. In fact, many administrators will delay in returning a banker's phone call, or perhaps not even return the call at all. The banker is thus put in the position of having to repeatedly call back.

Bankers become especially irritated when they are ignored by administrators who must confront a problem such as violation of a term loan agreement. Like any other business, medical organizations have unexpected problems, but this is no reason to disregard or discount a banker's concern. Bankers, like most other people, dislike unpleasant surprises. They expect to be kept apprised of negative as well as positive operating results. When problems occur, they need the client to take the initiative to lay the issues out on the table and, if possible, to propose remedial plans and actions. A medical organization's bank, in a sense, is its silent partner. The banker does not want to be shut out.

Administrators can improve the timeliness of communications with their bankers by simply delegating various functions to appropriate staff. Questions that a banker may have on financial statements or deposit accounts, for example, can be addressed by an able support staff member. The administrator only needs to be involved if the staff member is not equipped to handle the banker's request or concern. The administrator can also help build effective communications by periodically visiting with the banker over breakfast or lunch.

WHAT BANKERS LIKE TO SEE IN A BUSINESS PLAN

As stated earlier, written business plans are essential to guide the banker in understanding and monitoring the financial strength of the business entity. The format of the business plan, as described below, is primarily for the benefit of the lending institution and should not be confused with the strategic or detailed operating plans the entity may use for internal management purposes (see Chapter 2). The kind of business plan the banker looks for should provide broad-based financial and organizational information. It should be made available upon submission of the initial credit request and updated periodically thereafter. Lenders normally like to see the following components incorporated into the business plan.

Introduction. An effective introduction starts with a summary of the proposed loan request, specifying purpose, suggested terms, and the amount to be financed. If the credit request is to pay off existing debt, then some background on existing obligations should be included.

Organization. This section should include an overview of the entity's history, a description of the nature of the business, and a review of the organization's ownership, goals, and management structure. An outline of any subsidiary or affiliated entities should be provided here as well. Noting the relevant background and experience of the individuals who make up the management team is essential.

Market Environment. A discussion of specific markets served, by geography and demography, provides the banker with information to assess the entity's current market share and potential for growth. An overview of the market environment should also include a review of key competitors and other regulatory considerations and their expected impact on the entity.

Financial Information. Financial statements, together with management's analysis of financial performance, for the past three-year period are essential in this section. Explanations of any special circumstances such as lawsuits or loan agreement violations should be noted here. In addition, the lender will want to see financial performance projections for the coming two or three years. These projections should cover income, capital expenditure requirements, leasehold improvements, and anticipated growth in staffing and other operating expenses.

CONCLUSION

Bankers, by their very nature, want to play a role in helping the businesses they finance to grow and prosper. Although they have no desire to control a borrowing entity or interfere with its operations, they do wish to see their customers excel in their chosen fields. Bankers also realize that a business that advances towards its dream does so in steps. Meaningful and lasting success typically doesn't happen overnight. It takes clear vision, effective management, and sound financial strategies consistently applied over time.

The principles behind the banker-borrower relationship are not very different than those behind the physician-patient relationship. Both relationships require caring, open communication, and candor from each of the parties. Most of all, they require trust and good faith—trust in the skills and abilities of the professionals and faith in their desire to keep the welfare of those served uppermost in their minds. Medical organizations have a right to expect that a bank will offer this kind of relationship. The guidelines discussed above will assist the medical enterprise in seeking out and building a meaningful banking relationship.

Appendix 15-A

Glossary of Banking Terms

Below is a list of common banking terms generally used in loan agreement covenants. It should be stressed that each financial institution may have its own specific terms and methods of calculating ratios. Therefore, the following should be used only to increase general understanding. Individuals and entities seeking legal advice or other expert counsel should confer with appropriate professionals.

Accrual Basis of Accounting. A method of accounting in which revenue is recognized when earned, expenses are recognized when incurred, and other changes in financial condition are recognized as they occur, without regard to the actual timing of the cash receipts and expenditures. (*Banking Terminology* 1989)

Capital. (1) The amount invested in a business by the owners or stockholders. (2) The net worth of a business. (Berman 1983)

Capital Expense. An expense that has been recorded as a long-term asset. For example, the costs incurred in overhauling an x-ray unit are capitalized, while minor repairs to the machine are typically expensed. The treatment depends on when the benefits will be received. Benefits from a major overhaul will be received for several years. As a result, the expenditure is added to the cost basis of the machine and allocated by means of depreciation charges. In the case of a minor repair, the benefits are derived in the current period. As a result, expenditure is charged against current income and may not be considered a capital expense. Land, buildings, and equipment purchases are all capital expenses. (*Banking Terminology* 1989)

Definitions derived from: Berman, Ben. (1983) *The Dictionary of Business and Credit Terms.* New York: National Association of Credit Management; *Banking Terminology* (1989) 3d ed. Washington, D.C.: American Bankers Association; and Libkin, Ken. (1991) Senior Vice President, Imperial Bank.

Cash Basis of Accounting. An accounting system in which revenues and expenses are recorded and realized only when the accompanying cash inflow or outflow occurs, without regard to the actual period to which the transactions apply. (*Banking Terminology* 1989)

Cash Flow. (1) A company's funds available for working capital or expansion. (2) The expected timing and amounts of future net cash receipts from an investment. (3) The cycle through which a firm's cash passes as it is converted into raw materials, product, sales, receivables, and back into cash. (4) The income remaining from real estate operations after deducting operating expenses and debt service. (*Banking Terminology* 1989)

Cash Flow Coverage. Indicates the historical ability to repay long-term debt. Ratio of cash flow to the current portion of long-term debt. Cash flow can be defined as net income after taxes plus noncash expenses such as depreciation and amortization. (Libkin 1991)

Cash Management. Collection, disbursement (payment), concentration, and information services provided to a bank's customers to speed collection of receivables, to control payments, and to manage cash efficiently. (*Banking Terminology* 1989)

Compensating Balance. The balance that a customer must keep on deposit with a bank in order to ensure a credit line, to gain unlimited checking privileges, and to offset the bank's expenses in providing various services. (*Banking Terminology* 1989)

Corporation. A business organization that is treated as a single legal entity and is owned by its stockholders, whose liability is generally limited to the extent of their investment. The ownership of a corporation is represented by shares of stock that are issued to people or to other companies in exchange for cash, physical assets, services, and goodwill. The stockholders elect the board of directors, which then directs the management of the corporation's affairs. (*Banking Terminology* 1989)

Current Assets. Assets of a company (not including fixed assets) readily convertible to cash. Such assets include accounts receivable, securities, goods and materials in inventory, cash on hand, and cash in banks. (Berman 1983)

Current Liabilities. Money owed and payable within a short period of time, usually within one year. Includes debts owed suppliers and banks, notes, accrued salaries, taxes, and interest. (Berman 1983)

Current Portion of Long-Term Debt. The portion of long-term debt (i.e., debt with maturities exceeding 12 months from the date of the financial statement) that is required to be paid within 12 months of the date of the financial statement. (Libkin 1991)

Current Ratio. A measure of a firm's liquidity. Current assets divided by current liabilities. (Berman 1983)

Debt-to-Net-Worth Ratio. Debt (money owed to creditors) compared to capital (owners' money in the business). (Berman 1983)

Depreciation. (1) A decline in the value of property due to wear and tear, obsolescence, or the action of the elements. (Differs from deterioration, which signifies abnormal loss of quality.) (2) Account charges against earnings by which the costs of fixed assets are converted into expenses. A loss in value of a fixed asset over a period of time. (Berman 1983)

Gross Profit. The total income a company realized from sales, less the cost of the goods and services sold but prior to the deduction of selling, administrative, or general expenses. (Berman 1983)

Loan-to-Value Ratio. The ratio between the amount of a loan and the appraised value of the security for that loan, expressed as a percentage of the appraised value. (*Banking Terminology* 1989)

Net Profit after Taxes. The actual profit realized by a business over a specific period of time. Profit from a transaction or sale, after deducting all costs, expenses, miscellaneous reserves, adjustments from gross receipts, and income taxes. (Berman 1983)

Net Worth. The excess of assets over liabilities. The residual equity (or interest) of an owner after all debts have been paid. (Berman 1983)

Prime Rate. A benchmark that a bank establishes from time to time and uses in computing an appropriate rate of interest for a particular loan contract. The benchmark is generally based on numerous considerations, including the bank's supply of funds, cost of funds, administrative costs, and the competition from other suppliers of credit. Factors used in setting the prime rate and the circumstances in which it applies vary from bank to bank. This benchmark, however, is only one factor among several that banks use in pricing loans. For any specific loan, the interest rate actually charged may be above or below a bank's benchmark rate. The actual rate will be determined on the basis of several variables, including perceived risks, nature of collateral, length and size of loan, competition, and the overall relationship with the customer. (*Banking Terminology* 1989)

Receivables. Money due or collectible for goods sold, services performed, or money loaned. (Berman 1983)

Receivables Turnover. A measurement for the effectiveness of a practice's collection effort and the liquidity or quantity of receivables. (Berman 1983)

Retained Earnings. Earnings not distributed to partners or stockholders. Retained earnings are a part of the company's net worth. (Berman 1983)

Shareholder Distributions/Dividends. A periodic distribution of cash to the partners or shareholders of an organization as a return on their investments. (Berman 1983)

Working Capital. (1) Money used in conducting a business. (2) The excess of current assets over current liabilities. (Berman 1983)

Part III

Clinical Issues

16

Health Education

Paul E. Terry

INTRODUCTION

Medical practices in the 1990s will face greater challenges than ever in keeping pace with technological developments and remaining competitive in a volatile health care delivery marketplace. Business leaders have rated health care costs as their top concern, with 85 percent rating this issue as "very serious." They are more worried about health care costs than such issues as the federal budget deficit, productivity growth, and environmental protection (Kelly 1991). At the same time, purchasers of health care are seeking quality improvement from health care providers, including accountability for patient care outcomes, increases in patient satisfaction with clinical care, and consistency in patient care guidelines. Demographic statistics indicate the U.S. population is aging, which will result in more chronic health conditions needing medical attention. Each of these challenges creates opportunities for the type of multidisciplinary teams that provide educational services in managed care settings. Moreover, these challenges will require creative, multifaceted solutions. Health education can play an instrumental role in improving the quality of care while fostering innovation in a clinical setting.

This chapter addresses health education theory and practice in the ambulatory health care setting and presents a framework for integrating educational programs and approaches to patient care on an outpatient basis. Health education is treated as an ongoing system of needs assessment, intervention, relapse prevention, and evaluation.

Applying assessment findings to a medical practice's educational offerings and deciding among various instructional methods is a daily operational challenge for the health education program. In this chapter, program planning is described from a perspective that considers public health objectives as well as the clinical marketing contribution of educational initiatives. Several methods for assessing the health risks and educational interests of clinic patients are examined. Finally, the physician's role in education and the critical links between patient satisfaction and communication are addressed, along with future trends in patient education.

THE ROLE OF EDUCATION IN MANAGED CARE

With the growing influence of managed care delivery systems in health care, health education services are playing a greater role in addressing the needs of patients as well as insurers. In their formative years, prepaid systems were based upon tenets of primary prevention. Given the short-term financial results that have been demanded during the growth of the highly competitive managed care industry, few health care providers have demonstrated substantial evidence of long-term disease prevention or short-term health risk reduction. Still, the basis for supporting education and prevention as a viable component of managed health care is as scientifically sound as the basis for performing most other practices and procedures in medical care. Educational services are certainly no less worthy of prepayment than other medical services if purchasers of health care are intent upon reducing costs while improving health outcomes. Toward this end, ambulatory medicine–based educational programs play a role in ameliorating health risks (particularly those related to chronic illness), reducing unnecessary utilization, and inculcating a sense of personal responsibility for health improvement among health care consumers.

Risk Reduction

It is instructive to look at national campaigns that have used education to alter health-related behavior when considering the role of clinical providers in health education. However, the ultimate effect of health education on health status remains elusive (U.S. Public Health Service 1988). Perhaps the most progress creditable to education has resulted from the campaign of the National High Blood Pressure Education Program. Significant gains have been reported in the number of Americans who have controlled blood pressure.

Few would deny that the improvements in knowledge about hypertension are related to the achievement of blood pressure reduction. For example, a comparison of surveys taken between 1973 and 1979 shows that 16 percent more people knew hypertension was a serious disease at the later date, 66 percent more people knew normal blood pressure is less than 140/90, and 19 percent more people knew hypertension can cause strokes (U.S. Public Health Service 1987; Frederiksen et al. 1984).

Similar smaller scale educational efforts in clinic settings have demonstrated positive results in hypertension management. In a study of several combinations of educational interventions, a 12 percent average increase in blood pressure control was attained. The more intensive approaches resulted in a 24 percent increase in control (Levine et al. 1979). At Park Nicollet Medical Foundation, a study of a hypertension management program with a patient education and follow-up protocol showed the percentage of patients with blood pressure within controlled limits increased from 17 percent upon program entry to 44 percent at 12-month follow-up (Pheley et al. 1991). In a reference group, only 27 percent of hypertensive patients had their blood pressure under control (Kosecoff et al. 1985).

Studies with multifactorial designs have also shown promising relationships between education and the reduction of multiple risk factors. Communitywide health education efforts in North Karelia, Finland, and the Stanford Heart Disease Prevention program have focused on interventions relating to smoking, fitness, and cholesterol intake. Significant improvements in both knowledge and behavior were shown (Puske et al. 1985; Farquhar et al. 1977; Farquhar 1987). The Multiple Risk Factor Intervention Trial studied 12,000 men who were subject to concerted patient education. Results from this study also demonstrated decreased health risks (Multiple Risk Factor Intervention Trial Research Group 1982).

Aside from these more notable and intensive efforts in health education, evidence concerning the relationship between health behavioral interventions in clinical settings and health outcomes is scant (Lorig and Laurin 1985). For example, there are theoretical models for predicting the economic benefits of increasing the use of screening tests such as mammograms and colorectal exams (Kristein 1977; Warner 1987; Roccella 1976). However, a literature-based investigation of these tests showed that the evidence of their efficacy remains equivocal (U.S. Preventive Services Task Force 1989). It will be incumbent upon any serious clinically based health education program to include outcomes evaluation in the program design if such interventions are ever to share a place with more accepted approaches to medical care such as pharmacology. The elements common to the risk reduction successes reported in this section include multifaceted educational methods, programs targeted at susceptible patients, conscientious follow-up, and intervention by multidisciplinary teams. These elements are described in greater detail in later sections of this chapter.

Utilization Management

If health care cost savings result from risk reduction programs, the benefit to a managed care system will be seen only in the long term. However, education also plays a role in preventing unnecessary patient visits, which results in a shorter-term return on investment. Conversely, educational strategies for increasing compliance with therapeutic regimens—which in some cases means increasing utilization—have also been shown to be effective (Rosenberg 1971).

Patient education about medical self-care has focused on reducing patient visits for self-limiting conditions such as colds and sore throats. Several studies have demonstrated the effectiveness of such efforts in a managed care setting. Based upon a communications campaign using self-care books, newsletters, and brochures, an experimental group in an HMO had a 15 percent decrease in routine office visits compared to a control group. The experimental group in this study consisted of Medicare patients. The cost savings was estimated to be $2.19 for every dollar spent on intervention (Vickery et al. 1988). Similar studies using materials-based intervention showed significant reductions in visits in a small 6,000-member HMO (Kemper 1982) and a 21,000-member HMO (Zapka and Averill 1979). A follow-up study to determine if patients exposed to self-care information were late in visiting for necessary care showed no adverse health effects from self-care education (Vickery et al. 1989).

Marketing

Health education programs tend to need high visibility in order to succeed. Mass health screenings done for purposes of assessment, promotion of classes, educational brochures, and newsletters can serve both educational and marketing objectives. Patients leaving the clinic with professionally designed materials displaying the clinic's logo are apt to view these as an added value. Since attractively produced materials are more likely to be read and "splashy" promotions are more likely to attract participation in programs, health promotion and marketing are quite compatible. In a survey of HMOs, 35 percent of the respondents stated that health promotion was a very important part of their marketing plan. Additionally, 73 percent viewed health promotion as a method of retaining members, and 58 percent considered health promotion as important for attracting new members and increasing enrollment (Bernton 1987).

If health promotion is intended to serve a marketing function as well as a disease prevention role, strategic planning is needed to set priorities. This requires a process of market research, interdepartmental team building, and public relations expertise. Indeed, with a marketing orientation, it is unlikely that a clinic's educational efforts would be confined to the 10 percent of the adult population that typically attend classroom programs (Sofien and Graff 1986).

In a managed care setting, problems related to disenrollment of members may also be addressed, in part by a marketing approach to planning educational offerings. There is evidence to suggest that voluntary disenrollees are different from continuous enrollees with respect to their utilization of services (Griffith et al. 1984; Zapka et al. 1986). Although there is a need for more empirical evidence to understand the reasons for disenrollment, disenrollees tend to be higher utilizers of service. It may be that offering educational programs as an adjunct to clinical care would serve to satisfy the higher level of help-seeking behavior for this type of patient. Certain interventions such as group back care education or asthma support groups are also more cost-effective strategies for filling this need to utilize services. These offerings may also reduce the number of members who are dissatisfied with the amount of information they receive about their health condition (Pope 1978; Sofien and LeVan 1987).

PROGRAM PLANNING

Failing to plan is like planning to fail, according to pundits working in organizational development. In a competitive business environment, ambulatory care centers need to have a clear vision of their position in the community. Who are the customers? What do they want? Which of their needs can be met through education? At what cost? In what period of time? Planning in health education is similar to planning in other areas of service provision. The establishment of clear, realistic, and measurable goals is the hallmark of a well-managed health education program. Ideally, the education program plan should be derived from the mission statement of the medical practice. To be consistent with the philosophical posture and operational direction of the organization, program planners need to seek involvement with the broadest range of clinic constituents possible.

Perhaps the most widely used model for constructing a comprehensive health education plan is the "Precede" framework developed by Lawrence Green and his colleagues (Green et al. 1980). More in-depth applications of this planning approach in an ambulatory care setting can be found elsewhere (Sofien and Graff 1986; Kolbe 1988). Briefly, Precede stands for predisposing, reinforcing, and enabling causes in educational diagnosis and evaluation. It is a framework that attempts to compensate for the tendency toward disjointed planning in health education by offering a structured set of seven planning phases.

A Public Health Approach

The Precede framework is well suited to planning in a managed care setting. The first phase focuses on "quality of life" issues. Demographic characteristics of the patient population should be taken into consideration at the outset of planning. Given the past tendency to favor individualized clinical approaches to patient care, this is a critical step for adding a public health education perspective to the medical practice's planning process (Breslow 1990). Reducing the overall incidence of premature pregnancies or attaining a lower-than-average COPD rate among practice subscribers are examples of social goals that would be considered in this first phase.

Preparing To Measure Outcomes

Determining the health-related factors that might affect the achievement of the social goals is the second stage of planning. Consideration of the specific morbidity or mortality rates in the clinic population, along with information about how these rates vary according to demographic characteristics, is essential in this phase. Also, differences in rates according to clinical site, subspecialty, or practice physician could be germane. The first two phases require a deliberate use of data to support assumptions about the needs and interests of the patient population and about variations related to educational interventions among the health care providers. Assessment of the health risks and beliefs of patients will be discussed later.

Targeting Behaviors

Identifying those patient health behavior factors that affect the target health conditions occurs in the third phase of Precede. For example, the smoking rate of the clinic's patients would be pertinent to concerns about COPD and preterm pregnancy. A comprehensive set of behaviors, including the manner in which patients use the health care system, should be considered. A review of the Year 2000 Health Objectives for the Nation would be instructive during this phase. The Public Health Service provides useful comparative data as well as examples of risk reduction goals that have been proposed for the community level. For example, the 1990 pregnancy and health goals resulted in little progress—only 2 of the 19 objectives set are likely to be achieved (Anderson and Mullner 1990). Heeding these statistics, noting the changes in risk levels, and staying briefed on those problems that continue to be targeted at the national level can help the clinic keep track of the health behavior factors that most deserve attention.

Overcoming Barriers

In phases 4 and 5 of the Precede planning framework, factors that enable or predispose patients to engage in unhealthy behaviors become the focus. The knowledge, skills, and beliefs of the patients as well as the attitudes and values of health care providers are considered as they relate to the possibilities for intervention. Physicians vary in their attitudes about promoting health as part of their clinical practice. Some feel poorly equipped to counsel patients about life style-related issues and many are skeptical about the effect of advice on behavior change (Gemson and Elinson 1986). Accordingly, educational interventions that depend on physician involvement will need to focus on changing physician behavior and attitudes. Similarly, access to care, reimbursement for participating in interventions, and barriers to behavior change need to be addressed during these phases of planning.

Delivering Quality Programs

Phases 6 and 7 of Precede involve planning for implementation and program evaluation. Guided by the analysis done in the earlier phases, implementation strategies will be positioned for success. However, program delivery staff will need to remain flexible to respond to the evaluation components that should be presented in each phase. Many of the barriers to implementation of education programs in a clinical setting relate to the need for the involvement of interdisciplinary teams (Donaldson et al. 1987). When the multifaceted factors that predispose or enable a patient to sustain unhealthy behaviors are analyzed, a multifaceted approach to intervention is most appropriate (Mullen and Iverson 1982; Carlaw and DiAngelis 1982). However, with the strength of a team approach to care also come the difficult dynamics of coordinating allied health professionals. It has been suggested that the boundaries of authority in a medical practice can create irreconcilable differences between health professionals (Bartlett 1985). This possibility makes it even more important to enlist a broad range of organizational leaders in the health education program planning process.

FINANCING HEALTH EDUCATION

Budgeting follows planning. Assuming priorities have been established, the allocation of resources should directly support the goals and objectives that are of greatest importance to the organization. If the medical practice operates on a prepaid basis, capitation should reflect realistic support of educational strategies consistent with a managed care philosophy. A study of HMO payment approaches conducted in 1983–1984 showed per member per month capitated rates ranging from $.21 to $.53 for health education programs. Budgets were ordinarily adjusted on an annual basis, and funding for health education services was usually supplemented by copayments or full fees for select educational services (Zapka and Mullen 1985).

In contrast, when health education services are provided directly to employers, contracts usually cover the direct costs of educational materials and the delivery of educational services. Companies implementing employee health promotion programs will typically spend $15 to $25 per employee per year for limited health promotion events such as health screenings or select classes. Employers will invest as much as $150 per employee per year if they are implementing more comprehensive health promotion interventions.

ASSESSMENT AND EVALUATION

Whether assessment methods are used as a part of the overall program planning process or as a means of determining the needs of an individual program participant, assessment is the cornerstone of health education in a clinical setting. To identify what groups or individuals have the highest risks, to educate patients and health care providers about health habits related to risks, and to monitor progress in the attainment of goals related to an intervention all depend on effective and reliable assessment. In this section, three types of assessment are discussed. Health surveys designed to provide a representative picture of the patient population are among the most useful and underutilized tools for health education program development in a managed care setting (Terry 1990). Health risk appraisals, while having educational appeal and utility in mass screenings, are of somewhat more limited use in clinical settings. Nominal group process (focus groups) can garner information in an iterating fashion and provide patient feedback that is unlikely to be obtained from written surveys.

Patient Health Surveys

In spite of the methodological limitations of self-reported data, a questionnaire or phone survey remains one of the more economical alternatives for collecting data on the health behavior, interests, and beliefs of patients. Other sources such as claims data, medical records, or personal interviews can add depth to an assessment of health status, but they have other limitations of expense and reliability. The confidential nature of a questionnaire allows the health education providers to ask questions about individual health risks and to gather opinions about the value of program offerings. By using incentives and multiple waves of survey administration to ensure a high response rate, together with careful random sampling techniques, an accurate baseline of the health risks of the patient population can be established. In a managed care setting, understanding the distribution of risks is imperative given the likelihood of limited resources for intervention.

With a representative profile of the health habits and risks of the patient population comes the opportunity to deliver targeted interventions. In most instances, even when priorities have been clearly established, the range of interventions is still constrained by budgets and manpower. Accordingly, delivering services to those with the highest risk and the greatest likelihood for successful participation is the parsimonious approach. For such an approach to be workable, questionnaires need to be designed to capture information such as degree of health risk, program interests, likelihood of participation, instructional preferences, and satisfaction with existing services.

In a managed care setting, patients may be distributed throughout a number of geographic locations representing considerable variation in socioeconomic status. With this variation comes appreciable differences in patient readiness for educational services. Figure 16-1 shows the educational interests of patients

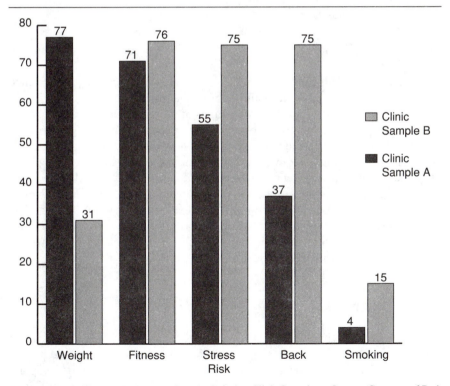

Figure 16-1 Differences in Program Interest between Clinic Locations. *Source:* Courtesy of Park Nicollet Medical Foundation, Minneapolis, MN.

of Park Nicollet Medical Foundation, a multispecialty group practice that serves a large metropolitan patient population, many of whom are HMO members. The dramatic differences between these two geographically separated clinic sites can probably be attributed to socioeconomic differences. Sample A represents a predominantly white-collar patient population. The patients in this sample expressed a much greater intent to attend weight control programs than the patients in sample B. These latter patients, of whom a large proportion were blue-collar patients, had a much greater interest in back-care education and smoking cessation programs than the patients in sample A.

Adjusting data according to risk level is another way to refine an intervention target group. Among those "at risk," interest in back-care and stress programs, for example, remains high. However, the percentage interested in weight and fitness programs is proportionately smaller (Terry et al. 1989). This indicates that many of those reporting an interest in attending programs to lose weight and exercise either consider themselves at risk or are interested in primary prevention. Anecdotal experience with relatively healthy but "worried" program participants would suggest they believe they are at risk.

Measuring Progress

For a mature health education program, survey assessments can be designed to measure improvements in health habits, changes in attitudes, or gains in knowledge. Additionally, patient evaluations of program offerings allow health education providers to reconsider priorities. Figure 16-2 shows the gap between what patients said they were interested in and how well they thought the clinic was doing in providing these programs. With respect to smoking programs, 26 percent more smokers reported approval of current offerings than reported an interest in attending these offerings. This suggests a potential overinvestment in smoking interventions. Conversely, 25 percent fewer of those having problems with stress reported approval of current programs than reported an interest in attending such programs. This suggests more must be done in the area of stress management to satisfy patient needs.

Health Risk Appraisal

Assessment activity intended to provide the patient with feedback about health risks is useful when there is a need for both data collection and patient motivation. The health education industry has generated a plethora of computer software programs designed to appraise individual risk and print out personalized advice. A number of medical practices used these programs as a part of the

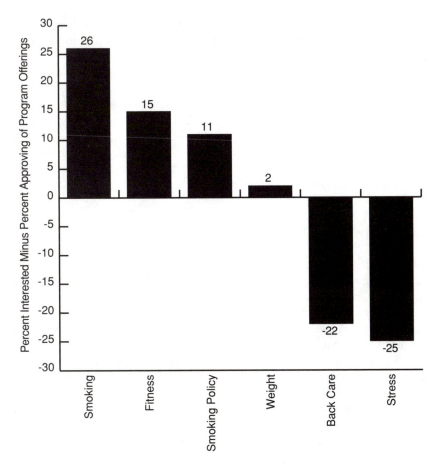

Figure 16-2 Program Performance versus Participant Need. *Source:* Courtesy of Park Nicollet Medical Foundation, Minneapolis, MN.

patient visit (Donaldson et al. 1987; Ellis 1985), but in their present form they are not likely to elicit broad physician acceptance.

As a catalyst for behavior change, individual risk assessments are critical. Dietitians use weigh-ins as a way to reinforce improvements in eating habits. Blood pressure or cholesterol measurements can serve as objective indices of progress or barometers of progressive decline in health practices. These measures, along with self-reported habits, provide a powerful set of input variables for health assessment software derived from epidemiological studies. The design of many health risk appraisals (HRA) is consistent with the tenets of the health belief model. This behavioral construct asserts that health behavior change is more likely to occur when the patients are cognizant of susceptibility to illness and understand that the consequences of succumbing to the illness could be severe (Becker 1974). However, many HRAs are so oriented toward providing probabilistic estimates of mortality that the messages relating to health habits are less noticeable.

In an ambulatory setting, a population-based HRA is clearly subordinate to individualized diagnosis and the physician's clinical judgment of health status. If an HRA is used, it should emphasize health habits rather than mortality statistics. Those HRAs with the ability to generate year-to-year result comparisons will also be of greater utility to clinicians, who may not often be able to find a history of health habits in the medical record.

Focus Groups

More traditionally employed in a marketing context, focus groups provide valuable insight into the strengths and weaknesses of intervention strategies. In particular, when programs depend on educational materials to convey health messages, these "products" need to be tested on the group they are intended to serve. Using a nominal group process may be instructive to the program developers. This involves equipping the focus group with several options for review and allowing them systematically to rate or grade each option from most preferable to least preferable. Many more members in a managed care setting prefer materials mailed to the home and convenient self-study alternatives than intend to participate in classroom activities (Terry and Pheley 1991). Maximizing the impact of these materials through focus group review is no less important than evaluating the effectiveness of instructors through classroom assessments.

MODES OF INSTRUCTION

Patients vary widely in their learning styles and their capacity for absorbing new information. They also vary widely in how much they already know about their health conditions and how much they need to know to comply with therapeutic recommendations. Those who design instruction for patients need to consider this variability if meaningful learning is to occur in the ambulatory setting. A widely used definition of health education is as follows: "Any combination of learning experiences designed to facilitate voluntary adaptations of behaviors conducive to health" (Green et al. 1980).

Having a broad menu of learning options available increases the likelihood that a patient will become engaged enough in the learning process to adopt new behaviors. Traditionally, this has meant offering individual counseling by allied professionals (e.g., dietitians), group classes taught by health educators or nurse specialists, and informational handouts describing medical condition. Increasingly this menu will include systems to integrate more intensive patient education during the physician visit, computer-based instruction, multimedia presentations, and "hypermedia" such as interactive videos. This section addresses issues related to designing a learning environment in a managed care setting. Three types of intervention strategies are discussed: physician-based instruction, group programs, and computer-assisted instruction. In an ambulatory setting, the physician's role is especially important in making education a part of the clinic's culture. Accordingly, most of this section is dedicated to discussing the role of the physician in patient education.

The Physician and Patient Education

Teaching has long been an acknowledged part of the physician's role. When considering the ambulatory health care setting, the critical mass of patients are seen by physicians one on one. Therein lies the greatest potential for increasing the impact of patient education and health promotion efforts in a managed care system. Indeed, with chronic illness consuming an increasing portion of the health care dollar (Breslow 1990) and clinical preventive services assuming greater importance among providers (U.S. Preventive Services Task Force 1989), the need for physicians to teach patients how to improve health habits is greater than ever. However, barriers such as lack of reimbursement, the disease orientation of physicians, time pressures, and lack of confidence in the outcome of their efforts continue to deter physicians from involvement in health promotion (Lawrence 1990).

There is considerable evidence that physicians spend little of their time teaching patients and, when they do give instruction or counseling, do it poorly (McClellan 1986; Ley 1982). However, there is also evidence that, when equipped with structured programs and materials or when trained in communication, physicians can have a significant impact on patient learning and health habit changes (Kottke 1988; Ley et al. 1973). Evidence linking patient satisfaction with physician communications skills is convincing. In turn, satisfied patients are more likely to comply with treatment regimes (Haynes et al. 1979). From a clinical as well as from a business perspective, involving the physician as an educator is essential.

Studies of patient compliance with medication regimens demonstrate the need for improved patient education. A review of a variety of methods for measuring compliance indicated patients fail to take antibiotics properly between 48 percent and 52 percent of the time, psychiatric medicines between 39 percent and 42 percent of the time, and antihypertensive medication between 43 percent and 61 percent of the time. Noncompliance with dietary advice occurs 49 percent of the time and other kinds of advice 51 percent of the time (Ley 1982). Compliance is positively correlated with patients' self-reported understanding of their condition and with their satisfaction with the amount of information received.

Increasing Patient Compliance

Patient understanding of information received is affected by the level of language used, by the use of materials to support the message, and by the readability level of materials provided. A number of studies have investigated the percentage of information recalled by patients after a visit. The amount recalled varies with the length of time since the visit and with the type of visit. For example, cardiac surgery visits created a much higher memory deficit than family practice visits. In general, though, studies indicate high recall failures ranging from 40 to 70 percent of the information presented within a short time after visits (Brody 1980; Ley 1982). Mistaken assumptions about the terminology that patients understand is partly responsible for the recall problem. Words commonly used by physicians such as *hypertension, tumor, virus,* and *pap smear* were misunderstood by from 24 to 72 percent of patients in one study (Spiro and Heidrich 1983). Although age and education level affect a patient's ability to understand medical terminology, certain terms are commonly misinterpreted. For example, Spiro found that 29 percent of those studied thought hypertension meant "extreme nervousness," and 72 percent did not know that people with hypertension have elevated blood pressure.

Physicians can increase their teaching effectiveness substantially by adopting several fundamental instructional techniques. Although it would be ideal if physicians were conversant with educational theory and the principles of public health education, even small changes in their teaching behavior could translate to large gains for a clinic's health education efforts. (Taking small steps is also consistent with the behavior change strategies that physicians need to become more comfortable professing to patients.) One problem relating to patient recall and compliance concerns the number of recommendations that are often run together during the presentation of information to the patient. A study by Ley and his colleagues demonstrated that "categorizing" information increased recall of information by nearly 50 percent (Ley et al. 1973). Organizing and clustering information is consistent with instructional design principles and is an important means of achieving patient behavior change objectives.

A Prescription for Physician "Health Educators"

During the typical office visit, a physician needs to assume many roles in caring for the patient. He or she might shift from interviewer to diagnostician to laboratory medicine expert to pharmacologist to counselor to health educator. All of these changes occur in a visit that is 10–12 minutes on the average. The proportion of time spent educating patients varies by specialty, with pediatricians tending to spend the most time. Observational studies indicate that from 20 percent to as little as 5 percent of the total office visit is spent on education (McClellan 1986). Thus, the physician, like the legendary "one-minute manager," has only a minute (or at best a few minutes) to teach and motivate the patient. The following are suggestions that busy physicians might do well to consider.

Preview the message. "Tell them what you are going to tell them." Patients will be better able to assimilate suggestions and directions if they know the scope and sequence of the information to be provided (Dick and Carey 1978; Ley et al. 1973). The preview might go like this: "First I am going to tell you what I think is wrong with you. Next, I am going to tell you what test you should have. Then, I am going to describe what treatment. . . ."

Present each category of information separately. "Tell them step by step what they need to be told." Avoid drifting from subjects such as testing to other issues such as treatment options or medication. Deliver information in "chunks" that are easily distinguishable. Make each transition to the next chunk obvious (e.g., "Now, the final thing I'd like to discuss is what you can do to help yourself").

Summarize major points. "Tell them what you told them." The use of repetition is at the core of instructional methodology. The patient is more likely to remember recommendations that the physician states more than once.

In addition to this outline for presenting information, the "two-minute health educator" should consider the following.

Use lay terms. Avoid professional terminology or any words that the average person is not likely to understand.

Supplement information with materials. However, providing readable materials is as important as avoiding medical jargon. For example, education materials developed at Park Nicollet Medical Foundation are usually targeted to an eighth-grade reading level.

Put it in writing. Alternatively, the patient could be instructed to take notes regarding certain directions. Brief notes will serve to engage the patient in listening to advice and as a reminder later on. Simple illustrations drawn by the physician are also likely to increase the patient's comprehension of his or her condition.

Supporting the Educational Efforts of Physicians

The health education staff can take an active role in providing physicians with tools to make them better teachers. Physicians who try to educate their patients develop an ongoing need for current materials that are readable. Group programs also can be a useful adjunct for physicians who see large numbers of the same types of conditions. Including a physician as a member of the faculty for class offerings is the surest way to ensure that group programs are an integrated part of patient care.

Structured systems for physician-directed patient education have also been shown to impact patient behavior. Reminder systems such as color codes in the medical record to indicate patient smokers and their quitting attempts or computerized cancer-screening triggers have been shown to improve physician counseling and subsequent patient behaviors (Kottke 1988). In spite of an understandable reluctance to use valuable clinical time educating patients about an intractable behavior such as smoking, physicians must realize that their advice may be cost-effective even when compliance rates are low (Cummings et al. 1989).

Group Programs

A survey of 340 HMO members of the American Medical Care and Review Association indicated group programs are the most broadly accepted component of health promotion in a clinical setting (Bernton 1987). Among the 60 percent of organizations responding, smoking programs were the most commonly offered (84 percent), followed by programs for weight loss (78 percent), stress management (75 percent), nutrition (74 percent), and hypertension management (43 percent). Although group programs are likely to remain the mainstay of the health education offerings of most organizations, they are a limiting strategy if offering them absorbs health education staff resources to the exclusion of other modes of instruction.

When considering the relatively small percentage of patients interested in attending classes (Terry and Pheley 1991; Sofien and Graff 1986) and the absence of compelling data to suggest that classes are more effective than other interventions, group programs should be positioned as one choice among many other educational options. Materials-based interventions, physician-directed interventions, media campaigns, and computer-assisted instruction all warrant equal consideration.

Computer-Assisted Health Education

A coordinated approach to health care requires tools for managing data about patients. The eventuality of an automated medical record makes consideration of computer-aided instruction and health behavior monitoring timely. Commercially available computer reference systems have grown to include extensive patient handouts that can be customized by clinics and accessed rapidly. Complete drug reference systems and on-line networks of medical information are also available. Acceptance of these services has been slowly developing. It is likely that when computerized systems for accessing lab results and radiology imaging are more broadly available, physicians' use of computer-based patient education resources will increase.

The potential for using the computer in patient health behavior change programs is yet unknown. Computers can serve as automated reminder systems that make recommendations specific to a patient's age, race, and gender. Patients due for routine clinical preventive services such as mammograms or immunizations can be automatically flagged. Personalized diet, exercise, and other health habit prescriptions can be developed and the computer can mark progress toward an individual's goals. Handouts that describe health conditions and the range of treatment options can be customized to teach patients about their health status. Such handouts can serve as both patient education forms and informed consent forms.

At Park Nicollet Medical Foundation, interactive computer programs have been developed that teach patients about health risks and generate a health risk profile to be used by hypertension nurse educators. Nutrition programs are also used by patients with high cholesterol. Using a touch screen, or via a point and click on the computer, patients take nutrition self-tests that provide immediate feedback about their awareness of low-fat food sources. Test results are stored for review by the physicians, who can assess trends in the knowledge of the patients participating in the program.

FUTURE TRENDS IN HEALTH EDUCATION

Health care delivery will become increasingly managed and increasingly accountable for outcomes of care. Among the strategies for containing costs, health promotion shows tremendous promise. However, with continued funding retrenchment by third-party payers, strategies for integrating health education into the fabric of an ambulatory care practice rather than positioning education as an add-on will be most effective. This will require greater involvement in preventive medicine among physicians, a trend that is consistent with the changes in health status expected in the aging population. This section addresses four issues that relate to the role of education in managing outcomes: (1) the need for improving the long-term prospects for behavior changes, (2) the need for greater involvement from health care consumers, (3) the implications of individual risk-based insurance rating, and (4) the importance of including health promotion as part of the minimum health care coverage.

Long-Term Compliance

Relapse is the Achilles heel of health promotion. Many educational programs can claim success in changing health habits. Few have long-term data (more than two years' follow-up) to support the effectiveness of interventions in reducing risks (Lorig and Laurin 1985). Health education programs committed to measuring outcomes need to structure programs that monitor the patient at the end of the critical three- and six-month periods, during which relapse to former behaviors is common. New skills related to sustaining new habits need to be introduced to the patient at regular intervals. A combination of follow-up methods such as phone reminders, materials-based campaigns, or support groups may be needed to sustain the progress made at the outset of interventions. Systems of reinforcement should be tested to determine which strategies are most effective for maintaining positive health practices.

Informed Medical Decision Making

The health care consumers' role in managing their own health care will also grow. Costs are likely to continue to shift to patients, and with this added burden will come greater scrutiny of treatment options. Shared decision making between physicians and patients assumes a greater amount of understanding among patients concerning the costs and benefits of treatment choices. This, in turn, will require that more sophisticated education resources are at the disposal of the health care team. Interactive videos are already being tested in some clinics to show patients the range of risks and benefits of selected surgical procedures. More patients are likely to decide against some types of procedures when faced with a clear impression of possible side effects and the reality of the data concerning treatment effectiveness.

Such educational technology will not diminish the physicians' role in medical decision making. Indeed, physicians already overestimate the desire of patients to make decisions (Strull et al. 1984). Rather, physicians will be pressed more than ever to describe and discuss options with patients who are intent upon being smart shoppers with their health care dollars, and they even now underestimate the amount of information desired by patients (Strull et al. 1984). The patients' need to weigh all of the options and understand the consequences of their actions will be felt more keenly than ever by physicians.

Individual Risk Rating for Insurance

Not only will costs continue to shift to the consumer, but insurance rating schemes will likely shift proportionately higher costs to individuals with greater health risks. Based upon assumptions that many health risks result from behaviors that are controllable, insurance premiums may be higher for those that need insurance the most. Aside from the "blame the victim" concerns that will need to be addressed if this trend is to continue, patients are likely to search for medical measures to ameliorate health risks. For example, patients who have to pay more if their blood pressure or cholesterol exceed certain levels will turn to physicians for solutions.

This departure from relying on health care only when one is sick could have both positive and negative consequences. If the physician is empowered as a patient ally by insurance companies so that being under a physician's supervision is sufficient to qualify an individual for the low-risk premium, then the doctor-patient relationship is not threatened. In this scenario, the physician can use insurance rating criteria as a tool to motivate patients to comply with treatment recommendations. Risk indicators for insurance rating provide a "teachable moment" for the patient hoping to avoid higher premiums. However, if insurance rating criteria are rigid and physicians are simply expected to provide an assessment of risk based on these rigid criteria, the physicians then become adversaries of their patients. The education and motivation of the patients would then be difficult to achieve.

Health education departments that provide health screening or health risk appraisal services may be in a position similar to that of the physicians if individual risk rating becomes prevalent. Opportunities for teaching risk reduction skills may increase, but the prospects for success may diminish if participation is coerced rather than truly voluntary. Continued study concerning the extent to which certain health risks are controllable and the extent to which illness subsequent to prolonged health habits is predictable will be needed.

Minimal Coverage in Health Care

The federal government and the state governments are likely to play a greater role in funding health care in the future. Managed care systems will be instrumental in moderating costs and assuring equal access to care. Debates about what is medically necessary will continue. The list of services that will be considered elective and beyond the purview of health benefits will grow longer. Health education services with proven success in reducing risks and managing utilization will be covered by even minimal health care insurance policies.

MEET MR. RISK

A forceful wind blew against him and he panted as he walked the short distance from his car to the clinic entrance. He had visited three different clinics in the past year about his shortness of breath, but he wasn't satisfied with any of the doctors. They didn't take the time to understand his problems. He was certain they must be missing something in their exams. Mr. Risk hoped this clinic could provide him with some answers as he entered and observed the sign, "Smoke Free Building for the Health of Our Patients." The waiting room racks caught his eye; there were neat displays of dozens of colorful educational pamphlets. He checked in with the receptionist, a cheerful young man who said the doctor would like some information about his health history and life style. He had two options—a computer assessment or a paper-and-pencil question-naire. Electing to be evaluated by the computer, he was impressed with how easy it was to use. By touching the screen, he received immediate feedback about his health habits. A printout at the end of the interview outlined his major health risks. The results form also indicated that he was overdue for his colorectal exam, an issue he should discuss with his doctor, according to the printout.

A nurse briefly reviewed his personalized risk assessment as he was ushered to an exam room. "I'm placing a red sticker on your chart, Mr. Risk," the nurse said, "It's a reminder for all of us at the clinic that you're still a smoker. I expect your doctor will be discussing this with you further."

Soon after the doctor arrived. "I see you are experiencing some shortness of breath, Mr. Risk," the physician said as he embarked on an interview that was quite unlike those of the previous doctors. The most noticeable difference was in the way he paused. He was really listening. By the end of the visit, Mr. Risk felt good about his treatment plan. The doctor had really gotten his attention when he started writing instructions and drew simple explanatory pictures on the health assessment form. "We need to prioritize some of these health habits you say you are ready to tackle," he had said, "and next month at this time you are going to look me in the eye and brag about your progress."

He learned that the red sticker on his chart would be replaced with different colors that corresponded to his quit attempts and the length of time he ab-stained. They had decided he wasn't ready to quit smoking yet, but they would discuss it at greater length at his next visit.

He also wasn't sure yet about the "sigmoidoscopic exam." The doctor agreed with the recommended interval for testing that was indicated on the health assessment feedback form, but he also explained some of the statistics about the effectiveness of colon cancer screening and the minor discomfort involved. Mr. Risk agreed to check out a video from the clinic's health education center to learn more about the costs and benefits of cancer screening. The doctor had indicated there might be other tests. It was a lot to remember, but the doctor had organized each piece of information in a logical order. It really helped to have the handout about the tests the doctor had given him and the risk assessment feedback form on which he had made notes. He knew he had some goal setting to do in order to be ready for his next visit. But he felt quite satisfied with this clinic and he said so on the "Tell us about your visit" form that he was asked to complete on his way out.

Mr. Risk noticed that he wasn't gasping on the walk back to his car. "Now the wind is at my back," he thought.

CONCLUSION

Those educational strategies that improve quality of life, particularly for patients with chronic health conditions, will be supported. Educational systems that reduce unnecessary visits by substituting reliable self-care knowledge and behavior will also be considered a medical necessity. Finally, health education programs that improve the efficiency and quality of the health care system will be sought. From improving physician communications to fostering patient compliance and preventing disease, challenges for education will arise as a result of both clinical and business necessities. Health education support services responsive to these needs will be an integral part of the evolution from a "medical care" to a "health care" system.

BIBLIOGRAPHY

Anderson, R., and Mullner, R. 1990. "Data Watch: Assessing the Health Objectives of the Nation." *Health Affairs* 9, no. 2: 152–63.

Bartlett, E. 1985. "Health Education and Medicine: Competition or Cooperation." *Health Education Quarterly* 12: 219–29.

Becker, M. 1974. "The Health Belief Model and Personal Health Behavior." *Health Education Monographs* 2: 4.

Bernton, C.T. 1987. "What Is the Future of Health Promotion in HMOs." *American Journal of Health Promotion* 1, no. 4: 24–27.

Breslow, L. 1990. "A Health Promotion Primer for the 1990s." *Health Affairs* 9, no. 2: 6–22.

Brody, D. 1980. "An Analysis of Patients' Recall of Their Therapeutic Regimens." *Journal of Chronic Disease* 33: 57–63.

Carlaw, R.W., and DiAngelis, N.M. 1982. "Promoting Health and Preventing Disease: Some Thoughts for HMOs." *Health Education Quarterly* 9: 81–95.

Cummings, S.R., Nowakowski, T.A., and Schwandt, J.R. 1989. "The Cost-Effectiveness of Counseling Smokers to Quit." *JAMA* 261: 75–79.

Dick, W., and Carey, L. 1978. *The Systematic Design of Instruction.* Glenview, IL: Scott, Foresman.

Donaldson, M.S., Schrott, L., and Frank, J. 1987. "Integrating Health Promotion and Medical Practice." *HMO Practice* 2, no. 1: 24–29.

Ellis, L.B. 1985. "Computer-Based Patient Education." *Primary Care* 12, no. 3.

Farquhar, J.W. 1987. *The American Way of Life Need Not Be Hazardous to Your Health.* Reading, MA: Addison-Wesley.

Farquhar, J.W., Fortman, S.P., and Macoby, N. 1977. "Community Education for Cardiovascular Health." *Lancet* 1, No. 8023: 1192–95.

Frederiksen, L.W., Solomon, L.J., and Brehany, K.A. 1984. *Marketing Health Behavior: Principles, Techniques, and Applications.* New York: Plenum Publishing.

Gemson, D.H., and Elinson, J. 1986. "Prevention in Primary Care: Variability in Physician Practice Patterns in New York City." *American Journal of Preventive Medicine* 2: 226–34.

Green, L., Krueter, M., Deeds, S., and Partridge, P. 1980. *Health Education Planning: A Diagnostic Approach.* Mayfield.

Griffith, J.J., Baloff, N., and Spitznagel, E. 1984. "Utilization Patterns of Health Maintenance Organization Disenrollees." *Medical Care* 22, no. 9: 827–34.

Hanson, S.A., Terry, P.E., and Fowles, J. 1989. "Is Smoking Consistent with Daily Practice at a Health Care Facility?" *Occupational Health and Safety* 58, no. 5.

Haynes, R.B., Taylor, D.W., and Sackett, D.L. 1979. *Compliance in Health Care.* Baltimore: Johns Hopkins University Press.

Kelly Communications. 1991. "Conference Board Ratings in Modern Health Care." *Health Action Managers* 5, no. 1.

Kemper, D. 1982. "Self Care Education: Impact on HMO Costs." *Medical Care* 20, no. 7: 710–18.

Kolbe, L. 1988. "The Application of Health Behavior Research." In *Health Behavior: Emerging Research Perspectives,* edited by D.S. Gochman. New York: Plenum Press.

Kosecoff, J., Fink, A., Brook, R.H., Dahlman, L., and Kirst, J. 1985. "General Medical Care and the Education of Internists in University Hospitals: An Evaluation of the Teaching Hospital General Medicine Group Practice Program." *Annals of Internal Medicine* 102: 250–57.

Kottke, T. 1988. "Attributes of Successful Smoking Cessation Interventions in Medical Practice." *JAMA* 261: 75–79.

Kristein, M. 1977. "Economic Issues in Prevention." *Preventive Medicine* 6: 252–54.

Lawrence, R.S. 1990. "The Role of Physicians in Health Promotion." *Health Affairs* 9, no. 2.

Levine, D.M., Green, L.W., Deeds, S.G., et al. 1979. "Health Education for Hypertensive Patients." *JAMA* 24: 1700–1703.

Ley, P. 1982. "Satisfaction, Compliance and Communication." *British Journal of Clinical Psychology* 21: 241–54.

Ley, P., Bradshaw., et al. 1973. "A Method for Increasing Patients' Recall of Information Presented by Doctors." *Psychological Medicine* 3: 217–20.

Lorig, K., and Laurin, J. 1985. "Some Notions about Assumptions underlying Health Education." *Health Education Quarterly* 12: 231–43.

McClellan, W. 1986. "Current Perspectives: Patient Education in Medical Practice." *Patient Education and Counseling* 8: 151–63.

Mullen, P.D., and Iverson, D.C. 1982. "Qualitative Methods for Evaluative Research in Health Education Programs." *Health Education* 13, No. 3: 11–18.

Multiple Risk Factor Intervention Trial Research Group. 1982. "Multiple Risk Factor Intervention Trial." *JAMA* 248: 1465–77.

Pheley, A., Fowles, J., et al. 1991. "Evaluation of a Nurse Based Hypertension Management Program as a Resource for Physicians: Screening, Management and Outcomes." Minneapolis: Park Nicollet Medical Foundation.

Pope, C. 1978. "Consumer Satisfaction in a Health Maintenance Organization." *Journal of Health and Social Behavior* 19: 291–340.

Puske, P.A., Nissinen, J., and Tuomilehto, J. 1985. "The Community-Based Strategy to Prevent Coronary Heart Disease." *Annual Review of Public Health* 6: 147–93.

Rocella, E. 1976. "Potential for Reducing Health Care Costs by Public and Patient Education." *Public Health Reports* 91, no. 3: 223–25.

Rosenberg, H.S. 1971. "Patient Education Leads to Better Care for Heart Patients." *HSMHA Health Reports* 86: 793–802.

Sofien, N., and Graff, W. 1986. "Marketing Health Promotion: Form and Substance." In *New Health Care Systems: HMOs and Beyond. Proceedings of the Group Health Practice Association,* 539–48.

Sofien, N., and LeVan, S. 1987. "Health Promotion: A Marketing and Cost Strategy." *HMO Practice* 2, no. 1: 20–32.

Spiro, D., and Heidrich, F. 1983. "Lay Understanding of Medical Terminology." *The Journal of Family Practice* 17, no. 2: 277–79.

Strull, W.M., Lo,C., and Charles, G. 1984. "Do Patients Want To Participate in Medical Decision Making." *JAMA* 252: 2990–94.

Terry, P.E. 1990. "Employers Scrutinizing Health Plans for Value and Impact on Employees." *Occupational Health and Safety* 59, no.3.

Terry, P.E., and Fowles, J. 1989. "Developing a Survey Strategy for Your Health Promotion Programs." *Business and Health* 7, no. 12.

Terry, P.E., and Pheley, A. 1991. "Health Risks and Educational Interests of Members of a State-wide HMO." *HMO Practice* 5, no. 1: 3–6.

Terry, P.E., Regan, M., Kallstrom, C., and Williams, D. 1989. "Health Education: Decentralization in a Large Multispecialty Group Practice." *Group Practice Journal* 38, no. 2: 18–24.

U.S. Preventive Services Task Force. 1989. "Guide to Clinical Preventive Services." Baltimore: Williams & Wilkins.

U.S. Public Health Service. 1987. *The 1990 Health Objectives for the Nation: A Midcourse Review.* Pub. No. 1987-191-691/70228. Washington, DC: U.S. Printing Office.

U.S. Public Health Service. May 1988. "Detection, Evaluation, and Treatment of High Blood Pressure." Report of the Joint National Committee, NIH Pub. No. 88-1088.

Vickery, D., Golaszewski, T.J., Wright, E.C., and Kalmer, H. 1988. "The Effect of Self-Care Interventions on the Use of Medical Services within a Medicare Population." *Medical Care* 26: 580–88.

Vickery, D., Kalmer, H., and Lowry, D. 1989. "A Preliminary Study on the Timeliness of Ambulatory Care Utilization following Medical Self Care Interventions." *The American Journal of Health Promotion* 3, no. 3: 26–31.

Warner, K. 1987. "Selling Health Promotion to Corporate America: Uses and Abuses of the Economic Argument." *Health Education Quarterly* 14: 39–55.

Zapka, J., and Averill, B. 1979. "Self Care for Colds: A Cost Effective Alternative to Upper Respiratory Infection Management." *American Journal of Health Promotion* 69: 814–16.

Zapka, J., and Mullen, P. 1985. "Financing Health Promotion and Education Programs in HMOs." *HCM Review* 10, no. 4: 63–71.

Zapka, J., Stanek, E., and Raitt, J. 1986. "HMO Disenrollment—Who Leaves and Why?" In *New Health Care Systems: HMOs and Beyond. Proceedings of the Group Health Practice Association,* 559–71.

17

Staff Education

Linda D'Angelo, Amy Bernard, Ann Casstevens,
Loretta Crowell, and Rebekah Jones

INTRODUCTION

Staff education is a vital component in assuring the provision of quality patient care in the ambulatory care setting. Direct benefits include a trained staff that functions effectively in an established setting; a knowledgeable professional staff; decreased liability concerns; and increased job satisfaction, which has the potential of diminishing employee turnover.

Staff education, which is defined as any effort undertaken to improve employees' skills or knowledge base, can be divided into three types: orientation, in-service education, and continuing education.

Orientation is concerned with acquainting the newly hired employee with organizational policies, personnel benefits, position requirements, and skill training. It also includes familiarizing the employee with some of the specific characteristics of each specialty unit or department. Orientation to standard policies and procedures ensures consistency among staff. Consistent understanding of and adherence to policies and procedures decreases uncertainty, errors, and duplication of effort.

In addition to orientation, specific skills and enhanced knowledge may be required for staff to fulfill job requirements. *In-service* or *continuing education programs* generally are developed to meet this need.

The term *in-service* refers to the type of educational programming that is procedure-oriented and job-specific. In-service programs can be designed, for example, to teach a revised ear irrigation procedure, to instruct staff on the operation of newly purchased sterilizers, or to acquaint staff with the operation of a new phone system.

The term *continuing education* refers to programming that provides information on a particular topic. It is generally designed to broaden and expand employees' knowledge base, and it is often used to introduce new concepts and current information on a subject. Some professional groups have mandatory continuing education credit requirements for licensure renewal. Examples include certain physician, nurse specialist, pharmacist, audiologist, dietitian, and radiologic technology groups. The national professional association for registered nurses, the American Nurses' Association, defines continuing education in the following way:

> The purpose of continuing education in nursing is to build upon varied educational and experiential bases for enhancement of practice, education, administration, research, or theory development, to the end of maintaining and improving the health of the public. The primary responsibility for obtaining continuing education lies within the professional but the employing agency may provide support in a variety of ways. (American Nurses' Association 1984)

The administrative leadership determines the presence and degree of staff education within an organization. Directly or indirectly it supports the philosophical concept of need for the existence of staff education and allocates funds to support the associated efforts. Some factors that determine the need for staff education include the number of staff who require training and the complexity of the requisite knowledge and skills. Other determining factors include the availability of appropriate educational programs and facilities within the community or region. Some education and training can be provided through junior college- or college-based programs. In the ambulatory care setting, resources for planning and providing education are often limited. The value of educational efforts is often difficult to quantify and may be viewed as an unnecessary cost. However, for most employees, the provision of appropriate ongoing educational opportunities functions to reinforce their existing skills, broaden their knowledge base, update their technical competency, and improve job satisfaction.

This chapter identifies considerations for the assessment of educational needs and the development of relevant programs, including examples currently being implemented in large multispecialty medical group practices.

The decision to centralize or decentralize the education function will vary among institutions and may depend upon the particular program. Regardless of the ultimate decision, it is critical that educational programs have the support of the administration and management of the organization and that policy decisions demonstrate that support. For example, if it is decided that cardiopulmonary resuscitation (CPR) skills are required for all personnel who work in patient care areas, it is essential for administration to provide the necessary personnel and resources, including time, space, and equipment, for the educational effort to succeed. In this example, centralizing the education program will maximize its efficiency, since there will be many employees in many different departments who will need CPR instruction.

Another example of an appropriately centralized staff education program is a management training program. In a large, complex ambulatory care facility, it is advantageous to ensure that all supervisory personnel are knowledgeable about the mission of the organization, particularly the management philosophy. Recurring management training courses provide new supervisors and managers with a consistent approach to their role. Although it is possible to hire skilled managers or send personnel to outside educational programs for management skills and knowledge development, in-house programs can also help fill the need for expert managers. Moreover, they have the advantage of promoting teamwork across departments, as new supervisors and managers learn together.

Alternatively, in some cases it might be more appropriate to decentralize the education and training functions to meet the needs of a specific group of health care workers. An example is teaching new medical receptionists skills that are relevant only within their work environment. In this example, the expertise required is role-specific. It should be noted, however, that medical receptionists interact with many other departments within a complex ambulatory care setting. It is important that training programs include procedural content that is consistent across the various departmental boundaries. Instructors of such programs must be knowledgeable in other departmental areas, and representatives of these other departments may actually assist in the didactic portion of the training process.

Preceptorship programs provide an excellent means for new personnel to gain support and guidance as they apply newly learned skills in the actual work setting. It is important to define the role of the preceptor and to educate the preceptor about specific support responsibilities. It is also essential that the preceptors be allowed adequate time to ensure appropriate guidance and coaching. The qualities possessed by preceptors should include expertise in a selected area, excellent communication skills, and a commitment to the educator role.

Ongoing staff education programs are also important to provide opportunities for those professional groups that are required to attain continuing education credits. Staff perceive these opportunities, when provided in-house, as a benefit that contributes to job satisfaction. While coordination of these programs may necessarily be a centralized function, it is important to provide program content that is important to staff. This can be done via elected or appointed committees or through the use of written surveys. It is desirable to plan program schedules and content far in advance to facilitate space allocations and speaker arrangements. A planning committee might be established to include volunteers from nursing, physician providers, and other staff. The involvement of the committee members in facilitating specific programs increases their commitment to ensuring quality instruction and also aids them in securing additional staff participation.

At times it may be necessary to provide opportunities for staff to participate in programs outside the particular institution. Many organizations have an administrative policy that defines the guidelines under which outside continuing education will be considered and supported. Department directors individually or through organized committees may make decisions regarding individual employee requests for outside program attendance. The criteria used for judging such requests would include relevancy to job requirements, need for technical skills development, and length of employment of the applicant. Support for approved programs can include paid time off, registration fees, and payment of travel and hotel expenses associated with the program. Such programs afford the supervisor or manager an avenue for directing employees who feel stymied by a particular job situation or who might benefit from further formalized education. Supporting growth opportunities for employees contributes to job satisfaction and is an important strategy for recruiting and retaining skilled health care workers for the organization.

TWO TYPES OF EDUCATIONAL PROGRAMS

Two types of educational programs may be offered within an institution: (1) programs designed for the enhancement of the skills and knowledge base of an educationally prepared group and (2) basic training programs formalized within the institution that are intended to ensure staff without formal professional education or training have the knowledge and support they need to be successful in their roles. Examples of each are discussed below.

A Telephone Triage Training Program

An example of the first type of educational program is a program designed to give nurses the necessary skills for telephone triage. Telephone triage traditionally has been limited to emergency room staff. Emergency room nurses acquired the requisite skills on the job, since most nursing school programs did not specifically educate nurses about handling patient problems by telephone.

Nurses, with their broad background and holistic approach to care, are uniquely prepared to respond to patients who call in. This new role of nurses has resulted in the emerging field of telephone triage. The word *triage* means "to sort." Telephone triage is the process by which nurses, through the use of phone conversations, apply their skills and knowledge to assess the patient's problem, develop a plan of action with the patient that is appropriate and agreeable to the patient, and assist the patient in carrying out that plan. Historically, the nurse's telephone role was that of a message taker, receiving information from the patient, forwarding it to the physician, and relaying the physician's response back to the patient. Such a routine was inefficient. Telephone triage maximizes use of the nurse's skills and knowledge and more effectively utilizes the physician's time.

Goals and Benefits of Telephone Triage Skills Development

The goals of nursing in ambulatory care include (1) meeting the patients' needs by providing direct nursing services within the nurses' scope of practice and (2) assisting the physicians in their medical practice. In today's environment, efficiency and cost-effectiveness are essential as well. An educational program designed to build on existing nursing knowledge and skills and give nurses a greater ability to use the telephone for patient care can result in improved efficiency and increased job satisfaction for nurses. This is important, since an ambulatory care nurse may spend up to 75 percent of his or her time providing nursing assistance over the telephone.

Patients benefit by accessing health care services at an appropriate level. Previously, patients who could have been treated at home were advised to visit the clinic. Now, many may be efficiently managed over the telephone. Patients seem to like the convenience of call-in services. They welcome the opportunity to talk with a trained individual who can assist them in determining the urgency of their health needs and often save them the time and expense of a doctor's visit. The health care organization benefits by having on the doctor's schedule only those patients who truly need to be seen.

Program Development

A telephone triage education program provides the professional nurse in the ambulatory care setting with the fundamental skills necessary for effective telephone triage and management.

Needs Assessment. In developing a program, the manager or educator must first assess the current functions of nurses in the patient care unit. This includes careful collection of data regarding the nurse's role and scope of practice. A committee of managers, educators, nurses, and physicians should identify outcomes expected and goals desired from the new telephone triage system.

Content. Once the desired outcomes are defined, the educator can develop program content to achieve the results. Since telephone protocols may involve medical advice, physician input is essential. Written guidelines documented and approved by medical staff provide triage nurses with needed support. Other areas to include in this training program are as follows:

- The nurses' role and responsibilities within their scope of practice. A critical component of the program is that professional nurses understand their scope of practice as it relates to telephone nursing. They must be familiar with the appropriate state practice act and the standards that establish what is allowed and not allowed by law.

- Basic principles of triage and case management. Emphasis is on critical thinking and decision making as opposed to responding by rote to patients' questions.
- Methods for data collection and documentation of telephone inquiries and responses.
- Effective communication techniques.
- Liability issues.
- Management of difficult cases.

Implementation. Principles of adult teaching and learning should be applied. The educational methods for presenting this material should be interactive. Workshops may include case studies and small-group exercises. Participants should have the opportunity to share and discuss telephone cases related to their work areas.

Evaluation Implications. Several methods for evaluating results of this type of continuing education program exist. A posttest, in essay form, can measure the amount of knowledge acquired. An essay allows the instructor to determine whether critical thinking skills are being applied appropriately. Patient feedback also can be indicative of training success, and physicians can evaluate the program's effectiveness by noting if and how their time is better managed. The telephone triage unit manager can measure how well the unit functions as a whole.

The best measure of training effectiveness is what actually happens in the different areas of the clinic. Nurses should be more productive, more challenged, and more satisfied. Managers should see more appropriate assessment and management of patients over the telephone. Physicians should be utilized more effectively, and patient satisfaction should increase.

A telephone triage training program is but one example of a useful in-house educational program that builds on existing skills and experience. In this time of health care competition and cost-consciousness, a well-run ambulatory care clinic will strive to implement staff educational programs that reflect the new roles its professionals have had to assume. Such programs should be cost-effective and result in improved patient care.

Training Medical Receptionists

The position of medical receptionist is an important one in the ambulatory care setting. Being in the "front lines," the medical receptionist is often the first and last contact a patient has with an organization during a typical office visit.

It is vital that the patient receive a favorable impression. The responsibilities of the medical receptionist vary considerably from one organization to another. They may include appointment scheduling, greeting and checking in patients as they arrive for appointments, filing lab results, sorting mail, answering phones, and performing an initial phone screening. In some organizations, medical receptionists may also help with cash collection, verify the eligibility of insured patients, and answer patient inquiries regarding billing and insurance.

Traditionally, the medical receptionist position is an entry-level position with a salary set accordingly. The average applicant has little or no experience in the medical field. Most are recent high school or college graduates who are looking for their first full-time position in a professional organization. Their work experience is usually limited to customer-service oriented retail settings.

Once hired, medical receptionists are assigned to clinical departments. They may be unaccustomed to the fast pace of many practices, the unfamiliar medical vocabulary, and the stress levels associated with ambulatory care settings. Usually, with the help of their supervisors, the receptionists are expected to learn the skills needed to perform their detail-oriented responsibilities while working. This on-the-job training system has several drawbacks: (1) It places stress on the medical receptionists, who are often expected to know and perform duties unfamiliar to them; and (2) it places stress and added responsibilities on the supervisors or trainers, who are also expected to continue as frontline workers. Many organizations have found that on-the-job training can produce negative results over a period of time. These include frustrated medical receptionists and trainers, high stress levels, departmental inefficiencies, and increased attrition rates. These organizations have found that a more structured training program yields better results and have developed what might be called a "medical receptionist school."

The following steps should be taken when an organization makes the decision to develop a structured training program for medical receptionists:

1. Set goals and objectives.
2. Develop a curriculum for the training program.
3. Define the role of preceptors.
   • Recruit appropriate preceptors.
   • Train the preceptors.
4. Implement the training program.
5. Document, evaluate, and revise the program.

Setting Goals and Objectives

The training of new medical receptionists must be role-specific and focus on skills that are relevant within their work environment. A committee of key employees should be formed to determine the relevance of specific skills and set goals and establish criteria for the program. This committee, made up of managers, supervisors, frontline medical receptionists, and a human resources representative, should also develop a plan of action. This action plan might include the following:

- Institution of a one- or two-week didactic classroom program to orient new medical receptionists to their roles and introduce basic concepts and skills prior to a departmental preceptored training program.
- Development of a current training manual to be used as a teaching tool by desk trainers and new medical receptionists and as a reference work by existing employees.
- Creation of a job description for the position of preceptor that lists expectations and responsibilities.
- Promotion of the concept of conformity of procedures and standards across departments to facilitate the training process (among the transdepartment standards should be specific performance and training standards, especially standards relating to service).
- Establishment of guidelines for an extended preceptored training experience following the classroom training.
- Formulation of policies regarding pay and benefits during the training period and screening criteria or tests to be used for determining acceptance into the program.

Committee members can be expected to contribute specific guidelines, procedures, and information segments, which when formatted could be organized into various sections. These sections would then be used to help form the curriculum.

Developing the Curriculum

After gathering ideas and suggestions from managers, supervisors, trainers, and medical receptionists, a list of skills and concepts to be dealt with in the training program should be compiled. It might include

- the role of the medical receptionist
- patient confidentiality
- appointment scheduling
- basic computer programs
- telephone etiquette, mechanics, and guidelines

- chart preparation and record maintenance for appointments
- basic forms
- desk procedures
- service standards

Defining the Role of Preceptors

In a small organization, the preceptor might be the more experienced of two receptionists. In larger companies, the preceptor for a given unit or department might be a supervisor. In any case, the preceptor should be an experienced medical receptionist who is knowledgeable and resourceful and has good communication skills and lots of patience. Each department manager should assess the qualifications of interested employees before designating a preceptor. Effective desk trainers must have "mentoring" qualities, which are so important when introducing new employees to their roles.

The role of the preceptor is complex and demanding. Preceptors are responsible for instructing, overseeing, supporting, and evaluating new medical receptionists during the designated training period. They should be made aware of all aspects of the position through in-service training. It is important that preceptors receive the support and resources needed to do their job effectively. For example, they need enough spare time to work one on one with new receptionists. The training program coordinator must prepare the preceptors for their role by providing appropriate resources and materials and by conducting appropriate training workshops. The topics of such workshops might include adult learning principles, motivational techniques, stress management, and individualized instruction.

Implementing the Program

Once the curriculum for the receptionist school is established, implementation planning may begin. Materials and resources will need to be developed or obtained. These might include classroom space, training manuals, workbooks, audiovisual aids and equipment, handouts, and skill tests. Guest speakers from within the organization and class instructors must be contacted to arrange for convenient course scheduling. Interested preceptors make excellent class instructors since they are very knowledgeable on the subject material. Using them as instructors also keeps them involved with the didactic portion of the training program. Sometimes an observation period of two to three days in the clinical department to which they will be assigned prior to participation in the offsite training program is beneficial to new receptionists. They will then have some understanding of the physical layout, the patient and chart flow, the vocabulary, and the responsibilities of the position when they begin the didactic portion of the program.

The didactic instruction is a combination of information dissemination through short lectures and hands-on activities where the participants practice specific tasks (e.g., basic appointment scheduling on the computer). The atmosphere should be conducive to learning, and the receptionist trainees should feel comfortable asking questions and interacting with each other and the instructor.

A designated training period of several weeks in the clinical department should follow participation in the offsite training. Each receptionist trainee works with a preceptor and receives further instruction during this time. It is here that the receptionist trainee practices those skills learned in the classroom. The program coordinator needs to meet regularly with the preceptors, medical receptionist trainees, and department managers to assess the progress of the trainees and to modify the training program content when needed.

Documenting, Evaluating, and Revising the Program

In addition to the skill testing done in the offsite training classes, further assessment of the new medical receptionists' progress must occur during the departmental training experience. This can be accomplished by providing each preceptor with a comprehensive core checklist to be completed by the end of this period. By using this checklist as a measuring tool, the preceptor and program coordinator can evaluate the success of the new employee's training and lengthen or shorten the training period accordingly. Accompanying the checklist might be a weekly progress form to be filled out jointly by the preceptor and the medical receptionist. This can provide a record of the trainee's progress and can be included in the employee's personnel file.

At the end of the designated training period, an overall formal evaluation may be completed by the preceptor in collaboration with the department manager. The organization's employee performance appraisal form might be useful for this purpose.

Although the program outlined above is specifically for medical receptionists, with appropriate modifications it can be used for other categories of employees. Unlicensed medical office assistants, for example, can be similarly trained but would require a longer period of classroom instruction. Traditionally, the aide or medical assistant has been hired untrained and has learned the skills needed to provide patient care while on the job. This practice has frequently placed considerable stress on the new worker, who is expected to perform with little or no preparation. The health care facility itself operates less efficiently while new employees are learning their jobs. Although programs are available to train medical office assistants, they are few in number, usually expensive, and not generally available in many geographical areas. As in the case of medical receptionists, outside training and experience does not often coincide with the specialized roles required by the larger medical groups. Many health care facilities, therefore, have found it to their advantage to provide initial training for their assistant workers.

Advantage of Initial Training for Medical Receptionists and Medical Office Assistants

Devoting time and resources to pretraining specific kinds of employees such as new medical office assistants and medical receptionists will entail a financial commitment but will also provide distinct advantages. If new employees are given initial training, they are better prepared to perform their jobs. The preparation will be more consistent than that provided by on-the-job training alone. New employees will have a better understanding of their roles, how they fit into the organization, and the value of their jobs to the overall mission of the ambulatory care facility.

CONCLUSION

Few effective outside programs are available to train individuals for health care positions in a modern group practice. A training program provided by the employing institution can provide a more consistent means to inform, instruct, and assess performance and can also increase productivity and improve employee retention.

REFERENCES

American Nurses' Association Cabinet on Nursing Education, Counsel on Continuing Education, and Task Force on Revision of Standards for Continuing Education. 1984. "ANA's Philosophy of Continuing Education in Nursing." In *Standards for Continuing Education in Nursing.* Kansas City, Mo.: American Nurses' Association.

Matherly, Sandra, and Shannon Hodges. 1990. *Telephone Nursing: The Process.* Englewood, Co.: Center for Research in Ambulatory Health Care Administration.

O'Connor, Andrea B. 1986. *Nursing Staff Development and Continuing Education.* Boston: Little, Brown.

18

Ambulatory Care Utilization Review

Thomas Mayer, Allan Korn, and Arnold Milstein

INTRODUCTION

Utilization Review (UR) evolved in the early 1970s as a mechanism for health care payers to control inpatient hospital costs. The UR process was designed to prevent unnecessary hospital admissions, keep hospital stays as brief as possible, and encourage patients to seek medical care in less expensive outpatient settings.

Hospital UR has changed significantly over the years, growing from retrospective review and second surgical opinion programs to incorporate precertification, concurrent review, discharge planning, and catastrophic case management. The effectiveness of UR has improved as well. In the first two decades of UR, the percentage of total health care costs related to hospitalization dropped from 70 percent to approximately 50 percent. An increasing number of procedures shifted to the outpatient setting or occurred in types of facilities that did not even exist prior to the widespread application of UR techniques such as ambulatory surgery centers and free-standing psychiatric and substance abuse rehabilitation facilities.

But UR generally did not control care in outpatient settings. During this period, the total number of medical and surgical procedures performed increased even as the number of inpatient procedures declined. This lack of control over outpatient care also impacted price and intensity as well as frequency, so that a procedure performed in an outpatient setting could be even more costly than the same procedure done on an inpatient basis.

Consequently, in spite of increasing utilization controls over inpatient care, the inflation-adjusted per capita cost of health care continued to increase. It became apparent that success in cost management required instituting utilization controls over outpatient care as well. Thus in the late 1980s, the need for outpatient utilization review became recognized.

THE UNIQUE UTILIZATION CONTROL CHALLENGES OF AMBULATORY CARE

Although inpatient UR systems are well defined and can be extremely effective when appropriately implemented, they are not adequate to address the unique features of care delivered in ambulatory settings. This is due to the very different nature of inpatient and outpatient services. Inpatient UR systems are focused on high-cost services provided to a relatively small number of people within a limited number of well-defined facilities. Ambulatory care UR, however, differs from inpatient UR in each of these parameters: cost, volume, and location of service.

Cost

The difference in unit price between inpatient and outpatient services is especially significant. The unit of concern on the inpatient side is a hospital day, which has an average price that exceeds $1,000. On the other hand, the average price of an outpatient encounter (an office visit) is less than $50, plus variable amounts of laboratory and x-ray charges.

This major cost differential strongly affects the cost-benefit ratio of ambulatory care UR. The expense of programs to reduce hospitalizations and shorten lengths of stay through precertification, concurrent review, discharge planning, case management, and second surgical opinions can be easily offset by relatively small percentage reductions in costly hospital days. However, the considerably smaller price tags of ambulatory services require much greater UR-based reductions in service volume for UR to be cost justified. It makes no sense to expend $50 worth of UR activity to eliminate a $40 outpatient charge.

Volume

The average individual under age 65 has about a 10 percent probability of being hospitalized in any given year. But that same individual may well have four or five outpatient visits each year, with each visit generating additional requests for laboratory and x-ray services, prescription drugs, medical equipment and supplies, and various other ancillary services. Although outpatient claims represent only 50 percent of total health care cost, they constitute approximately 89 percent of all health care claims.

The dramatically higher volume of claims generated in the outpatient setting creates a unique challenge for UR systems. Increasing the number of UR judgments five- or tenfold would demand a tremendous administrative effort. It is unlikely that program costs would be offset by the savings.

Location of Service

Although inpatient hospital claims include a vast array of different services, each of them occurs within a hospital, and there are thus a limited number of contact points with which a UR system must coordinate for preservice UR. In contrast, outpatient claims include a vastly increased number of contact points and, accordingly, provide a much greater administrative challenge.

Inpatient UR systems have traditionally relied upon preservice and/or concurrent review activities. The administrative costs exceed $50 per review interaction. The design of cost-effective ambulatory care UR systems, on the other hand, depends upon an understanding of the wide range of $80 to $120 episodes that make up ambulatory care and that therefore require less expensive review procedures.

Communication

For any control system to be effective, patients must understand and be a part of the utilization control process. Communication materials for patients can help them develop a new understanding of their benefits and can result in a change in their expectations about the benefits obtainable from their individual medical plans.

Comprehensive medical benefit plans and their associated managed care programs often convey a sense of "entitlement" to patients, and consequently the provision of health care services is expected as a right or as the return on premium dollars. Consequently, utilization management systems may be interpreted as an infringement of patients' rights rather than as a technique for controlling costs and monitoring events that may impact the outcome of care. Educating patients about the importance of UR systems on the overall cost and quality of their health care system aligns their goals with those of the system.

A REVIEW OF UTILIZATION CONTROL METHODS FOR AMBULATORY CARE

Although the range of ambulatory health care services is wide, these services fall into eight discrete categories:

1. primary care visits
2. specialty referrals and visits
3. ambulatory surgery
4. office-based procedures

5. laboratory and x-ray procedures

6. prescription drugs

7. physical rehabilitation

8. mental health and substance abuse care

Each of these areas of service has unique characteristics that must be considered in order to develop effective utilization management systems in an outpatient setting.

Primary Care Visits

Although one of the most overlooked areas of ambulatory care, primary care visits are the stock in trade of the physicians who provide the majority of outpatient services. They include most office visits to general practitioners, family physicians, pediatricians, and general internists for common ailments such as coughs, colds, flu and fevers, earaches, back pain, sprained ankles, and headaches as well as visits for routine physical examinations.

The lack of utilization control in the outpatient setting allows primary care physicians to create their own demand for services. Routine follow-up examinations such as blood pressure checks or well-baby examinations can be recommended at any frequency that a physician chooses. Preventive care procedures such as breast examinations and Pap smears may be performed at shorter intervals than is typically considered medically necessary. In general, the frequency and intensity of patient interactions with the health care delivery system should be a function of the physiology of the patient and outcome research and not a function of individual physician preference.

One mechanism for establishing utilization control in primary care is through the use of utilization guidelines. With specific utilization guidelines to define an optimal approach for each clinical situation, an ambulatory care UR program to prevent inappropriate utilization can be implemented in a claims payment environment by using postservice, prepayment claims screens. This is necessary in an uncontrolled clinical environment and helpful even in systems that rely on primary care "gatekeepers."

Primary care gatekeeping is an approach favored by many managed care systems to control the utilization of inpatient and outpatient services. But such an approach is only as effective as the gatekeepers are in their ability to encourage limited utilization. Primary care gatekeepers directly provide a substantial portion of all outpatient services and may not be objective about appropriately managing their own care. Therefore, primary care gatekeepers should be regarded as candidates for ambulatory care utilization education and for review of their own care.

Capitation has been extensively employed, especially in gatekeeper settings, as a mechanism of controlling the utilization of resources. In a few well-managed programs, costs have been effectively controlled with this strategy. In many instances, however, physician gatekeeper behavior has not been appropriately impacted by the capitation process. For a physician to internalize the discipline necessary for successful utilization control,

1. the economic impact of poor utilization control on each physician must be apparent and sufficient to encourage compliance
2. the cause-and-effect relationship between an individual episode of care and the total plan cost must be visible
3. peer behavior must be consistent and supportive within the provider community, sending clear and persistent messages to the patient population

Most capitated gatekeeper systems currently in place fail to consistently meet these criteria.

Specialty Referrals and Visits

The use of specialists either by referral or by spontaneous visit is one of the more commonly monitored areas of ambulatory care, since it is a relatively easy component to identify and often is a source of substantial cost. Most managed care systems rely on primary care gatekeepers to control this aspect of utilization, with the gatekeeper functioning as the access point for services throughout the remaining network. In such managed care systems, if the patient is not referred to the specialist by the primary care physician, the patient's insurance plan will not cover the visit. Other managed care systems offer patients an option to self-refer to specialists, bypassing the gatekeeper function, but this is often associated with higher costs to the patient.

The gatekeeper system places the burden for controlling referrals on primary care physicians. The actual rate of referral will vary depending on the skills and experience of the gatekeeper. For this reason ob/gyn physicians do not often make satisfactory gatekeepers, even though they do act as primary care physicians. Their training has not prepared them to provide the variety of primary care services needed outside their specialty, and consequently they have very high referral rates.

Reimbursement structure is another factor determining the effectiveness of primary care gatekeepers in controlling referrals. An HMO may capitate its primary care physicians for all physician services, so that any referral represents negative income to the gatekeepers. This tends to limit even desirable referrals. A PPO, on the other hand, may pay all physicians under a discounted fee-for-service arrangement, thus offering no economic incentive for the gatekeeper to effectively manage, and thus control, referrals.

In some managed care settings, precertification is required for specialty referrals. This means that a primary care gatekeeper who wants to refer a patient to a specialist must have that clinical decision authorized by the UR system. The referral is further controlled by limiting the number of authorized visits to the specialist and by requiring that any further services, tests, or procedures that the specialist might wish to perform must also be precertified.

Regardless of the approach used, the area of specialty referrals is an important one for ambulatory care UR. The success or failure of precertification as a mechanism to control utilization is a function of how well the discipline has been internalized by all physicians in the network and how consistently the message is transmitted to patients.

A referral control system that does not take into account the patient relations and marketing aspects may also prove counterproductive. The negative effect on patient satisfaction of constant delays in treatment as various review processes occur can adversely impact reenrollment in the health plan. Utilization procedures must work smoothly, rapidly, and effectively and be virtually invisible to patients.

Ambulatory Hospital Surgery

Outpatient surgery has been one of the most common targets of ambulatory care UR, since it is an extension of inpatient services and has a high cost per incident of care. It is, therefore, amenable to control by the traditional approaches of precertification and/or second surgical opinion. Data in this area are incomplete. In an era in which virtually all surgery was performed on an inpatient basis, a UR program would capture data on almost all surgical procedures. Today, however, with up to 50 percent of all surgeries occurring on an outpatient basis, a traditional UR program would only be made aware of outpatient surgical procedures that appeared on a "second surgical opinion" list or were specially targeted for review. Consequently, universal outpatient surgery review remains an important focus for ambulatory care UR.

Office-Based Procedures

This area, which comprises an expensive and expansive array of services, has been virtually uncontrolled by existing ambulatory care UR systems. It encompasses all office-based procedures (many surgical in nature) provided by primary care and specialty physicians, including cortisone injections of joints and tendons, skin biopsies of moles and other lesions, casting of traumatic injuries, and minor surgeries like vasectomies, breast biopsies, and uterine curettage. Physical therapy and chiropractic visits as well as medical devices also fall within this area.

Until ambulatory care UR is applied to the doctor's office setting, it is not unreasonable to assume that the clinical approach used may often be the most expensive rather than the most appropriate one. However, the lack of a cost-effective method for performing UR at this level has resulted in essentially unchecked utilization of outpatient procedures. The developing research on outcomes, as well as focusing on "episodes of illness" rather than individual visits, may enhance effective control in this area.

Laboratory and X-Ray Procedures

This area is responsible for a significant component of outpatient expense, but there are very few systems in place to control utilization. It comprises a large number of procedures, with an even wider range of charges. The variation extends from several dollars for a simple blood or urine test to hundreds of dollars for sophisticated imaging procedures like computerized axial tomography (CAT) scans or magnetic resonance imaging (MRI).

Some attempts have been made to apply traditional utilization review techniques to this area. For example, some managed care systems require precertification of "big ticket" items like CAT scans or apply such a requirement to any procedure or combination of procedures that exceeds a specific price threshold. However, the bulk of the expense in outpatient care is caused by a large number of low-cost services. For these, traditional UR techniques have not been very effective. The insecurity and inexperience of newly trained physicians, as well as the fear of legal action, also contribute greatly to the overuse of these supportive procedures.

Significant additional benefit can still be attained by the implementation of effective ambulatory care UR techniques. Clinical models (e.g., "critical pathways") may be developed that link tests, procedures, and consultants to diagnoses. Such models will permit a "screening" process through which possible inappropriate patterns of care could be identified for more detailed review.

Prescription Drugs

With more managed care and insured programs covering prescription drugs, the cost of this component of ambulatory care is becoming a concern as well. In 1990, some plans reported that prescription drug costs exceeded 15 percent of medical benefits paid. As with other outpatient services, there is a wide variation in cost and virtually no guidelines for optimal therapy. This has resulted in rapidly escalating costs. Also, until recently, even prepaid plans had not put physicians at risk for pharmacy costs.

Control of this aspect of outpatient service may be aided by the introduction of a fourth party, the pharmacist. The pharmacist is a naturally occurring control point for prescription drug utilization mechanisms such as generic substitution, formularies, or limitations in dispensing lot size. Managed care systems have used generic drugs, mail-order pharmacies, and prescription card services in an attempt to gain control over utilization of prescription drugs. Success has thus far been limited. (See Chapter 22 for further discussion of the current status of these and other methods of drug utilization control.) Again, physician education and awareness of drug costs and benefits are vital to achieve control in this area.

Physical Rehabilitation

Rehabilitation following trauma, neurologic insult, or surgery is increasingly used to speed recovery and enhance the clinical potential for optimal function. Rehabilitation services may be performed on an inpatient, day-program, outpatient, or home-care basis. The challenge of UR in this environment is to ensure (1) that treatment is rendered in the most efficient setting, and (2) that the treatment procedure is a "medical necessity" as defined by the benefit plan.

Some examples may help illustrate the challenge. An athlete undergoing an orthopedic procedure is directed to a postoperative rehabilitation program by the surgeon or perhaps by the athlete's coach. Once the athlete has achieved a functional level sufficient to accommodate activities of daily living, is further therapy medically necessary or is it more properly considered athletic training?

A stroke patient, recovering well, has achieved the ability to independently accommodate activities of daily living. The patient's return to work, however, will require significant therapy directed at specific fine motor skills. Most states define such treatment as occupational rehabilitation and financially support such care. At what point, therefore, does rehabilitation cease to be medically necessary under the terms of a benefit plan? Although such treatment might continue to benefit an individual patient, the role of UR is key in defining the interface between care that is necessary under the terms of a plan and care that is desirable, but excluded from coverage.

Mental Health and Substance Abuse Care

Outpatient UR in the area of mental health care must take into account that many problems are not easily identified as medically necessary. However, if social and behavior problems are left untreated, they may soon result in severe and expensive physical illness and disability. A caring and intelligent approach will not define "medical necessity" too exactly. It will liberally allow access to the system but then shift the focus of care to family, friends, and other community resources when feasible. Community resources include some of the most successful programs (e.g., Alcoholics Anonymous) for dealing with substance abuse.

FOCUSING AMBULATORY CARE UTILIZATION REVIEW

Since such a broad range of ambulatory care services must potentially be controlled, it is useful to decide on basic targets for utilization review efforts. These targets may include cost, volume, patients, providers, and specific procedures and referrals. An elegant approach to UR would focus on episodes of care and would include a review and measurement of clinical outcomes. Current models for defining episodes of outpatient care and for measuring outcomes require substantial refinement.

Since the goal is to control cost, focusing on high-cost items would seem to be a logical approach. Some carriers have identified lists of very expensive outpatient procedures and require precertification of these procedures before accepting responsibility for payment. A recent study demonstrated a 40 percent reduction in outpatient MRI scans when a review agent asked the ordering physician, during the preprocedure review, if the result of the scan would alter the treatment plan.

High-volume, low-cost, easily obtainable tests (blood counts, urinalyses) do not lend themselves to UR given the processes and tools currently available. Such items are, at this time, best addressed by clinical protocols, practice standards, and physician education.

One focus for an ambulatory care UR system might be specific procedures and referrals that are universally observed frequently to be inappropriate. Another might be specific physicians who are observed to use health care resources less efficiently than their peers. Since providers control about 80 percent of the health care dollar (even though they only receive about 25 percent of it collectively), they are an obvious target for ambulatory care utilization controls.

An attempt may be made to upgrade utilization awareness across the entire physician population or to focus efforts on physicians whose practice patterns deviate from established norms. If the latter method is used, the involved physicians must be identified.

Aggregate utilization data for procedures and referrals can be collected by provider and plan. Incentives and disincentives can be created to reward necessary utilization and discourage inappropriate utilization. They may be applied universally or when dealing with a particular physician, specialty, or contracted entity on a focused basis. Using incentives serves as a more comprehensive approach to ambulatory utilization management. The data necessary to implement this approach are generally not available to provider organizations, although many payers have the necessary management information systems.

AMBULATORY CARE UTILIZATION REVIEW SYSTEMS

Ambulatory care UR systems now evolving must address the breadth of the delivery system for ambulatory services.

They must also recognize that the acceptable range of clinical practice is wide but that inappropriate utilization must be identified and eliminated. Furthermore, these ambulatory care UR systems must at least preserve the present level of quality while maintaining a reasonable cost-benefit ratio.

As previously discussed, the differences in the cost, frequency, and location of outpatient services in comparison with inpatient ones pose special challenges for an ambulatory care UR system. Successful ambulatory care UR combines three core ingredients: (1) precertification, (2) individual claims review, and (3) multipatient and multiphysician profiling. Although retrospective approaches such as claims review and profiling have not been effective in changing utilization behavior in the inpatient setting, they are central elements of ambulatory care UR.

Important applications of these core ingredients include

- multiphysician procedure profiling (e.g., tracking MRI scans or endoscopies)
- multipatient service profiling (e.g., frequency of extended or comprehensive visits)
- individual patient-physician profiling (e.g., concurrent care, duplicative prescriptions)

Also important in controlling ambulatory care utilization, although independent of the actual utilization review system, are the benefit design and delivery systems that create the structure within which the UR system functions. Benefit design is important, since utilization controls alone can hardly compensate for a patient who has no financial investment in the services used. Deductibles, coinsurance, and copayments are mechanisms for patient risk-sharing that directly impact the degree of medical services required.

Likewise, modifying the reimbursement systems for providers of outpatient services can affect the overall cost of those services. The resource-based relative value scale (RBRVS) being implemented for Medicare Part B reimbursement attempts to change a physician reimbursement system that rewards the use of costly diagnostic tests and procedures to one that rewards diagnostic acumen and therapeutic skill. In addition, transferring the risk of paying for medical services to physicians and hospitals through managed care techniques such as capitation provides another level of control that complements utilization review.

Precertification

A precertification requirement entails that a utilization review must occur before a service is performed. It allows a second opinion with respect to the clinical decision of an attending physician and may be applied to whatever procedures or services appear to be in need of such review. Precertification might be required prior to expensive procedures like MRI scans, referral to potentially overused specialties such as dermatology, or any diagnostic test or procedure that exceeds a specific dollar limit. Precertification may be appropriate for any outpatient surgery. Most outside UR organizations already have programs for the precertification of many (10–20) surgical procedures such as knee arthroscopy, dilatation and curettage (D & C), cataract removal, and tonsillectomy—as do many IPAs and group practices.

The typical precertification process requires the patient or provider to notify the UR organization or in-house committee before having any of the specified outpatient procedures performed. These procedures are usually listed in a patient booklet explaining the health plan benefits. Once notified, the UR organization obtains medical information from the patient or the attending physician performing the procedure.

If that information meets the UR organization's clinical criteria for the specific procedure, it is certified. If the UR organization's criteria are not met, the case may be referred to the attending physician or surgeon for further information. If the two parties cannot negotiate a treatment plan, certification is withheld pending a formalized process of appeal or a second opinion exam.

Although this precertification process is essentially identical to that used for inpatient care, it has limited application to the ambulatory care setting. Let us assume that approximately 25 percent of all dollars spent on ambulatory care arise from procedures that are expensive enough and have sufficient inherent abuse potential to warrant precertification. Even if one-third of those procedures might be felt to be medically unnecessary, only about half of this one-third could realistically be avoided by effective utilization review. Therefore, only about four percent of ambulatory care services costs could be eliminated through precertification alone. Obviously, other approaches to ambulatory care UR will be necessary if there is to be any significant impact on rapidly increasing total health care costs.

Individual Claims Review

The retrospective approaches of claims review and physician profiling are considerably less costly than prospective and concurrent review processes. Accordingly, they offer a greater opportunity for cost-effectiveness across the entire spectrum of ambulatory care services. These approaches depend heavily on data systems that track and display a variety of outpatient claims information. In addition, they require a normative data base for comparison. Again, the sophistication of this data base makes this type of claims review only suitable for outside UR organizations and payers.

Traditional claims review has focused on identifying overutilization and potential fraud and abuse problems by using claims audits that screen for inappropriate combinations of codes, upcoding (code creep), and unbundling of services (code fragmentation). Although such screening remains an essential component of claims review, newer claims screening programs search for patterns of potentially inappropriate medical services to single out those claims for closer review. The challenge for an ambulatory care UR system is to develop an outpatient claims screening program that is sufficiently specific (free of false positives) to not interfere unduly with the timely payment of most claims.

The newer claims screens embody either global or practice-specific norms ("norms" are descriptions of minimal, average, or optimal anticipated clinical behavior by diagnosis). Global norms are derived from a large data base collected from many sources and a variety of practice settings. Practice-specific norms may be derived from a specific health care practice or setting or from a broader data base. Thus, they may take into consideration regional variations and local idiosyncracies of practice style. The intensity of the review process, as well as the intensity of the desire to reach "best achievable" UR results, determines whether to use one type of norm or the other. In any case, each physician is actually compared only with true peers and along specialty lines.

Claims are accumulated per patient by diagnosis, and when the accumulated claims, through the addition of a new claim, exceed the typical pattern present in the normative data base, the new claim is considered an outlier and scrutinized more closely prior to payment. Outlier claims are more likely to be associated with inappropriate utilization than claims that conform to the norms. Therefore, this claims review system helps to focus the UR system's attention on the areas at high risk for overutilization. Closer review is necessary, however, to determine whether the outlier reflects overutilization or an atypical clinical situation. For example, the diagnosis for iron deficiency anemia may have a norm of two "limited" office visits per quarter, with a limit of seven visits per year, one of which is for a thorough physical exam. As soon as a third visit for iron deficiency anemia occurs in any three-month period (or an eighth visit occurs in a one-year period), the claim becomes an outlier and is pulled for review. Although this approach has several advantages over traditional claims screening, it also has several potential shortcomings.

If the screening criteria are rigidly applied, then the number of claims requiring review becomes excessive and the timeliness of claims payment falls. However, if the criteria are loosely applied, a significant proportion of unnecessary medical care will go undetected. The example, cited earlier, of an approach to the review of comprehensive levels of service illustrates the point. By varying the threshold of review by diagnosis and site of service, the selection of claims for individual review can be focused. Individual claim review may also be stratified such that (1) technicians may be able to pay a claim based on written, physician-derived criteria; (2) nurses may be able to resolve payment decisions based on clinical interpretation of claims information (e.g., patient age or secondary diagnosis); or (3) physician peer review would be the highest level of individual claim review and might produce one of three outcomes—pay the claim, deny or reduce the claim, or request additional medical information.

A significant concern generated by this approach is the problem created by claims denial based on inappropriate or unnecessary medical services. Since the service has already been rendered, denial of payment merely shifts the responsibility for the cost onto the patient, who generally will be billed for the outstanding balance. Although this may reduce health care costs from the third-party payers' perspective, it does little to change provider behavior. Further, it penalizes the patient, who has little control over the ambulatory care services provided. This problem, however, can be mitigated through the use of appropriate contract provisions as well as effective patient relations and education.

Physician Profiling

The physician profiling approach is much more appealing to physician providers. It has much more potential to be effective in changing physician behavior and controlling the associated costs. Physician profiling is a relatively new ambulatory care UR technique that uses both inpatient and outpatient claims data to compare the practice patterns of physicians within the same specialty. If the comparison reveals that specific physicians' patterns of practice are outside the range of the expected norms, then the UR organization can focus attention on those physicians to determine which activities account for their outlier status.

Those physicians with practice patterns on the high end of the utilization spectrum should be more closely reviewed from a utilization control perspective, whereas those on the low end should be examined from a quality control perspective. In either case, the profiles help identify physicians who are of concern, and who are likely to be good candidates for cost-effective ambulatory care UR.

Because this form of UR requires a substantial amount of data for each physician, it lends itself best to self-administration by focused networks of physicians like those found in managed care systems (e.g., a PPO or HMO network) rather than broadly dispersed, unstructured provider organizations. In order to draw adequate conclusions, it is critical that the available data are accurate, the data base is large enough to assure statistical significance of differences, and the "denominator" used is significant.

For the time being, practice profiling is limited to more generalized descriptions, such as norms that broadly describe typical practice patterns within a specialty. These norms may define the average number of visits to primary care physicians; the proportion of visits involving laboratory testing, x-rays, or surgical procedures; the typical number of referrals to be anticipated; the expected number of rechecks; or drug prescribing patterns. When the same practice patterns are evaluated for more specifically defined populations, the resulting physician profiles can be more detailed.

In the future, norms may be developed around specific diagnoses. Such a process anticipates that outpatient claims data can be specifically linked to a diagnosis. Mechanisms to do so are presently under development. A leading approach is to use ambulatory patient groups (APGs). These would be the outpatient equivalent of the DRGs used to categorize inpatient Medicare claims data.

Physician profiles developed using internally established practice-specific norms capture a wealth of information comparing individual practice patterns within particular practice settings. Practice-specific norms allow a more focused analysis of practice patterns so that primary care physicians can be meaningfully compared by the number of referrals, by specialty, or by the dollars spent per patient or per visit on laboratory tests, x-rays, or office procedures.

The precision with which such differences in practice patterns define poor utilization practices depends upon the ability to risk-adjust the patient data. Patients, after all, have a certain level of clinical need relative to their diagnosis. A diet-controlled diabetic will have less need for medical services or procedures than a blind, azotemic, insulin-dependent patient. Each patient's claim form, however, may indicate only a diagnosis of diabetes.

At present, risk-adjusted outcome measurements are available through several computerized systems but are applicable only to inpatient care. The future, however, holds great promise for the application of this technology in the outpatient environment. A search into the claims history, for example, for evidence of care by a nephrologist or ophthalmologist for other than an annual routine exam would differentiate the diabetic at high risk from the one at low risk. Specialists could be profiled by the cost of a referral or by the number of visits per referral.

Once typical physician practice patterns are reliably established, they can be used in a variety of ways to modify physician behavior and improve outpatient utilization. At a minimum, practice profiles are provided to attending physicians and consultants as educational tools to modify outlier behavior. Often, that alone is effective in bringing physician practices within achievable, acceptable norms. In addition, incentives can be developed to reward the physicians with efficient practice profiles while disincentives can be used to discourage the outliers. In network settings, physician profiling may be used to eliminate those doctors who are consistently outside the norms without clinical justification.

This retrospective analytic information has other useful applications as well. The pattern of specialist referrals suggests which specialties to recruit for the network or where to target continuing medical education for the primary care physicians. The clinical efficiency and cost-effectiveness of specialists identifies with whom to contract within the managed care program as well as whom to consider for disenrollment from the network. Finally, the cost per visit, visits per physician, and visits per patient can all be factored into the budgeting of future health care costs in order to set realistic capitation levels and thus determine premiums.

At present, the only substantial evidence that physician profiling can be effective in changing physician behavior comes from HMOs that have implemented such systems to manage their risk better. Eventually physician profiling may prove to be the most effective form of ambulatory care UR, for it deals with the basis of the inefficiency: physician practice behavior.

CONCLUSION

The importance of ambulatory care utilization review for the control of health care costs has become increasingly apparent as more services are shifted into the outpatient setting. Furthermore, inpatient-style preservice UR systems are often not applicable to the unique demands of the ambulatory setting.

In order to control utilization in all areas of ambulatory clinical activity, an ambulatory care UR system must consider

- the breadth of the delivery system
- the range of acceptable clinical treatment
- the degree of inappropriate treatment being provided
- the access points available for implementing changes in utilization behavior

Finally, ambulatory care UR not only must maintain quality within the outpatient setting but must also operate in a cost-effective manner so that savings from the system exceed its administrative costs. Although eventual savings from outpatient UR may approach 5 to 8 percent of total health care costs, ambulatory care utilization review still has a lengthy process of development before achieving its potential.

19

Clinical Guidelines for Ambulatory Care

Jeffrey V. Winston

INTRODUCTION

Clinical practice guidelines may be defined as standardized descriptions of care, developed by consensus, that incorporate the best scientific evidence of effectiveness and are consistent with expert opinion. They are written standards that suggest how individual physicians should evaluate, test, and treat patients for a variety of clinical indications. Evidence indicates that the quality and consistency of ambulatory health care may be increased, and costs reduced, by the use of clinical practice guidelines. It is probably also in the interest of managed care providers to design and implement workable, cost-effective clinical guidelines before the government or the insurance industry imposes them by default. Finally, the public will ultimately benefit if clinical guidelines help prevent overutilization of valuable health care resources.

Spiraling health care costs have led to a period of fiscal constraints. Over the past several years, the previously uncontrolled allocation of health care resources has been questioned by state agencies, Medicare, and private insurance companies. In one effort to curb health care costs, many state governments restricted the ability of hospitals to acquire CT scanners and other high-cost items. Medicare required increasingly stringent justification for hospital services. Medicare then developed a prospective payment system based on DRGs in an effort to force hospitals to accept some of the financial risk in health care. Similar constraints and regulations are now being imposed on the ambulatory sector.

In this restrictive atmosphere, clinicians are under increasing pressure to provide high-quality health care at a lower cost. Medicare is developing health care guidelines and a relative value payment system for determining reasonable reimbursements to physicians. American business, which pays for employee health care through private health insurance as well as taxation, is demanding a greater role in determining both the quality and cost of health care. Government and industry have begun to demand that providers of outpatient care document clinical outcomes, reduce employee time off, and contain costs. The American

Medical Association is working with the Rand Corporation to develop guidelines for a more effective utilization of common medical procedures. In a study published in 1989, for instance, Robert Brook, professor of medicine and public health at UCLA and deputy director of Rand Corporation's health program, found that 30 percent of coronary angiographies were inappropriate. Professional organizations such as the American College of Physicians are debating their role in developing guidelines for their member physicians. The thrust of much of this activity is ultimately to reduce cost by reimbursing on the basis of treatment outcomes as well as to provide incentives for superior performance in the provision of care.

Clinical practice guidelines based on sound clinical data should enable physicians to avoid expensive, low-yield tests and instead perform only those studies that might be needed to confirm a suspected diagnosis. In training, physicians are taught to order many tests in order to learn the utmost about the patient, with little thought given to the cost or the logical sequencing of those studies, and these habits are carried forward into practice. The attempt to please patients and the fear of litigation are further motivators for excessive patient workups. David Tennenbaum (1989) of Blue Cross examined guidelines for common diagnostic tests and observed, "The practice of performing every test possible, whether guided by unrealistic patient expectations or fear of malpractice suits, threatens to make health care unaffordable."

Clinical practice guidelines also have the potential to increase the quality of health care by making the practice of medicine more consistent. As a general rule, patients with advanced disease require more expensive therapy than patients in the early stages of the same illness. Mass cancer screening imposes great costs but may pay for itself by reducing the number of patients presenting with advanced disease. Decisions to impose mass screening for cancer are difficult for an individual physician to make. But a group of physicians may reach a clear consensus after objectively reviewing the literature and/or a screening procedure for cancer. Daniel McLaughlin, administrator of the Hennepin County Medical Center in Minneapolis, noted a 30 percent decrease in colon rectal surgery after guidelines for endoscopy were implemented (Koska 1990).

In a time of increasing technological complexity, with new diagnostic and treatment tools introduced regularly, it is difficult for physicians always to be fully informed. Individual physicians may not be able to assess accurately the point at which a new technology increases a patient's lifespan or improves his or her quality of life. Guidelines, updated in a timely fashion, can also serve to help manage these problems.

This chapter explains the process of designing and implementing clinical practice guidelines. It shows how guidelines fit into a managed care environment and then considers the legal issues. It shows how a group of clinicians may develop and continually refine guidelines. Finally, it outlines the components of good clinical practice guidelines and presents specific examples of both clinical practice and workup guidelines in use today.

MANAGED CARE

The applications of practice guidelines differ between third-party payers and providers. Third-party payers desire guidelines to allow nonpayment for nonindicated procedures. In a managed care group, clinicians will utilize guidelines to ensure the quality and consistency of medical care and to restrict unnecessary procedures. In fact, the prepaid managed care setting is ideal for utilizing clinical guidelines. An efficient managed health care system mandates the creation and implementation of a thoughtful general plan covering all the basic aspects of patient care.

Some progressive hospitals already have inpatient guidelines (sometimes called "critical paths") analogous to outpatient clinical guidelines. Critical paths are similar to standard orders or standing guidelines for a particular problem signed by physicians in advance for the entire period of hospitalization. They allow nurses the flexibility to move patients from step to step as tolerated without waiting for specific physician intervention at each stage. This system provides a consistent care plan that is understood by the entire health care team, and it often allows earlier patient discharge.

Successful managed care groups are ideally suited to develop and implement ambulatory clinical practice guidelines, because they have superior organization and discipline compared to individual practicing physicians. They also have more incentive to control costs. In fee-for-service systems, on the contrary, physicians quickly learn that the more tests they order, the greater their income. Physicians working without supervision in this environment receive no criticism for ordering excessive tests or performing unnecessary procedures. Many do not know at precisely what point an evaluation is adequate. Often, a physician finds it is easier to order additional tests than to admit to the patient that there are no other tests to do. In prepaid managed care settings, physicians are generally not financially motivated to overutilize tests and procedures.

Generally speaking, good guidelines should include documentation of medical history and a recommended pertinent physical examination. Explicit directions for appropriate laboratory and radiology tests must be included in the guidelines. A stepwise approach to treatment and required follow-up of the patient must also be present. Physicians outside the managed care environment find these steps onerous intrusions into their practice and denigrate them using terms like "cookbook medicine." But prepaid managed care groups, with compensation based on salary and cost reduction, can achieve physician acceptance of the premise of clinical guidelines, often without resorting to disciplinary measures.

LEGAL ISSUES

Fear of litigation is a major reason for ordering excessive studies. Physicians fear missing a diagnosis and not meeting the legal standard of care. "Standard of care in the community" is a term widely used by the legal profession, although physicians are now held to national standards rather than community standards. In terms of the law, this phrase is quite restrictive and implies negligence and malpractice if certain standards are not followed explicitly. Malpractice defense attorneys prefer the term "practice guidelines," which implies suggested rather than mandatory rules of care. Current standards of care define only minimum care, not excessive care.

Fear that clinical practice guidelines will increase liability in a malpractice case should not be a major concern. Practice guidelines could be used as evidence in a malpractice case but would be of marginal value compared to expert testimony, authoritative medical textbooks, and medical journals. Clinical practice guidelines might corroborate the experts' testimony but would not justify a lawsuit by themselves.

In fact, there is evidence that good practice guidelines improve both patient care and documentation and therefore decrease the number of legitimate malpractice suits. As an example of this, guidelines adopted by the American Society of Anesthesiology have improved monitoring during anesthesia. Guidelines for anesthesiologists have dramatically reduced the number of malpractice cases, which has resulted in significant reductions in malpractice insurance costs. When clinical practice guidelines are followed and quality care is given, the guidelines may actually assist in defending against a malpractice suit based on a bad outcome. Many malpractice defense attorneys believe that the benefits of good practice guidelines far outweigh any potential liability.

A further advantage of clinical guidelines in the legal context is their enhancement of documentation. Because of time constraints, many clinicians rush through paper documentation of their findings. Although a physician cannot be expected to write by hand all the details of an examination, documentation is nonetheless crucial, especially when the patient is seen by others in the same group practice. Practice guidelines can specify the important and pertinent positives and negatives requiring documentation. Many parts of the history, for example, can be elicited by a well-trained medical assistant when guidelines are in place. Proper documentation also helps to avoid duplication of tests and provides an excellent malpractice defense.

MONITORING OUTCOMES AND COMPLIANCE

Even in a good managed care system, it is difficult to monitor the quality and efficiency of physicians objectively. Physicians who order excessive tests or see patients more tend to rationalize by claiming they deal with more difficult patient care problems. But the study of patient outcomes using clinical practice guidelines allows continued feedback to physicians as well as continual improvements in the guidelines, and hence it potentially increases the real productivity of the group.

Once a practice guideline is implemented, it becomes possible to monitor patient outcomes. If there are too many poor patient outcomes, then the practice guideline can be modified. Perhaps additional studies or earlier referral to specialists can be added to the guideline. If certain laboratory tests are found to have no influence on patient care or outcomes, they can be deleted. With outcome data, the managed care group can objectively measure physicians' compliance with the guideline. Thus, the implementation of clinical practice guidelines should improve productivity, decrease overutilization of laboratory and other ancillary procedures, and improve patient outcomes.

WORKUP GUIDELINES

Guidelines, for practical purposes, can be classified as either workup guidelines or treatment guidelines. Clinical practice guidelines may be developed for any specific diagnosis, but often a patient presents with a list of complaints and symptoms and with no clear diagnosis. This type of presentation is dealt with by using workup guidelines.

Workup guidelines may be developed to suggest how to proceed logically with diagnostic tests and how to implement interim therapy. They should list the most likely diagnoses and indicate how to select the correct one based on the history, the physical, laboratory tests, or the response to initial therapy. When the diagnosis is clear, the clinician can then follow the appropriate treatment practice guideline. Physicians cannot be expected to perform a complete physical examination every time a patient visits the office. The examination needs to be directed to the patient's complaint, although the physician must be careful not to miss other important clinical clues. Practice guidelines can specify which parts of the examination are necessary, increasing productivity by saving the physician time.

Workup guidelines require a plan or outline to reach the correct diagnosis efficiently with the minimal number of visits and the least testing. Sometimes a panel of inexpensive tests is most expedient; at other times, tests may be too expensive and even hazardous and should be done only when the less expensive and safer studies are abnormal. Intelligent laboratory panels can be developed that involve drawing blood only once, with indicated tests performed as needed in a logical fashion. While awaiting test results, it is sometimes useful to begin interim therapy, which may provide a therapeutic trial or provide symptomatic relief. The result of this trial of therapy can then be used in the process of determining the diagnosis.

For complicated workup guidelines, a branching flow chart is helpful. Evaluation of thyroid nodules, for instance, has become a complicated process that may require multiple laboratory tests and procedures. Instead of ordering all possibly needed laboratory tests, workup guidelines would allow a few tests to be performed based on the history and physical examination. After the results are received, more expensive or invasive tests, such as needle biopsy, could be performed if necessary.

GUIDELINE DEVELOPMENT

Clinical guidelines can be extremely simple or extremely complex. At the University of Wales, for example, data indicated a wide variation in the number of follow-up visits and tests ordered by specialists (Hall et al. 1988). This simple set of guidelines proved effective in reducing the number of follow-up visits and eliminating unneeded laboratory tests:

- New patients should be seen only once and then referred to the primary doctor.
- Follow-up appointments should only be made
  —if there is diagnostic uncertainty
  —for purposes of monitoring a complex disease
  —if there is a serious disease requiring further investigation and treatment by a specialist
- Follow-up appointment should not be made for lab results.
- The referring physician should be called or written.
- Diagnostic tests should be ordered only if the results will change patient care.

Dr. Lawrence K. Gottlieb, director of the Clinical Guideline Program at the Harvard Community Health Plan (HCHP), has formalized the process of designing and implementing clinical practice guidelines. This process is called the Algorithm Based Clinical Quality Improvement Process (ABCQIP). The stated goal of the program is

> to improve the ability of clinicians to provide medical care to HCHP patients that is consistently of the highest quality by: (1) developing, disseminating, and continually updating uniform, state-of-the-art guidelines for the optimal cost-effective evaluation and management of important clinical problems; and (2) incorporating the guidelines into clinicians' daily practice routine in a manner that facilitates, rather than complicates practice management. (Gottlieb et al. 1990)

The development of effective practice guidelines can be broken down into five general stages:

1. project planning
2. consensus algorithm development
3. algorithm review
4. implementation
5. auditing, review, and revision

Project Planning

Initially, a planning process is required to select not only the clinical areas suitable for guideline development but also the personnel and methods to be used in developing a consensus. A list of the most common diagnoses identified by the number of patient visits is a good starting point. Diagnoses in which there is great variation in workup or treatment patterns will produce useful practice guidelines. The list of areas selected can be prioritized before study groups are formed and topics assigned.

After a review of the relevant literature, the assigned study group identifies the key points to be considered and possible areas of disagreement. Algorithms can then be written as flow diagrams. These may be simple or complex but should be as concise as possible. Editors of the guidelines should check for conformity, spelling, conciseness, and clarity. The initial results should be reviewed by the physicians who will follow the guidelines and should be modified using their suggestions. For legal purposes, the completed guidelines should be carefully documented in a manual as to source and authority.

Guidelines are most effective when medical jargon is held to a minimum. Medical history questions, for example, can be designed so that they may be asked by a medical assistant. Input from pathologists, radiologists, and operations and accounting personnel is also valuable in determining the lowest-cost options consistent with good patient care. Guidelines should be designed so that peer review audits can be done by nonmedical personnel. For example, they could be listed on a computer spreadsheet that allowed results of audits to be tallied on the right side of the page.

Consensus Algorithm Development

In developing consensus algorithms, factors pertaining to the demographics and illness patterns of the particular patient population must be considered.

Physicians who will use the guidelines should have the opportunity to review them early in the process because of their past experience dealing with the particular patient group.

When reviewing the literature, the possible bias of the authors should be considered. For example, some cancer-screening recommendations by the American Cancer Society may be excessive, since their focus is on one particular disease process. Screening tests that are not sensitive and specific are not helpful for mass screening. The ethnicity and geography of the patient population should also be taken into account, as some groups are at higher risk for some clinical conditions than others. Cancer screening should be more aggressive for the cancers of higher incidence. When early diagnosis significantly improves prognosis, as in breast cancer, more aggressive screening provides better patient care and will be more cost-effective. Screening for untreatable disease does not improve patient care. In addition to the cost-benefit ratio of tests, the cost of follow-up studies when false positives occur needs also to be considered. Tests that do not affect medical care should not be performed.

Among other important considerations is the effect of clinical practice guidelines on physician-patient relations. The expectation of patients to be given antibiotics for viral syndromes, for example, may make it too consuming to adhere to the guideline. In this case, these expectations may make it cost-effective to dispense clinically unnecessary antibiotics.

Algorithm Review

The review process should ensure that the chosen paths are based on documented history, physical examination, or laboratory tests. Expensive and potentially risky procedures should have indications that can be easily audited. A quality assessment committee must review the guidelines before distribution to determine if they are specific, well documented, and easily audited. This committee needs to look at the guidelines from an auditor's point of view. Audit scoring and criteria can be developed concurrently. Successful outcomes need to be defined. The guidelines should also be edited to ensure they are stylistically consistent with other guidelines.

Implementation

Some physicians initially react to the idea of clinical practice guidelines with anxiety and reluctance. Education and the utilization of input from those physicians who will be using the guidelines are important keys in calming fears. Physicians should learn to appreciate the importance of clinical practice guidelines to the group instead of continuing to feel that guidelines are basically punitive. Department meetings at which new guidelines are presented should include scheduled time for answering physician questions. Data from compliance studies on each guideline should be presented to the physicians. This provides them with feedback on how they can improve their compliance.

A study of adherence to practice standards in a community hospital oncology program showed that even the participation of physicians in the development of guidelines did not automatically guarantee compliance. For instance, compliance was only 33 percent for staging of breast cancer. Younger physicians were somewhat more compliant with guidelines, probably because they learned the appropriate care in their residency. Also, physicians in a managed care group are generally better able to achieve compliance than individualistic fee-for-service providers.

The most convenient method of distributing clinical practice guidelines to physicians is to put them in a loose-leaf notebook, which can be easily updated. When patients call for appointments, trained personnel can identify which workup guideline is appropriate. A longer appointment time may be reserved for certain clinical practice guidelines. The specific guideline form can be attached to the patient medical record prior to the patient's meeting with the physician. If records are computerized, the appropriate practice guideline form can be displayed on the monitor.

Auditing, Review, and Revision

A system of continuous quality improvement is a necessity for workable clinical guidelines.

Clinical practice guidelines must not be regarded as static but should be allowed to evolve. After an initial guideline is developed and implemented, compliance and patient outcomes must be measured and used as tools for further refinements. Based on these results, guidelines can be reevaluated and modified in order to improve patient outcomes. Laboratory and x-ray tests and medication regimens that do not contribute to patient care can be eliminated.

COMPONENTS OF PRACTICE GUIDELINES

There are a number of important components in constructing good clinical practice guidelines. These components may be logically arranged as follows:

1. history
2. physical

3. laboratory and radiology
4. differential diagnosis
5. therapy
6. patient education
7. expected outcome
8. follow-up
9. indications for referral

History

A medical history is necessary for each problem and must be documented to establish legal proof that appropriate questions were asked. These inquiries may be written so they can be asked and documented by a medical assistant, saving the physician valuable time and increasing productivity.

Physical

The components of the physical examination should be directed to the patient's complaint and history. Cues should be established so that clinically or legally important parts of the physical exam are not forgotten. As an example, a test of vision must be recorded for any patient with any eye injury.

Laboratory and Radiology

For both practice and workup guidelines, indications for ordering laboratory and radiologic tests must be developed. The input of radiologists and pathologists, plus a review of the literature, can help determine which tests improve patient outcomes and are cost-effective. National health organizations such as the American Cancer Society and the Canadian Task Force Study have developed guidelines for routine health exams such as Pap smears, mammograms, and rectal examinations. Interestingly, far fewer routine physical examinations, chest x-rays, and blood chemistry tests are recommended by these organizations than are now advised by most physicians.

Differential Diagnosis and Therapy

In many cases, treatment guidelines should include therapeutic trials and time to allow healing before the ordering of laboratory tests, radiologic studies, or imaging procedures. Observation of viral syndromes is appropriate before ordering tests for mononucleosis or Epstein-Barr virus. After an appropriate physical examination, low back pain should be treated conservatively before ordering lumbar x-rays or magnetic resonance imaging (MRI).

When medication is required, the least expensive and most effective drugs should be used first. An alternative should be listed if the primary drug is not tolerated or proves ineffective. The antibiotic selected should be the one expected to kill the most likely involved organisms at the lowest cost and with the least side effects. Sometimes a medication may be expensive but still be cost-effective because it has fewer side effects or because fewer visits are needed to monitor its performance.

Patient Education

Since extensive discussions by the physician are time consuming, practice and workup guidelines should recommend how much information should be given to the patient. Important information to share with the patient should be listed and documented. Patient information brochures or videotapes can be used as well as instructions from nonphysician staff. Guidelines should also indicate a back-to-work interval as well as provide instructions regarding activity or diet restrictions. If a follow-up visit is not recommended in a guideline, the patient needs to be warned when to return if symptoms worsen or do not improve. When emergency care for a problem may be required, pertinent warning signs should be given to the patient.

Expected Outcome

Practice guidelines should define desirable outcomes and undesirable outcomes. Physicians, patients, and quality assurance personnel need to be informed of expected outcomes and risks. Informing a patient with viral conjunctivitis that recovery will be complete in three weeks prepares the patient to await that outcome and prevents an unnecessary return visit. If symptoms persist longer than three weeks, then the patient should understand that the original diagnosis may need to be reconsidered. Goals of therapy can also be defined in the guideline. In the guidelines for hypertension shown in Exhibit 19-1, the stated goal is to reduce the diastolic pressure below 90.

Follow-Up

Follow-up of patients varies tremendously between clinicians. In a large group practice, stable hypertensive patients may be seen as often as once a month or as seldom as once a year. Unnecessarily frequent follow-up visits are costly for a managed care group as well as for the employee and employer. When a physician's schedule is filled with recheck appointments, there is no room for patients with urgent new problems. Certain aspects of follow-up may be done by a physician's assistant or nurse practitioner, and this may be designated in the guideline.

Indications for Referral

Certain aspects of the history or the physical may indicate the need to refer the patient to a specialist. Practice guidelines should stipulate when the referral should be immediate, urgent, or routine. Timely referral is essential to good patient care. Clinical practice guidelines should specify which specialist should be seen first. In some groups stroke patients are evaluated by an internist and in other groups by a neurologist. The referral depends on the availability and skills of the specialists. Clinical practice guidelines should refer to the specialist most likely to reach a diagnosis and avoid referral to the other specialists.

Sample Workup Guidelines for Hypertension

In Exhibit 19-1, the first section is devoted to the patient history. The questions included there are designed for a family practitioner. A longer list of pertinent negatives may be required for a specialist. The "Frequency" column on the right informs the physician how often the particular question should be asked and documented. Some important items in the history that are more likely to change between visits may be asked at every visit (they can be marked *EV*). Most historical questions need to be documented on the chart only once.

Section II, the physical, lists items that must be checked during the physical examination. Again, some parts should be done every visit, some just once, and others on an annual basis. Findings that may change the diagnosis or management should be listed specifically.

Section III deals with laboratory tests, which tend to be overutilized. Some screening tests may be appropriate for anyone who meets the criteria for the practice guidelines. Other laboratory tests should only be done if indicated by the history or physical examination.

Expensive laboratory tests should only be indicated after less expensive screening tests are done first. Invasive laboratory tests should only be performed after referral to a specialist.

Section IV, the differential diagnosis, is provided as a reminder to the physician. The corresponding CPT code is written in the adjacent column. Not

Exhibit 19-1 Workup Guidelines for Hypertension

	Primary Type	Specialist Type	Frequency
I. History			
1. Blood pressure on 3 visits	R	R	O
2. Family history	R	R	O
3. History of hypertension	R	R	O
4. Exercise, diet, smoking	R	R	O
5. Past history of medications/side effects	R	R	O
II. Physical			
1. Weight	R	R	EV
2. Heart, lungs	R	R	EV
3. Funduscopic exam	R	R	1Y
4. Blood pressure and pulse, both arms	R	R	O
5. Height	R	R	O
6. Peripheral pulses	R	R	O
7. Abdominal masses, bruits	R	R	O
8. Thyroid	R	R	O
III. Laboratory Tests			
1. Electrolytes, BUN, creatinine 80004/ 84540/82565	R		O
2. Cholesterol 82465	R		O
3. Hemoglobin/hematocrit	R		O
4. Urinalysis 81000	R		O
5. Electrolytes if on diuretics as follow-up 80004	R	R	1Y
6. EKG (40 yrs of history coronary artery disease) 93000 & 99090	I		O
7. Uric acid (if history of renal insufficiency, gout) 84560	I		O
IV. Differential Diagnosis			
1. Essential hypertension	401		
2. Cushing's disease	255		
3. Renal artery stenosis	440.1		
4. Borderline hypertension	401.1		
V. Therapy			
1. Begin with the following as indicated:	R		O
A. Exercise			
B. Weight reduction			
C. Salt reduction			
D. Alcohol reduction			
E. Smoking cessation			

2. Stepwise (4 classes of drugs)—use 1 drug of one class; if not successful, increase dosage or add a drug from another class
A. ACE inhibitors
B. Calcium channel blockers
C. Diuretic
D. Beta blocker

continued

Exhibit 19-1 continued

	Primary Type	Specialist Type	Frequency
VI. Patient Education			
1. Stop smoking on own and/or smoking cessation class	I		
2. Low sodium diet	I		
3. Exercise program	I		O
4. Stress reduction classes	I		
5. Weight reduction	I		
VII. Expected Outcome			
1. Diastolic 90 or lower within 2 months			
2. Systolic 140 or lower within 2 months			
VIII. Follow-Up for Patient on Drug Therapy			
1. Diastolic 90—6 months			
2. Diastolic 90–104—2 months			
3. Diastolic 105–114—2 weeks			
4. Diastolic 115–129—2–3 days			
5. Diastolic 130—referral			
IX. Indications for Referral			
1. Diastolic 130			
2. Any hypertensive crisis (chest pain, pulmonary congestion, papilledema, encephalopathy, eclampsia)			
3. Not controlled with 3 or 4 drugs			
4. Refer back to family practice when BP stabilized			I
Type			
First visit	F		
Recommended	R		
Do not do test	N		
When indicated	I		
Frequency			
Every visit	EV		
Once in chart is adequate	O		
Every x days	XD		
Every x weeks	XW		
Every x months	XM		
Every x years	XY		

considering the possibility of certain diagnoses is the most common cause of an incorrect diagnosis.

In Section V, therapy, the life-style changes at the top of the list are often very effective therapeutically, as they have minimum risk and can dramatically improve the health of the patient. On the other hand, medications should only be recommended after considering their cost and chance of success. Therefore, a stepwise approach to treatment with drugs is presented. Second- and third-line drugs should be listed if there are drug allergies or first-line medications fail.

Section VI reminds the physician to educate the patient about the disease and its treatment. Many physicians and groups have written their own time-saving instruction forms or have purchased published information sheets. Standardized forms contain more information than physicians can convey and should be used routinely when available.

Section VII defines and quantifies the expected outcomes and treatment goals. It is important that both the patient and physician are aware of the anticipated time for recovery. If no improvement occurs by the expected time, the patient should return for evaluation. From time to time, the physician may need to reconsider other items in the differential diagnosis. This section is also important because it allows quality assurance committees to measure treatment outcomes and to evaluate the success of the clinical practice guidelines.

As noted before, the timing of follow-up visits often varies widely between physicians. A consistent interval should be selected for the guidelines. In Section VIII of the hypertension guidelines, the follow-up time interval is determined by the diastolic blood pressure reading. More frequent follow-up is required for the uncontrolled patient.

The final section outlines the indications for referral to a specialist. In this example, referrals are made for very high diastolic blood pressures or a sudden increase in pressure that requires urgent treatment and possible hospitalization. Because hypertensive patients can develop complications rapidly, they should perhaps be under the care of an internist. After control is achieved by the internist, the patients may be referred back to the primary care provider. Although primary care providers vary in their abilities to handle more difficult cases, all should have clinical guidelines for referral.

Sample Practice Guidelines for Diabetes

Clinical practice guidelines for diabetes are shown in Exhibit 19-2. The guidelines in the first two sections, the medical history and physical examination, are similar to workup guidelines, except that some items must be documented only once whereas items such as weight loss should be documented on every visit. A detailed neurologic examination is to be done once a year (indicated by "1Y"), with the specific items of concern.

The frequency of routine blood tests for diabetes is listed in Section III. Blood sugar tests must be done consistently for all diabetes patients by all physicians. Note that home glucose monitoring by the patients on insulin is required by this guideline. The differential diagnosis in Section IV directs the physician to look for potential complications of diabetes such as urinary tract infections. The remaining sections concern chronic care and follow-up.

Exhibit 19-2 Practice Guidelines for Diabetes—Adult Onset

	Primary Type	Specialist Type	Frequency
I. History			
1. Weight loss	R	R	EV
2. Polyuria	R	R	O
3. Polydipsia	R	R	O
4. Polyphagia	R	R	O
5. History of recurrent infection	R	R	O
6. Family history of diabetes	R	R	O
7. History of visual problems	R	R	1Y
8. History of paresthesia	R	R	1Y
II. Physical			
1. Weight	R		EV
2. Blood pressure	R		EV
3. Funduscopic exam (hemorrhages or exudates, A/V ratio)	R		1Y
4. Presence and strength of pulses in feet	R		1Y
5. Examination of feet (color, ulcers, coldness)	R		1Y
6. Neurosensory examination (peripheral neuropathy)	R		1Y
7. State of dehydration	*		1Y
8. Tachypnea (respiratory rate)	*		
III. Laboratory			
1. Urinalysis (dipstick) 81000	R		1Y
2. Fasting blood sugar till stable 82948	R		1M
3. Fasting triglyceride, cholesterol 84478/ 82465	R		1Y
4. BUN, creatinine 84540/82565	R		1Y
5. HGB A1C (Q 4–6 months, NOT essential if controlled) 83036	I		4–6 M
6. Glucometer purchase for patients on insulin	R		
IV. Differential Diagnosis			
1. Urinary tract infection	599		
2. Diabetes insipidus	253.5		
3. Incontinence	788.3		
V. Therapy			
1. ADA diet and weight reduction initially 90699	R	R	EV
2. Oral hypoglycemic agents if dietary measures fail	I	I	
3. Insulin if oral hypoglycemics fail	I	I	
VI. Patient Education			
1. Foot and skin care	R		
2. Dietary consultation	R		
3. Glucometer instruction	I		

continued

Exhibit 19-2 continued

	Primary Type	Specialist Type	Frequency
VII. Expected Outcome			
1. Normalization of plasma glucose (FBS 120)	R		EV
2. Treatment of complications (e.g., laser therapy for retinopathy, revascularization for arterial occlusive disease, etc.)	I		
VIII. Follow-Up			
1. Blood glucose monthly until level normalized	R	R	1M
2. Routine blood glucose when stable	R	R	4M
3. HGB A1C when indicated	I	I	4–6 M
IX. Indications for Referral			
1. Routine diabetic education referral	R*		
2. Routine diabetic eye exam referral and following after diabetes x 7 years	R		1Y
3. I.M. referral if diabetes not well controlled	I		
4. Vascular surgery referral if severe peripheral vascular occlusive disease	I		
Type			
First visit	F		
Recommended	R		
Do not do test	N		
When indicated	I		
Frequency			
Every visit	EV		
Once in chart is adequate	O		
Every x days	XD		
Every x weeks	XW		
Every x months	XM		
Every x years	XY		

CURRENT STATUS OF PRACTICE GUIDELINES

A recent study of eight prominent group practices in the process of developing clinical practice guidelines showed that the development and implementation of practice guidelines is still in its infancy. Guidelines too often lack specific goals. "Improving health care," for instance, is not a specific goal. A more specific goal would be a "10 percent reduction in laboratory expenses without decreasing successful patient outcomes." Developing effective practice guidelines involves a review of the literature, consultation with outside experts, and practical input from experienced physicians who will use the guidelines.

Reliance on outside experts alone for guidelines may not produce the best results. Outside experts cannot take into account the organization's unique characteristics and the particular patient demographics. Many groups, moreover, lack the resources or will to implement guidelines effectively. Many disseminate the necessary information but fail to provide incentives for compliance.

Systems that evaluate outcomes under clinical practice guidelines are also still rudimentary. Certainly, a major commitment of resources is required. A large staff of chart reviewers or computer-automated records is critical for the quality improvement cycle. Some methodology for identifying consistent episodes of illness and measuring recovery may also be required for meaningful outcomes data.

Although the benefits have yet to be completely proven, the implementation of clinical practice guidelines should increase the consistency of patient care. Guidelines can be expected to enable physicians to deliver a higher quality of ambulatory care at a reduced cost.

REFERENCES

Gottlieb, L.K., Margolis, C.Z., and Schoenbaum, S.C. 1990. "Clinical Practice Guidelines at an HMO: Development and Implementation in a Quality Improvement Model." *Quality Review Bulletin* 16(2): 80–86.

Hall, R., Roberts, C.J., Coles, G.A., Fisher, D.J., Fowkes, F.G.R., Jones, J.H., Kilpatrick, G.S., Lazarus, J.J., Scanlon, M.F., and Thomas, J.P. 1988. "The Impact of Guidelines in Clinical Outpatient Practice." *Journal of the Royal College of Physicians of London* 22(4): 244–47.

Koska, M.T. 1990. "Will Clinical Care Guidelines Cut Costs in MN?" *Hospitals* 64(7): 54.

Tennenbaum, D. 1989. "Blue Cross and Blue Shield Association's Perspective on the Common Diagnostic Testing Guidelines." *Journal of General Internal Medicine* 4(6): 551–52.

BIBLIOGRAPHY

Audet, A.M., Greenfield, S.G., and Field, M. 1990. "Medical Practice Guidelines: Current Activities and Future Directions." *Annals of Internal Medicine* 113(9): 709–14.

Brook, R.H. 1989. "Practice Guidelines and Practicing Medicine: Are They Compatible?" *JAMA* 262: 3027–30.

Denolin, H., Feruglio, G.A., Gobbato, F., and Maisano, G. 1988. "Guidelines for Return to Work after Myocardial Infarction and/or Revascularisation." *European Heart Journal* 9 (Supplement L): 130–31.

Ford, L.G., Hunter, C.P., Diehr, P., Frelick, R.W., and Yates, J. 1987. "Effects of Patient Management Guidelines on Physician Practice Patterns: The Community Hospital Oncology Program Experience." *Journal of Clinical Oncology* 24(3): 504–11.

Leape, L.L. 1990. "Practice Guidelines and Standards: An Overview." *Quality Review Bulletin* 16, no. 2: 42–49.

McGuire, L.B. 1990. "A Long Run for a Short Jump: Understanding Clinical Guidelines. *Annals of Internal Medicine* 113(9): 705–08.

Robinson, M.L. 1988. "Medical Practice Guidelines May Affect Payment." *Hospitals* 62(22): 30–31.

Shewhart, W.A. 1931. *Economic Control of Quality of a Manufactured Product.* New York: Van Nostrand Reinhold.

Shortell, S.M., and McNerney, W.J. 1990. "Criteria and Guidelines for Reforming the U.S. Health Care System." *New England Journal of Medicine* 322(7): 463–67.

20

Health Information Management: The Medical Record

Nicolet A. Handy

INTRODUCTION

Quality, legal, and regulatory interests in the past few decades have compelled the ambulatory health care organizations to establish and maintain excellent medical record management systems. Record management, largely ignored in the medical practices of the past, has had to quickly come of age. It has had to establish systems to compile and track vast amounts of administrative and clinical data and make them available rapidly and accurately to all those with a legitimate interest in them. A quality medical records management system must not only provide support to clinical practitioners in the form of efficient data retrieval but must also make data available for analysis and for legal defense in the advent of professional liability suits.

No doubt, medical records will eventually be maintained in real time using computerized paperless systems. Although numerous vendors are working on various aspects of such systems, the vast number of records and entries necessary for a busy ambulatory practice makes total computerization still futuristic. Nevertheless, the day may come when all doctors will be able to type and all exam rooms will contain a computer terminal. Until then, however, ambulatory care medical records will be dependent on paper systems, with their apparent drawbacks and liabilities.

DEVELOPING MEDICAL RECORD FORMS

When developing the system for documenting patient care, much consideration must be given to the forms that will be used. Creating forms specific to the users' needs will allow for efficient and effective collection and retrieval of patient information. Two forms that greatly facilitate a physician's documentation and access of medically useful information are the patient care summary sheet (or problem list, as it is often referred to) and the physician's progress notes.

The patient care summary sheet is a multidisciplinary form. Physicians from multiple specialties, as well as nurses, use this form to summarize the patient's chronic medical problems, prior surgeries, long-term medications, vaccinations, past physical exams, and other pertinent medical information. In order to best serve its purpose as a quick-glance refresher for caregivers, this form should be located in a highly visible area in the medical record (e.g., the inside cover of the medical record folder). It can aid in the ready recall of existing conditions and prior surgeries and prevent untoward drug interactions, allergic reactions, and overdoses of medications.

Perhaps the major difficulty with summary sheets is that physicians often do not maintain them. Relying on a summary sheet that is not up to date can be worse than having no summary sheet at all. Generally nursing must also play a role in the maintenance of summary sheets to ensure their validity. Especially in multispecialty group practices, where many different physicians make chart entries, it is essential to have a well-maintained summary sheet that pulls all aspects of patient care into a coherent whole.

A physician's progress record form should be generated each time a patient is seen. Various regulatory agencies dictate the content of this form. All entries in the progress notes should include

- the date, department, and provider
- current vital data such as age, weight, blood pressure, medications
- the purpose of the visit (chief complaint)
- the impression (diagnosis)
- the tests ordered
- the treatment rendered
- the patient's disposition, including recommendations and follow-up instructions.

This document should be signed by the initiating practitioner.

In most organizations these notes are handwritten by the practitioner due to the cost and lack of availability of transcription staff. Some organizations transcribe the physician's progress record. The benefits of transcription include more complete documentation and better legibility. Transcribed documentation can also be read with greater speed and ease.

The main disadvantages of transcription is the almost inevitable delay in getting the signed transcribed notes into the record. Causes of such delays include procrastination on the part of physicians in dictating and then later reviewing, correcting, and signing the notes, the unavailability of transcribers to transcribe the notes immediately, and the additional "chart pull" needed to get the dictated notes into the medical record.

Either type of documentation—handwritten or transcribed—should provide an effective means of communication among all health care providers in the organization. The contents of the patient record in either case should be analyzed in terms of completeness and accuracy to ensure continued quality of care. A careful review of the entries should be made to check that they are legible and concise and include only those abbreviations approved by the organization. Each entry should be signed and dated by the originating practitioner.

To ensure the highest standards of professionalism in regard to quality of care, the medical staff should periodically become involved with quality assurance review of the health information record. Set criteria for patient care have been published and can serve as a baseline tool in the screening of medical records. Although these criteria exist, time and effort should be spent by the medical staff in creating performance standards that are specific to their organization. The standards should include screening criteria such as treatment requirements based on severity of illness, indicators to identify incomplete treatment, and adequacy of documentation.

The findings of the quality assurance review should be communicated to the professionals in the organization with the goal of continuously improving the quality of patient care. The information should not just be gathered, presented, and then left to rest, but there should be a plan for follow-up evaluation to determine if changes have occurred based on the data. (More information on quality assurance may be found in Chapter 21.)

The medical record is a prime source of data used in the compilation of health care statistics. These data are vital to the health care practitioner, the health care organization, and many other outside agencies. Medical staff performance can be evaluated, differences in practice standards between peers can be examined, and treatment effectiveness can be identified. The health organization's viability in the marketplace can be determined, the effectiveness of marketing efforts can be reviewed, and resource utilization can be compared to that of other organizations. Outside organizations also use health information abstracted out of the medical record to ascertain the effectiveness of the organization in caring for its patients, to determine trends in disease, and to ensure compliance with government and other regulatory agencies' requirements.

No matter who the requester is, the likelihood is that the medical record will play a key role in the ability of the health care organization to assemble, abstract, and disseminate health information. The need for completeness, conciseness, accuracy, and availability of the data contained in the record cannot be ignored. The data extracted could greatly affect long-term health care decisions being made by the organization or could be used for marketing the practice to health plans, employers, and individual patients.

THE MASTER PATIENT INDEX

Any health care organization must have a mechanism to capture and maintain basic information about its patients. A master patient index is a reference listing of all patients who have ever been treated by the organization. There is wide variation as to the data captured in this file, but there are several data elements that are essential, including

- patient name
- address
- telephone number
- date of birth
- medical record number
- dates of treatment
- attending practitioner

This information should be collected upon the patient's initial visit to the organization and continually verified and updated as necessary.

The master patient index is a key tool in tracking the patient population and is used in conjunction with the identification and retrieval of any preexisting medical record information. In most group practices, this information is kept on index cards, which are often arranged alphabetically by last name. Many of the larger practices have found it necessary, due to space constraints, to microfilm the master patient index. This allows continued retrieval but alleviates the burden of large, cumbersome manual files. Another method of capturing and storing this information is with data processing programs that permit the computerization of the master patient index. The master patient index can then be tied into the registration system (if computerized) to allow immediate updating of the index with each patient registration.

It is advisable that the master patient index be maintained permanently. Depending on the size and volume of the medical group, this may not be feasible. If permanent maintenance is not feasible, the data should be kept for at least the period of time required by the statute of limitations for that state.

The master patient index is a vital tool in the verification and retrieval of valuable health care information maintained by the organization. As a consequence, it should be kept in a safe and secure place. Quality patient care, legal liability, and efficient flow of information require that this file be maintained in an accurate format, alphabetical or otherwise. Adequate attention given to these details will ensure the practice's ability to function effectively.

Mention should also be made of the practice of utilizing family charts, where all family members' records are contained within a single folder. This system, widely employed by family practices and some multispecialty groups in the past, is no longer a tenable system. Legal constraints of patient confidentiality compel the segregation of information on each family member into an individual medical record.

FILING, STORAGE, AND RETENTION

In order to ensure the smooth flow of health information, efficient systems for filing and retrieval must be established. It is most common to use an alphabetical or numerical arrangement. Many medical record filing systems begin as alphabetical due to the ease of use for most individuals and the fact that no cross-referencing is required. In today's society, however, it is not uncommon for individuals to have several different last names, which adds to the difficulties associated with an alphabetical file system based on patient name. Confidentiality of information also becomes an issue when using alphabetical systems. Visibility of the patient's name for filing purposes, when the file is located in public access areas, can become a violation of the patient's right to privacy. Add to these problems the many misfiles due to incorrect alphabetizing and the weakness of the system becomes apparent. Numerical filing systems have proven to be more efficient with respect to filing and retrieval of health information. Among the advantages of a numerical system is that unique patient numbers are assigned to each individual, which increases confidentiality, makes filing quicker, and reduces errors. A numerical system is also more compatible with a data processing system. These clear-cut advantages make a numerical system the best choice for all but the smallest practices.

There are basically three types of numbering systems used in health care organizations: serial, serial-unit, and unit. In the serial numbering system, the patient receives a new number with each visit, thus having more than one unique number. The drawback is that several different numbers have to be tracked in order to ensure that all of the patient's medical records are retrieved for visits. The serial-unit numbering system also assigns the patient a new number with each visit, but all the information filed under the old number is pulled forward and assigned to the newly created number. The drawback of this type of numbering system is that it is labor- and resource-intensive.

The most effective numbering system is the unit system. In this type of system, a unique number is provided for each patient, and all visit information is filed under this number. The system allows for ease of retrieval and ensures that all patient data are made available to the health care provider at each visit. The unit numbering system provides the health care professional with a complete cumulative picture of the patient's medical information while eliminating the labor-intensive task of gathering separately filed portions of the patient's medical record from different sources.

Historically, one of the most popular adaptations of the unit numbering system was the straight numerical system. The filing was done in chronological order based upon the number assigned to the patient at registration. The advantage of this system was the ease with which staff could be trained. Because the numbered charts appeared in sequence on the file shelf, the staff needed only to know how to count to use the system. However, there are several disadvantages of this system. The misfiling of records increases with patient volume because the clerk must consider all digits of the patient number at once when filing. Another drawback is that quality control checks become difficult to perform because the heaviest and most recent activity is concentrated all in one area. The area with the most recently assigned numbers will require the largest concentration of effort and makes record maintenance more difficult.

The best filing system in terms of accuracy, even work distribution, and quality control is the terminal digit system. This is especially true in large practices. In a terminal digit filing system, a unique six-digit number is usually assigned to each patient. This number is then divided into three sections of two digits each (e.g., 22-33-45). The chart filing area is then divided into 100 primary sections ranging from 00 to 99. The last two digits, or primary digits, are the first to be considered by the clerk when filing. Once the corresponding primary section is located, the middle two (secondary) digits are matched accordingly. Finally, the first two (tertiary) digits are reviewed for correct filing. An example of terminal digit sequencing is as follows:

17-10-52	05-20-52	47-00-53
47-10-52	77-20-52	02-13-53
62-10-52	40-00-53	02-14-53

This type of numerical filing system allows for more even distribution of workload because only 1 medical record out of every 100 will be filed in a given primary file section. This division of filing also creates an even dispersal of work by dividing the responsibility for primary section ranges among the filing staff. Quality control is more effective with this type of system because of the lack of congestion in each section. Educational efforts can be focused on those staff members responsible for sections identified as not being adequately maintained.

The next area of concern is how best to house the medical records. The area chosen must have adequate space and lighting. Although there are several options available, from five-drawer file cabinets and automated carousel cabinets to open-shelf file units, the recommended storage is open shelving. Two of the major advantages of open shelving are its cost- and space-effectiveness. Open shelving can be purchased in both stationary and movable versions. Movable files increase efficiency and allow for more file space than conventional stationary units. Filing equipment specifically designed for various department sizes, volumes, and budgets can be purchased through medical record equipment vendors. Purchasing the equipment from these trained professionals should assure buyers that their specific needs will be met and that the safety codes and seismic codes will be abided by.

No matter what kind of storage system, patient confidentiality must be a prime concern. Medical record locations must be secured and locked when not in use, and care must be exercised that only approved personnel have access to these areas. When patient records are delivered to patient care areas, they must also be protected from perusal by nonmedical individuals. The orientation and training of all medical records personnel must include clear rules for the protection of patient confidentiality.

The location of the health information files can vary from group to group. In most instances, centralized record storage proves more efficient, because it allows a complete record of the patient's care to be maintained. Fragmented histories tend to result when different visits are filed in separate areas. Centralization provides more consistency in the processing and handling of health information due to the standardized policies and procedures, the proficiency of personnel, and the consistency of supervision.

The ideal situation would be to provide ample storage space for all the medical records for an indefinite period of time. Unfortunately, overcrowding of records inevitably occurs. Therefore, medical record professionals must develop a system for formalized record retention and destruction. The retention policy must be in keeping with the needs of the health care providers while taking into consideration the legal requirements dictated by individual state laws.

Several approaches to handling inactive records are available: The records can be stored in an offsite warehouse, microfilmed, or destroyed. Before any of these approaches is chosen, the definition of an inactive record must be ascertained. As part of this process, the medical staff should review patient activity trends. The space constraints of the medical records department as well as legal requirements should also be considered. Whether the final decision is made to store inactive records offsite, microfilm them, or destroy them, effective control of the process is essential. Medical records can play a crucial role in malpractice suits and should not be disposed of too quickly or without thought.

LEGAL ISSUES

Public health laws and statutes in every state dictate the type of information that a health care organization must record and report and the length of time that information must be retained. The responsibility to maintain the information falls on health information professionals. They are entrusted with the duty of ensuring that the medical records contain complete, accurate, and timely information. Stringent guidelines must be enforced for both medical and administrative purposes. The legal climate in today's society also mandates excellent records. In malpractice cases, where settlements can range up into the millions, the admissible business record of health care (the medical record) can serve as the deciding factor.

The medical record can be the health care professional's best friend or worst enemy. Entries in the medical record should be

- factual (not speculative)
- specific (not vague)
- complete (not half-done)
- timely (not written two weeks later after a reminder notice from medical records has been received)
- legible (not scrawled so as to be only decipherable by the writer)

In a trial situation the information documented in real time (while the actions were being taken) will usually weigh heavier than the dimming memory of the practitioner who perhaps treated thousands of other patients in the interim.

Alterations, deletions, and omissions to the medical record can also prove devastating in the costly malpractice arena. Alterations should be made only when absolutely necessary. The individual making the alterations should follow these guidelines:

- Draw one line through the inaccurate entry.
- Date and sign the alteration.
- Note what the correction is and why it is being made.

Omissions are extremely hazardous in that the burden of proof falls on the practitioner. The law assumes that if it isn't documented, it probably didn't happen. Regulations regarding required entries protect not only the patient but the health care professional as well. Deletion of information through the use of white-out or a felt-tip marker, through retyping, or through the removal of the document must be avoided. It becomes very difficult to disprove the allegation of negligence when supporting documentation has been obliterated. The practitioner might find it necessary to make a change, but if not done correctly, the change will be considered tampering. Sophisticated methods of detecting alterations such as chemical or spectroscopic examination are often employed to detect the falsification of records.

It is the health care professional's responsibility to ensure not only the complete and accurate content but also the confidentiality of the health record. The accessibility of the information contained within the medical record is regulated to some extent by the laws and regulations of each state. To help decipher the complex legal language used in the statutes, health information professionals should turn to the publications specific to their state. In California, for example, the California Association of Hospitals and Health Systems manual is an excellent resource. It provides clear and concise guidelines for handling questions regarding the release of information to certain outsiders while preserving confidentiality, and it also contains sample authorization forms that can be used by the health care organizations to govern the release of information.

Patient information is commonly released to the patients themselves and to third parties. Although technically the medical record is the property of the medical organization, patients have a legitimate right to the information contained in their records. State statutes should be consulted if patients request medical records. Restrictions on patient access should apply only to documentation that would be detrimental to the patient. Even though the release is to the patient, an authorization form should be filled out describing what is being released and why, and this form should be signed by the requesting party.

There are many third-party payers who have a legitimate need for the information contained in the medical record such as attorneys, insurance companies, and government agencies. Each request must be reviewed carefully to ensure that the inquiries are legitimate and follow the guidelines for request and release of confidential patient information. Health care professionals should never hesitate to question the legitimacy of a request and should consult all resources necessary to make certain that the patient's right to privacy is not breached. The requester must supply a release of information form signed and dated by the patient or other responsible party.

CONCLUSION

The medical record of today is not the traditional one-line description of the patient's primary problem. It is now a sophisticated document that serves as a detailed analysis of the patient's medical history, a communication tool to assist the multidisciplinary health care team in providing quality medical care, a resource for statistical analysis, and a potential means of defense in a legal suit. Creating, maintaining, and housing patient information is a time-consuming and detailed task, but, when accomplished, it can greatly enhance the efficiency and the effectiveness of an ambulatory health care organization.

BIBLIOGRAPHY

Fox, Leslie Ann, and Imbiorski, Walter. 1989. *The Record That Defends Its Friends,* 4th ed. Chicago: Care Communications.

Huffman, Edna K. 1981. *Medical Record Management,* 7th ed. Berwyn, IL: Physicians' Record Company.

21

Managing Quality Health Care

Gloria Gilbert Mayer, Judith M. Bulau, and Thomas Mayer

Ambulatory health care organizations face significant challenges as they experience competitive demands to demonstrate their delivery of quality health care services in a cost-effective manner. The rapidly evolving health care environment confronts ambulatory health care providers with economic, political, and regulatory incentives to control escalating costs without sacrificing quality and safety.

The ability of an ambulatory health care provider to address quality health care issues is significantly affected by the provider's quality assurance (QA) program. An effective program relies on (1) a written QA plan implemented through the use of QA policies and procedures and (2) a process for evaluating the implementation.

COMPONENTS OF A QUALITY ASSURANCE PROGRAM

The ambulatory QA program might consist of the following components written into a QA plan:

- objectives (see Exhibit 21-1)
- scope
- QA committee
- continuous QA activities
- special QA studies
- confidentiality policy for QA information
- documentation methods for QA activities
- system for communicating QA information
- QA program evaluation method (Bulau 1990)

Implementing the administration control component of the QA plan is extremely important and can be accomplished by writing guidelines that determine

288

Exhibit 21-1 Objectives of an Ambulatory Care Quality Assurance Program

Objectives

1. To develop, implement, and evaluate standards to measure medical, nursing, and therapy practice and delivery of ambulatory health care services.
2. To develop, implement, and evaluate effective quality assurance activities according to the ambulatory health care provider's mission statement, philosophy, and objectives.
3. To develop effective systems for problem assessment, identification, selection, study, corrective action, monitoring, evaluation, and reassessment of nursing/interdisciplinary team practice and ambulatory health care services.
4. To provide focus and direction for quality assurance activities.
5. To develop effective verbal/written information systems to communicate quality assurance activity outcomes to appropriate individuals and committees.
6. To provide educational opportunities for all ambulatory health care staff members to increase their knowledge and participation in quality assurance activities.
7. To correlate the findings of quality assurance activities with the content of ambulatory health care provider continuing education programs.
8. To encourage input and participation of all ambulatory health care staff relative to quality assurance activities.
9. To coordinate and integrate ambulatory health care provider interdepartmental/ intradepartmental quality assurance activities with overall provider quality assurance activities.
10. To ensure administrative commitment and support for quality assurance activities.

Source: Reprinted from *Quality Assurance Policies and Procedures for Ambulatory Health Care* by Judith M. Bulau, pp. 116–117, Aspen Publishers, Inc., © 1990.

how the QA program will be organized. These guidelines define staff areas of responsibility concerning QA activities. They clearly specify that the ambulatory health care provider's governing body and administrative staff maintain administrative control and establish lines of authority for the delegation of responsibility concerning QA activities. An example of the incorporation of QA into an ambulatory health care organizational chart is presented in Figure 21-1.

EVALUATING A HEALTH CARE SYSTEM

The QA program is instrumental in evaluating a health care system. The focus of evaluation may include three classic approaches: structure, process, and outcome.

Structure

The structure of an organization comprises the physical environment, the personnel, the equipment, and the operational systems that are established to

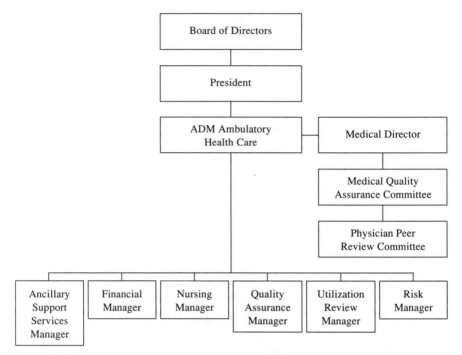

Figure 21-1 QA Organizational Chart. *Source:* Adapted from *Quality Assurance Policies and Procedures for Ambulatory Health Care* by Judith M. Bulau, p. 15, Aspen Publishers, Inc., © 1990.

meet the needs of the patients. Items to be assessed in a QA structural evaluation would include building and fire safety, the appointment system, the credentialing of personnel, the committee structure, and policies and procedures. The adequacy of the medical records system is a key structural issue. Methods for assessing structural adequacy include environmental checklists, patient surveys, focused studies of selected systems, personnel interviews, and formal accreditation. In fact, the current state-of-the-art accreditation for third parties is primarily structural in nature.

Process

The process focuses on the actual care and services provided to the patients. QA process studies might evaluate whether diabetic patients are tested in a timely manner, whether patients' vital signs are taken, whether appropriate x-rays are performed, and whether patients are given appropriate instructions about their treatment. Chart audits are usually process-oriented, and certain studies of follow-up care can also measure process.

Outcome

The outcomes are the actual results of the care and services provided. They are especially difficult to assess. Focused chart audits, patient interviews and surveys, statistical analysis of relapses, readmissions, and increased office and emergency visits can all be used in outcome QA.

Structure, process, and outcome are vital components of QA. These three elements not only constitute an appropriate framework for QA activities but also provide an operational focus for those activities. No one method of measurement has evolved as the sole standard of measurement. For example, a patient who stopped smoking only for six months may not be considered to have a successful outcome after completing a "no-smoking program."

Provider Credentialing As an Example

An example of structure, process, and outcome can be examined by provider credentialing activities. Evaluating the *structure* of the credentialing program includes the interval for reviewing credentials as well as the credentials being reviewed such as state licensure, board certification, malpractice experience, and continuing medical education courses. Assessing the *process* of provider credentialing involves the methodology for determining the status of those credentials. The procedures used can vary significantly. For example, the following are possible methods for verifying credentials:

- Ask the individual provider to attest personally to his or her status.
- Ask the provider to submit unverified copies of the credentials.
- Ask the provider to submit verified copies of the credentials.
- Obtain verification of the credentials from the primary source.

Finally, an evaluation of *outcomes* obtained from the provider credentialing process includes a summary of the information obtained and what actions were taken because of it. The outcomes might include the following:

- One hundred percent of the providers had 50 continuing medical education credits within the past three years.
- Sixty-seven percent were board certified in a specialty recognized by the American Board of Medical Specialties.

- Seventeen percent have one or more malpractice suits pending.
- Five percent have had one or more malpractice settlements.
- One and a half percent were not recertified for lack of compliance with credentialing specifications.

The credentialing example was used to demonstrate all three aspects of a QA program's evaluation of structure, process, and outcome.

Identifying Quality Concerns

There are several ways of conducting ambulatory QA activities that assist in the identification of appropriate quality concerns.

Auditing Clinical Activities

One way involves auditing clinical activities. Although this auditing most commonly involves medical record audits, it may also include other sources of clinical information such as laboratory reports of abnormal test results or compliance with outside referrals. Patient satisfaction surveys provide another means of identifying potential QA concerns. Also, patient complaints should be tracked and trended. (Both patient surveys and complaints tend to focus more on service quality rather than quality of care.)

Auditing Medical Records

Medical record auditing can be done in a variety of ways, each with differing outcomes.

Random Screening. One way is to use random screening. For example, 10 charts from every physician might be reviewed each quarter. A specific format must be developed so that the charts are reviewed in the same fashion. The format might include items such as these:

- Did every patient have his or her vital signs and weight recorded?
- Were the notes legible?
- Did the record denote the chief complaint?

This approach has the advantage of including all the organization's physicians within its scope.

Specific Screening. Medical record auditing can also use specific screening, with targets identified from various internal and external sources. These might include

- patient accident or incident reports
- medication error reports
- infection control reports
- patient complaints
- patient letters or comments regarding ambulatory health care services
- patient surveys
- staff concerns
- patient deaths
- utilization review reports
- drug utilization review reports
- accreditation, licensure, and certification survey reports
- contracting managed health care organizations
- ambulatory research studies
- financial reports (Bulau 1990)

Occurrence Screens. Common occurrence screens are also useful in targeting audits.

Diagnosis or Procedure-Specific Audits

Another way of frequently identifying quality problems is to perform diagnosis- or procedure-specific medical record audits. Immunizations, Pap smears, and screening mammography are examples of commonly audited procedures. "Red flag" hospital admissions can also be the focus of ambulatory medical record audits. These admissions signal a high probability of inappropriate ambulatory care (Solberg 1987). The diagnoses to be flagged might include

- diabetic acidosis
- perforative appendicitis
- gangrene
- hypokalemia
- pulmonary embolism or infarction
- cellulitis

- upper G.I. perforations
- stroke or transient ischemic attack (if patient under age 65)
- primary breast cancer
- drug toxicity
- endometrial uterine cancer
- asthma
- prematurity
- ectopic pregnancy
- toxemia of pregnancy

The Quality Loop

The ambulatory QA program requires an informational feedback loop. The ultimate goal of ambulatory QA activities is to improve outpatient care. Outcomes are patient sensitive and should improve patient care. After the audit, the outcome phase of QA answers the question, "What's next?" Data must be transformed into information and changes in systems and provider behavior must be based on this information in order to close the quality loop (see Figure 21-2). Structure, process, and outcome affect each other and the ability to make meaningful judgments about quality of care.

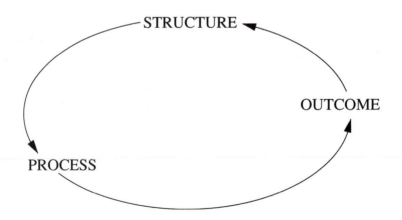

Figure 21-2 The Quality Loop

CLINICAL VERSUS SERVICE QUALITY

The preceding paragraphs have focused mainly on clinical aspects of QA. This is because ambulatory care QA practices and procedures have generally been transposed from the hospital environment. But quality care is more than good outcomes and cost-effective processes; it must also give rise to patient satisfaction. Because ambulatory care generally involves more selective procedures than hospital care, patient satisfaction and service issues become increasingly important as a component of QA in the outpatient sector.

Techniques for measuring patient satisfaction and quality of service are still being developed, and current ones have never achieved universal acceptance. Yet the challenge of obtaining meaningful indicators for this aspect of quality and of translating these data into superior service still remains. Although perhaps more administrative than clinical, service issues rightfully belong in a comprehensive ambulatory QA program.

Service areas measured by some practices as part of their QA program include

- waiting time on the telephone
- waiting time to make appointments
- next available physician appointment (by specialty, if a group practice)
- waiting time in reception area
- waiting time on telephone hold
- next available appointment for routine diagnostic procedures (i.e., mammography, CT scanning, and ultrasonography)

Areas that are more subjective and still require tools for identification and evaluation include the doctor-patient relationship, the satisfaction of patients' emotional needs, and the need of patients to be adequately informed.

STANDARDS FOR QUALITY

Practice standards are the basis for measuring quality. Structure standards are reflected by the policies, procedures, and systems needed to provide quality care. Process standards specify series of actions and behaviors necessary for performing and measuring the quality of care, whereas outcome standards measure the goals achieved and reflect the actual patient care provided.

Standards can be developed internally or be adapted from other sources. HMOs, PPOs, and medical association groups provide standards for both practice and service. For example, many HMOs provide access standards for primary care physicians as well as specialists. They may also audit physician credentials and provide QA guidelines.

National medical specialty groups publish general practice guidelines. These are usually diagnosis-based and may be somewhat generic in character, but they serve as an excellent resource in establishing basic standards.

National and local accrediting agencies also provide standards for QA. The Joint Commission on Accreditation of Healthcare Organizations is the major national agency that accredits ambulatory care organizations. Provider-based voluntary organizations also may accredit ambulatory medical groups. They are usually considered credible with their QA programs accepted as meeting all QA requirements.

CONCLUSION

Continuing concern over the quality of health care despite increasing expenditures of health care dollars has created an opportunity for the ambulatory health care industry to share individual and collective expertise, experience, and leadership for the refinement of ambulatory health care QA programs and activities. It is hoped that the material presented here will be useful for professionals and providers who are striving to deliver quality ambulatory health care services in an increasingly competitive health care environment.

REFERENCES

Bulau, Judith M. 1990. *Quality Assurance Policies and Procedures for Ambulatory Health Care.* Gaithersburg, Md.: Aspen Publishers.

Solberg, Leif I., Peterson, Kent, E., Ellis, Ronald W., Romness, Kenneth, Thell, Terry E., Rohrenbach, Elizabeth, Smith, Angela, Routier, and Wermuth, Mary. 1987. *The Minnesota Project: A Focused Approach to Ambulatory Care Quality Assurance.* Minneapolis, Minn.: Group Health Plan, Inc., HMO Minnesota, and Share Health Plan.

SUGGESTED READING

Batalden, Paul B., and O'Connor, J. Paul. 1980. *Quality Assurance in Ambulatory Care.* Gaithersburg, Md.: Aspen Publishers.

Gould, E. Joyce, and Wargo, Joan. 1987. *Home Health Nursing Care Plans.* Gaithersburg, Md.: Aspen Publishers.

Joint Commission on Accreditation of Healthcare Organizations. 1991. *Ambulatory Health Care Standards Manual.* Chicago: Joint Commission on Accreditation of Healthcare Organizations.

Meisenheimer, Claire Gavin. 1985. *Quality Assurance: A Complete Guide to Effective Programs.* Gaithersburg, Md.: Aspen Publishers.

Schroeder, Patricia S., and Maibusch, Regina M. *Nursing Quality Assurance: A Unit-Based Approach.* Gaithersburg, Md.: Aspen Publishers.

Spath, Patrice. 1990. "Ambulatory Care Requires Meticulous QA Plan." *Hospital Peer Review,* October, 160–63.

22

Risk Management of Prescription Drugs

Elan Rubinstein

In recent years, HMOs, insurers, and self-insured employers have become concerned about rapidly escalating prescription drug expenditures for their beneficiaries. To counteract this, drug benefit restrictions have been applied by increasing numbers of payers and have become incrementally tighter. While these restrictions impact some medical groups' finances and operations, internal operating systems and personnel are not always available to manage drug prescribing nor are financial systems available to track it.

Typical examples of benefit restrictions are increasing beneficiary cost sharing, mandating generic dispensing, excluding various drug categories from coverage, and developing pharmacy preferred provider organizations. In some HMO environments, restrictions include using drug formularies, mandating prior authorization for nonformulary products, reviewing drug utilization, sharing the financial risks with contracting medical groups, and, less frequently, delegating full financial and operational responsibility for provision of drug benefits to medical groups.

Medical groups which accept risk for prescription drug benefits, whether financial risk alone or operational risk as well, should be prepared to manage this risk to ensure a satisfactory outcome. And groups' risks are magnified as payers' prescription drug restrictions become tighter and ever more complex. This chapter suggests steps through which these risks may be managed.

DEFINING THE NEW MANAGEMENT CHALLENGES

It is challenging for a medical group to manage delegated financial responsibility for a single prescription drug benefit against a prescribed drug formulary and a per member budget. But competitive metropolitan areas where managed care is strong present additional challenges. In such areas, medical groups are confronted with inconsistencies in delegated responsibilities, types of beneficiary coverage, claims administrative requirements, levels of HMO claims reporting, and HMO clinical pharmacist support. In the absence of standardization of these factors, the additional challenge is to obtain medical group physician compliance with the sometimes contradictory array of administrative constraints regarding prescribing behavior.

FINANCIAL AND OPERATIONAL RISKS

A medical group may be placed at financial risk for exceeding a per beneficiary annual drug budget or capitation amount. On the other hand, the group may share in the savings if expenditures are lower than budgeted, or these penalty and bonus arrangements may apply together.

HMOs may support contracting medical groups in their effort to remain within budget. Support may take the form of managing the pharmacy PPO, providing useful claims reports and drug utilization reviews (DURs), and targeting the interventions of their clinical pharmacists at certain pharmacist and physician providers. Unfortunately, many HMOs are weak in this area, and some do not provide sufficiently detailed claims reports to enable monitoring of prescribing behavior.

An HMO may also delegate operational responsibility for the drug program to the medical group. The medical group may arrange for the provision of prescription drugs via physician dispensing and through contracted retail pharmacies. Management and monitoring may include the use of claims reviews, pharmacy claims audits, DURs, physician prescribing "report cards," and educational programming targeted at certain group physicians or contracting pharmacists.

In the face of inconsistent and sometimes contradictory signals from contracting HMOs, medical group physicians may develop prescribing habits that meet the most prevalent requirements or may simply ignore all prescription drug–related guidelines.

EVALUATING DRUG BENEFITS–RELATED RISK

Understanding medical group financial and operational risk for prescription drugs is an important first step in the management effort. An evaluation of these risks across all HMO contracts would include the following tasks:

- *Quantifying the medical group's risk.* For what fraction of the managed care patient base is the medical group subject to financial risk (or financial and operational risk) for prescription drug benefits?
- *Assessing the group's risk-based experience.* What is the medical group's financial experience with each risk-based prescription drug benefit ar-

rangement? Has an analysis been done of each arrangement to determine why it was successful or unsuccessful?

- *Assessing the adequacy of payment.* Were the assumptions on which the financial risk and operational arrangements were accepted realistic in the first place? Is the medical group's negotiating position based on an analysis of these assumptions and of the group's experience with these arrangement over the past year? If operational responsibility is delegated, does the payer's formula provide for the medical group's administrative costs in managing the benefit and for lesser retail pharmacy discounts than the HMO would enjoy in its own pharmacy PPO?

- *Determining the HMO's role in risk management.* What support does the HMO give to the medical group to enable it to manage the delegated risk? Are timely drug utilization and cost reports available, identifying physicians, pharmacies, patients, and drugs for special attention? Does the HMO make available clinical pharmacy staff to interpret these reports and to recommend, develop, and implement interventions?

- *Assessing medical group's risk management system.* Does the medical group have a system to monitor the prescription drug benefit program in terms of per member per month costs against budget and in terms of individual physician prescribing compliance with requirements? Is this the pharmacy and therapeutics committee's responsibility? Is someone delegated to be responsible for prescription drug–related use and cost analysis and for interfacing with the payer's staff regarding it? If operational responsibility for the prescription drug benefit is delegated to the medical group, has the group assigned someone to manage it? Is someone assigned to work with physicians to maximize compliance with drug-related administrative requirements?

MANAGING PRESCRIPTION DRUG BENEFITS–RELATED RISK

The following suggests an organized approach to managing the risk associated with a prescription drug benefits program.

The Pharmacy and Therapeutics Committee

A pharmacy and therapeutics committee should be established to be responsible for reviewing drug prescribing by group physicians, medical clinic drug floor stock policies, and physician dispensing. On the basis of its ongoing review, including the results of targeted audits, the committee may determine that it is necessary to develop prescribing protocols for particular indications or drug therapies. Pharmacist input should be solicited to support the committee in all of these functions, with the degree of involvement dependent on the size of the group, and on its drug-related risk.

The Pharmacist's Responsibilities

The following suggests responsibilities for a pharmacist devoted to drug risk management at the medical group on a full-time basis. Some of these will not apply if the pharmacist is available to the group only part-time or on a consulting basis.

- Act as permanent secretary of the pharmacy and therapeutics committee.
- Implement decisions of the group's pharmacy and therapeutics committee under the guidance of its director, including the performance of drug utilization audits and the institution of educational programs and other approved interventions intended to enhance physician prescribing quality and maintain cost control.
- Act as the group's primary interface with clinical pharmacists at contracting HMOs, understand utilization trends, and request special HMO reports and services.
- Determine appropriate interventions that will best manage the group's financial risk given conflicting drug formulary requirements and incentives, variable HMO report quality, variable HMO clinical support, and any of the group's own practice protocols.
- Work with HMOs to upgrade available clinical services and reporting and alert the group's managed care contracting department of any lack of HMO cooperation or quality of service.
- Review utilization and cost reports to ensure that prescriptions are appropriately charged against group experience in terms of patient eligibility, drug coverage, group affiliation of the prescribing physician, and drug pricing.
- Initiate monthly "drug rounds" that focus on high-cost, high-utilization, or frequently misused pharmaceuticals. Work with HMOs and with pharmaceutical manufacturers of products on the drug formularies to schedule, coordinate, develop, fund, and implement high-quality and attractively presented drug rounds.
- Represent the medical group at any local or regional association of medical groups that offers pharmacy-related services to members.
- Interface with contracting retail pharmacies serving the group's enrollees, particularly with respect to their actions when faced with nonformulary

prescriptions and with respect to the need to review patients' drug profiles prior to filling prescriptions to avoid inappropriate combinations of medications or too frequent refills.

- If the group owns or is affiliated with a hospital, work with the hospital pharmacy and therapeutics committee to identify, audit, and correct problems. Possible issues include protocols supportive of a continuum of care between inpatient and outpatient care and speeding the transition of inpatients to outpatient care through the application of outpatient oral or intravenous pharmaceutical therapy, including home care support as necessary.

- Consult with group physicians, upon request, concerning patient-specific outpatient prescription drug issues.

- Together with nursing, and subject to the approval of the pharmacy and therapeutics committee, develop standards for floor stock medications in medical group patient care areas.

- Establish policies and procedures regarding ordering, inventory, stocking, dispensing, checking for outdated products, and monitoring for pilferage. Special attention should be paid to narcotics.

- Develop and maintain a drug-ordering relationship with a wholesaler and bargain for the best prices possible given the group's purchasing volume.

- Supervise the ordering, receiving, storage, and distribution of floor stock pharmaceuticals and the processing of wholesaler drug billing statements.

- Support the group's managed care contracting department in establishing and periodically reevaluating the retail pharmacy network to provide pharmaceuticals under full-capitation and full-delegation contracts.

- For contracts that include full drug capitation and full delegation of operational responsibilities, review and manage drug utilization and cost through the group's contracted pharmacy network and periodically reevaluate the adequacy of the capitation payments to cover the group's costs for drug ingredients, dispensing, claims administration, and risk management services.

- Support the group's managed care contracting department in its periodic re-evaluation of HMO contracts up for renewal.

Drug Utilization Review

According to the American Pharmaceutical Association and the American Medical Association, drug utilization review (DUR) is a formal program for assessing data on drug use by means of explicit prospective standards and, as necessary, introducing remedial strategies. The three primary objectives are (1) to improve the quality of care, (2) to conserve program funds and individual expenditures, and (3) to maintain program integrity (e.g., control problems of fraud and beneficiary abuse).

Each of the objectives of DUR requires the periodic availability of detailed drug utilization claims data organized so as to allow thorough, targeted, and efficient review. The following list outlines suggested reports that the HMO should provide to the medical group, preferably on a monthly or quarterly basis, to support DUR efforts:

- The number of prescriptions and prescription drug expenditures per medical group assigned member per month compared with the same statistics for other HMO contracting medical groups in the geographic area.
- The medical group's compliance with the HMO drug formulary, in terms of the ratio of formulary to nonformulary drug use, compared with the compliance of other HMO contracting medical groups in the geographic area.
- Top-ranked and ordered listings of members, primary care physicians, and pharmacies, by drug expenditure per month received, prescribed, or dispensed, respectively. Listings should also show the number of prescriptions and identify the drugs involved. (This would involve a series of reports, not a single report.)
- Top physicians by expenditures for nonformulary drugs.
- Top-ranked and ordered listings of drugs, by number of prescriptions and dollar expenditures, with notations as to formulary or nonformulary status.
- Drug claims-level dispensing detail, sorted by member, rank-ordered by total member drug expenditures over the period, and possibly limited to the top-ranked 50 to 100 members. Dispensing detail should include the prescribing physician's name, the date the prescription was filled, the medication and dosage, the quantity of drug dispensed, the period of the supply, the ingredient cost, and the pharmacy's identification.

Changing Drug Prescribing Behavior

Identifying therapeutically or economically inappropriate prescribing behavior is only the preliminary objective of DUR. Changing physicians' prescribing behavior is the second and more difficult goal.

A review of published studies of nonregulatory and noncommercial programs aimed at improving drug prescribing in primary care settings summarized its findings on the postpayment DUR-type of intervention as follows:

Based on one randomized controlled trial and several inadequately controlled studies, we conclude that ongoing feedback reports of physician-specific prescribing performance may be effective in improving certain types of prescribing practices, such as use of generic drugs, in academic group practice settings. No well-controlled study has been conducted on the effectiveness of this approach directed at private office practitioners, who may be more resistant to influence from influential colleagues or authority figures than hospital-based or group-practice physicians. In addition, private physicians may be suspicious of such attempts at intervening in their practice and rating their performance. (Soumerai, McLaughlin, and Avorn 1989, pp. 294–95)

Soumerai and Avorn (Soumerai, McLaughlin, and Avorn 1989) have done studies to determine the impact on physicians' prescribing practices of one-on-one and face-to-face educational meetings with specially trained pharmacists or physicians. Their findings support the idea that brief one-on-one educational outreach visits are effective in substantially reducing inappropriate prescribing of a wide range of medicines, including use of contraindicated or expensive antibiotics, ineffective drugs for geriatric patients with peripheral vascular disease or senility, potentially addictive analgesics, and psychoactive drugs.

In an economic analysis of one of these studies in a Medicaid population, the Soumerai study concluded that targeted education of moderate to high prescribers of certain drugs would lead to government drug savings at least two to three times higher than the operating costs of such a program, not to mention the likelihood of positive spillover effects to these physicians' non-Medicaid patient practice.

FUTURE PERSPECTIVES ON DRUG RISK MANAGEMENT

Point-of-sale (POS) systems have become ubiquitous in retail pharmacies and are beginning to make their way into physician offices and hospitals. Pharmacies are increasingly tied to one another and to HMOs they contract with via real-time point-of-sale prescription drug claims systems. Through these systems, patient eligibility, copayment responsibility, plan design, and various dispensing requirements and limitations can be made known to the pharmacist prior to dispensing a medication to a patient at the counter. Through POS systems, medical groups may be able to integrate pharmacies more clearly into their drug cost management efforts.

Drug utilization review is in its infancy but has been given a political push (and the promise of a large infusion of capital) by the 1990 Omnibus Budget Reconciliation Act (OBRA) Medicaid provisions. Medical outcomes-based appropriateness standards are being developed in various research settings (e.g., United Health Care) and entrepreneurial settings (e.g., Value Health

Sciences). Integration of drug, medical, and hospital claims data with patient demographic information and "appropriateness of care" standards will lead to the ability of HMOs, potentially on a real-time basis, to oversee case management. With respect to prescription drugs, this may mean more intervention by third parties into physician-prescribing and pharmacist-dispensing decisions than is now the case, and additional management challenges to the group.

Some HMOs have developed special programs in order to manage high and increasing costs of cancer therapy drugs injected in physician offices and clinics. One relatively common type of program "carves-out" payment for these drugs from medical group capitation arrangements, and instead pays for them on a shared-risk basis. HMOs may, for instance, agree to pay their portion of the shared-risk pool only for drugs which they preapprove for use on a case-by-case basis. Thus, to the extent that HMO's drug preapproval procedures are interventionist rather than ceremonial in intent, medical groups may face this additional financial and operational risk.

REFERENCE

Soumerai, S.B., McLaughlin, T.J., Avorn, J. 1989. "Improving Drug Prescribing in Primary Care: A Critical Analysis of the Experimental Literature." *Milbank Memorial Fund Quarterly* 67, no. 2.

23

Home Care Services

Helga Bonfils, Denise E. Stanton, and Sharon Guller

INTRODUCTION

Home care before the late 1890s consisted primarily of house calls by physicians for the affluent and nursing care by charity organizations for the poor. Initially, communicable diseases and child health and nutrition (with an emphasis on prevention) were the focus of home care visits. The Visiting Nurses' Association was the first formally organized home care network, funded and designed by the community and charitable funds to service the needs of the community. The enactment of Medicare legislation in 1966 provided for federal insurance reimbursement for home care services. The beneficiary of home care services paid no out-of-pocket fees for covered services. Providers of home care services were paid based on cost reimbursement. It was not until the early 1980s that hospitals rapidly expanded into home care programs to help offset the newly instituted cost-containment measures of the Medicare DRG guidelines. Private insurance carriers and health maintenance organizations (HMOs) only recently have offered coverage for home care services in order to reduce hospital utilization.

Independently owned home health agencies proliferated during this time as intermittent home care was viewed as a lucrative area of health care. Other home health providers altruistically saw home health as a way to improve the quality of care and the quality of life for clients who were being discharged from hospitals earlier due to DRG regulations. This rapid growth in home care, however, meant that many home care providers were without adequate experience or even state licenses. This led to the closure of many Medicare-certified agencies. The current trend for home care companies is to provide profitable ancillary services such as pharmacy services, durable medical equipment services, and private duty nursing and to decrease dependency on traditional Medicare services.

HOME CARE SERVICES

The most traditional as well as most common service provided in the home is nursing. The purpose of intermittent nursing care is to augment or complete the nursing care program required by the client and to ease the transition from clinic or hospital to home. Nursing services include wound, intravenous, catheter, ostomy, drainage tube, and tracheostomy care and management. Nurses also assess patients' physical status and psychosocial environment, as well as monitor new disease processes and response to new medications. Education of clients and their families regarding medications, disease processes, nutrition, skilled nursing care procedures, skin care, and bowel regimes is an important part of the medical team effort. All nursing services are under the direction and guidance of the patient's personal physician. Intermittent services are those performed at the patient's home over a period of time. The duration and frequency of visits is dependent on the patient's needs and the physician's orders.

Specialty nursing services are becoming more available to the patient in the home setting. Enterostomal therapists, for example, are available to provide management of clients who have undergone an ostomy or have skin problems. Some home health agencies also offer the services of pediatric nurse specialists to deal with the specific and complex needs of pediatric patients and their parents. Perinatal and neonatal services are being offered as an alternative to extended hospital stays and as an adjunct to early postpartum discharge. These services include instructions on neonatal care, postpartum checks, and management of equipment such as bili-lites and apnea monitors in the home. Rehabilitative nursing services focus on bowel, bladder, and skin problems and the regaining of maximum function by the neurologically impaired.

Hospice services emphasize the emotional and physical comfort of the terminally ill patient. They focus on pain control, body function control, and support of the client and family so as to maximize the quality of life remaining.

Private duty nursing or shift care provides round-the-clock care for patients who require or desire continuous nursing care. These services are generally available to patients who are unable to care for themselves, have no caregiver available, or have chronic conditions that require skilled nursing care.

Among the most popular home care services are those provided by home health aides. These services include bathing, nail and hair care, meal preparation, bedmaking, and some light housekeeping to ensure a clean and safe environment. Home health aides can also assist with a range of motion exercises, ambulation, and transfer activities and are available on an intermittent or shift basis.

Therapy services can also be provided in the home on an intermittent basis. The types of therapy available through home health agencies include physical therapy, occupational therapy, and speech therapy. The most frequently ordered service is physical therapy. The diagnoses for which physical therapy is most commonly prescribed are fractures, total-joint replacements, CVAs, and neck and back pain. Physical therapy services are also utilized for patients with medical conditions that decrease function and mobility and raise concerns about safety. Physical therapists can provide education for clients and their caregivers regarding the use of orthotics, transfer techniques, and body mechanics. Therapy services are available under the direction of a physician and are prescribed for a period of several weeks or until the patient reaches maximum function.

Occupational therapy focuses on activities of daily living such as dressing, grooming, bathing, cooking, and self-care. Occupational therapists also aid clients with upper extremity difficulties, teach energy conservation and work simplification to patients affected by pulmonary and cardiac limitations, and provide splinting and adaptive equipment management to maximize independence. Occupational therapy visit frequencies, which are similar to physical therapy frequencies, are dependent on the diagnosis and on physician directions.

Speech pathologists work with clients who have communication and swallowing difficulties. They most frequently work with patients who have a brain tumor or are recovering from a CVA, head injury, or neck or throat operations. Speech therapy treatment continues over a longer period of time than physical or occupational therapy treatment because it deals with the higher brain functions.

Social workers are available on an intermittent basis to assist with securing community resources, including Meals on Wheels, transportation, homemakers, and skilled nursing facility or board and care placement. Social workers also provide counseling for family problems, grief counseling for terminal patients, and counseling for depression, and they can help patients deal with body image adjustments resulting from medical problems. Providing financial assistance information and making appropriate resource referrals to meet family needs are important functions of social workers in the home. Social workers generally visit a patient two or three times over a period of several weeks.

Durable medical equipment (e.g., beds, wheelchairs, walkers, oxygen, commodes, and respiratory aides) is generally ordered by physicians to maximize quality of care and provide safety in the home. Such equipment can be provided by private durable medical equipment companies or home health agencies, but its provision should be coordinated by the home health agency supplying the other services.

Home care pharmacy services include infusion therapies and supplies, enteral feedings and supplies, and injectable medications. Infusion therapies available in the home include antibiotics, hydration, chemotherapy, pain management, and total parenteral nutrition. Pharmacy services must be closely coordinated with physician and nursing care to ensure proper clinical management of intravenous and central line infusions. Integration and communication of laboratory testing is also important for ensuring successful home infusion therapy.

The various home care services mentioned above are provided under the direction and guidance of the patient's personal physician. The nurse's responsibility is to report any changes in the patient's condition to the physician and implement any modifications in the plan of care.

UTILIZATION OF HOME CARE SERVICES

Client Utilization

Home health care is still one of the best kept secrets in the health care system. In a recent poll (Scemons 1990), 72 percent of clients who know about or have had home health nursing prefer remaining at home to receiving nursing care in an institution. Client satisfaction surveys reveal that patients feel they have a better understanding of their illness due to home nursing care. Home care patients also feel that they are more involved in and have more control over their own plan of care. The primary purpose of home care is to educate the patient and family and prevent complications related to the disease process. Nursing assessment at home allows for early detection of possible complications, which are reported to the physician before the patient or the family experiences a medical crisis. Early detection of impending medical problems can prevent costly emergency room visits and rehospitalization.

Not only is home care preferred by patients, but there are substantial cost savings to payers and providers. For the average patient, one day in the hospital is more expensive than one month of intermittent home care services. Because of the variety of home care services, virtually every hospitalized patient could be discharged earlier if provided with home care follow-up. A good example is the patient with osteomyelitis. After diagnosis and the initiation of antibiotic therapy, the patient can complete the necessary six to eight weeks of I.V. antibiotic therapy at home for a small percentage of the cost of an equivalent hospitalization. Instead of remaining in the hospital, diabetics can receive daily insulin injections, blood sugars, and instruction at home.

In fact, home care services can also be utilized in lieu of hospitalization. Diabetic patients can be started on insulin in the home, with daily monitoring provided by home care. Changes in chronic medical conditions can be assessed in the home by trained nursing personnel and reported to the physician, who can then determine the necessary treatment adjustments. Terminally ill patients can be managed at home through skilled nursing assessment and symptom management as their condition warrants.

How home care follow-up can significantly reduce rehospitalizations can be illustrated by the following case study.

> Mrs. Newman was an 80-year-old woman with a history of recurrent episodes of acute congestive heart failure (CHF), and she required hospitalization every three to four weeks over a six-month period prior to having home care. After the physician ordered home care, the nurse's initial visit and assessment revealed congestion in both lungs and swelling of the legs. Mrs. Newman lived alone and prepared her own meals. The nurse examined Mrs. Newman's cupboards and refrigerator and found that she had only easy-to-prepare foods containing large amounts of sodium. The nurse first educated Mrs. Newman on the relation between her high-sodium meals and her fluid retention. The nurse then arranged for home meals to be delivered and asked Mrs. Newman to weigh herself daily and record her weight on a chart. The nurse instructed Mrs. Newman on how to take her multiple medications properly, what side effects to look out for, and the importance of each medication. Mrs. Newman was given further instruction on using a low-sodium diet. The nurse also repeatedly instructed her on what signs and symptoms to look for and when to contact her physician. Mrs. Newman, at the end of an eight-week treatment period, was able to have some control over her disease process, her CHF was stabilized, and she no longer required frequent hospitalization.

There are many factors that account for the success of home care. When given a choice, patients for the most part will voluntarily choose the home setting to recover. This accounts for the shorter recovery time seen in home care patients. Not only are patients in familiar surroundings, but they have family and friends to support and assist them. The hospital setting connotes illness and sickness, whereas being at home promotes an attitude of wellness.

Home care provides nursing care and support. There is no substitute for the personalized one-on-one care received in the home. In the hospital, patients are often seen by several specialists and nurses without care coordination. The home care nurse acts as a case coordinator or manager and orchestrates and integrates the patient care. Home care evaluates the physical, social, and emotional needs of patients and responds to them. Often patients are confused about their medical regime. Medical doctors and hospitals can be intimidating, and important questions are not asked or answered. The nurse in the home setting is able to explain the patient's medications, disease process, and diet to the patient at a level that is understandable. Patients can be taught to be knowledgeable about and responsible for their health care needs.

Physician Utilization

In a prepaid managed health care system, cost savings is of primary importance. The cost savings when home care is provided in lieu of hospitalization is obvious. Home care services help prevent inappropriate and costly emergency room visits, ambulance transportation, and possible rehospitalization.

There are a variety of home care agencies that provide limited services. However, one of the most time-consuming activities of those assigning home care services to patients is calling several specialized agencies and repeating the referral information. Agencies that provide a variety of services or coordinate additional services for the referral source can be very valuable in terms of time and cost savings. The better agencies offer in-hospital or in-clinic consultation for specialties such as enterostomal therapy or other complex home care services. These factors need to be taken into consideration when choosing the most suitable home care provider. Once a home care provider has been selected, familiarity with the referral source's systems and staff will facilitate the client's transition from the medical practice site to home.

The quality of services provided in the home should be consistent with the referral source's philosophy and values. Communication between the home care providers and the physician is essential for the continuity of care. Home care providers should be considered part of the health team and should provide feedback on client status. Home care agencies should be utilized as a resource regarding the suitability of patients for home care and should also furnish providers with updates on new treatments and equipment available in home care.

There are, of course, some limitations to home care services. Nurses who do intermittent home health care see an average of six patients per day. The time spent with an individual patient varies according to needs but rarely exceeds two hours. Private duty nurses provide care for patients who require extended nursing services (four hours to round the clock). Payer sources often dictate the length of time that patients can receive home care benefits.

Home health services are limited by the fact that they are provided offsite. Physician availability is limited by the schedule of the patient's personal physician. Home care does not provide services in life-threatening situations. Home care agencies must abide by state and federal guidelines and mandates, which can limit services to be provided in the home.

Most often, however, home care services are underutilized due to a lack of physician understanding. One factor is the recent rapid expansion of home health care and the lack of physician education about its utilization and capabilities.

The final limitation is the scarcity of experienced home care staff. There is some interest in including home care education in formal health professional educational programs, but for the most part the agencies themselves must provide on-the-job training.

There are two basic ways of providing home care services. The most cost-effective and simplest way is to contract with an established Medicare-certified intermittent home care agency. It is important to evaluate the credibility, quality, and integrity of the agency. The evaluation should include an examination of their reputation in the community and an analysis of staff turnover (the turnover of both administrative and field staff). State licensing boards have information regarding home health agency deficiencies that might be detrimental to patient care. To find potential agencies, consult the phone book under "Nursing" and "Home Health Services." It is also advisable to contact state home health associations for a "shopping list." Other sources include the social service, discharge planning, and utilization review departments of community hospitals. It is important to investigate services that the agencies offer to determine their "fit" with referral source needs. Home health agencies vary dramatically in the types and quality of services they provide. It is important to find an agency that is willing to work with, and within the structure of, the group practice. The agency should not only have the interests of patients in mind but also have an awareness of cost-effectiveness issues.

Another important consideration in looking for the right home health agency is the cost of services. Cost does not necessarily reflect the quality of service. As a general rule, community-based home health agencies are more cost-effective than hospital-based home health agencies. In part this is due to the fact that Medicare allows hospital-based agencies an additional 20–28 percent in reimbursement, which may artificially increase their charges. One of the best ways to evaluate an agency is to refer several patients with various diagnoses on a trial basis and then assess the results in terms of patient and physician satisfaction as well as overall cost.

The second way of making home health care available to large groups is to create a home health agency. This requires state licensure and, in some states, a certificate of need. Information as to what the requirements are can be found through the state home health association. Federal or Medicare conditions of participation must also be met, not only in order to service Medicare patients but often as a measure of quality used by private payers. The application procedure can be cumbersome and complex. Manuals specific to home care are required. It is imperative that the new agency start with administrative personnel experienced in home care. Administrative personnel requirements are determined by state and federal guidelines, which may preclude otherwise qualified candidates. For selecting the most talented home care administrative personnel, specialized knowledge of home care is invaluable. Consultant services for the interview procedure are highly recommended for those inexperienced in home care.

All home health staff must have home health experience or be trained specifically in the provision of home care. There is a shortage of experienced home health staff due to the recent rapid growth in home care. Nurses not trained in home care need to have a broad base of medical and surgical experience. Home care is a multispecialty area of health care. Field staff need to be independent, flexible, organized, reliable, and self-motivated. Home care is very specialized and differs substantially from hospital or outpatient care. Recruitment and retention are important factors in any health care organization, but they are especially important in home care because of the shortage of experienced staff and the cost of training.

Home care is very labor-intensive, as all services are provided on a one-on-one basis. Personnel costs (e.g., benefits and malpractice and workers' compensation insurance) are much higher than in other health care settings.

Billing procedures and regulations for home health are diverse and complex. Medicare has rigid guidelines that are interpreted by fiscal intermediaries. Documentation required for Medicare payments is extensive and based on cost reimbursement as defined by Medicare and interpreted by the fiscal intermediaries. Medicaid has more stringent documentation requirements and covers fewer services. Reimbursement for Medicaid home care is frequently below cost.

HMOs have cumbersome preauthorization procedures and constraints on the services they will allow under risk-sharing programs. Private insurance companies also vary in the services they will allow and the amount of coverage they will provide. In fact, many private insurers still do not have home care coverage in their policies. Insurance verification procedures are also labor-intensive. It is frequently necessary to negotiate rates and restructure policies in order to meet patient needs while working within the cost constraints imposed by insurers.

Quality assurance is an integral and necessary component of home care. There are inherent difficulties in monitoring quality in an offsite setting, especially in regard to risk management and liability concerns. Utilization review and justification for services provided are more important in home care than in outpatient or even hospital settings because of the variety of payer source guidelines. Joint Commission accreditation for home health providers is an option and may be required by specific payers and referral sources as a confirmation of the existence of quality control measures.

In evaluating the pros and cons of contracting for home health as opposed to starting a new home health agency, close attention should be given to the issues of expense, control, quality, responsibility, and liability and to the amount of business needed to offset costs.

Home care is becoming a major part of the health care system. There is a need to educate many health professionals about home care and its value as a quality, cost-effective alternative form of care provision.

REFERENCE

Scemons, D. 1990. "Home Health Care Today: Restructuring the Delivery System for Quality Patient Care." In *Home Health Care Nursing,* Stump, D. (ed.), (pp. 1–5). Danville, CA: Contemporary Forums.

24

The Telephone Challenge: From Costly Nuisance to Profitable Tool

Sandra C. Matherly and Shannon Hodges

TELECOMMUNICATIONS IN THE AMBULATORY CARE ENVIRONMENT

Each and every person working in the ambulatory care environment experiences problems with the telephone: the frustration of too many calls chasing too few providers; the feeling of being pulled away from one's "real job" in order to handle callers' questions and concerns; the inconveniences caused by telecommunications equipment that does not satisfy either patients' or providers' needs; and the (sometimes uncounted) costs, both in time and personnel, of providing adequate telephone support. People at every level of the ambulatory care organization, including physicians, administrators, nurses, and receptionists, have their own set of difficulties with the telephone, especially with regard to how the telecommunications system influences the ease with which providers can interact with patients and with one another.

The use of the telephone to assist and inform patients has achieved dramatic growth in recent years. Because of the volume of calls and the importance of the telephone in providing health care, there is an obvious need for an organized approach to the provision of information (including advice, appointments, and referrals) via the telephone. But for a variety of reasons, telecommunications remains an area in health care operations that has yet to be dealt with in a systematic way. By and large, solutions are created that fix the most obvious problems (the "firefighting" approach) but that do not systematically address the long-term needs of the organization, its physicians and staff, and its patients. We believe that a "systems" approach is the only way to arrive at telecommunication solutions that proactively anticipate and address problem areas. In such an approach, the organization needs to examine and then describe desirable solutions for the following areas (see also Figure 24-1):

1. equipment
2. personnel training and telephone roles

3. policies and procedures
4. information and documentation tools

Because of rapid changes in technology, new equipment-based solutions are continuing to evolve. But without a problem-solving approach that takes all relevant factors into account, these technological solutions will not have the desired effect, since other necessary elements of a well-planned telecommunications system such as personnel training and support will be left to chance.

The telephone and its role in ambulatory care services is a given. It will never just "go away." With the rise in patient consumerism and changes in reimbursement mechanisms, the telephone is being used more than ever before as a means of economically matching patient needs to provider services. Its role will continue to grow as health care resource conservation becomes more important.

TELEPHONE ROLES

Physicians, administrators, nurses, and receptionists can each contribute to or reduce the telephone system's effectiveness. Their different clinical or administrative roles, combined with the patients' differing expectations regarding their behavior, mean that each specialty's unique telephone problems must be evaluated if a comprehensive telecommunications solution is to be found.

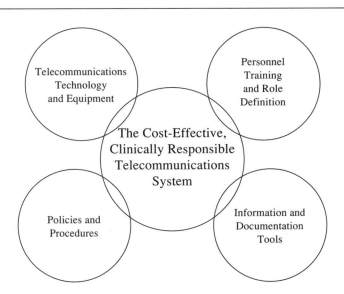

Figure 24-1 Telecommunications: A Systems Approach

Physicians

Patients often call their physicians when they are unsure about whether or not to come in or how to cope with symptoms at home. Pediatricians, for example, spend more than one-quarter of their practice time on the phone with patients (Zylke 1990). But physicians are not typically trained to deal with patients over the phone. Studies have shown that patients are typically looking for reassurance and advice when they call a physician but that physicians are oriented toward diagnosis and act accordingly (Zylke 1990). Because it is impossible to offer a medical diagnosis to a patient not evaluated in person, this mismatch of expectations results in frustration for both parties and may also influence patient compliance. Clearly the role of the physician in telephone management, and the amount of training necessary to fulfill that role, should be evaluated by the organization. Zylke observed that the amount of attention devoted to developing and evaluating teaching programs is slight compared to the amount of time spent on the telephone and potential effects on patient outcome (Zylke 1990).

Receptionists

Receptionists, though not trained to offer clinical assistance, are often placed in the role of triaging patients. In some organizations, receptionists operate in this role without a minimal safeguard of physician-approved guidelines. Even with guidelines, receptionists must rely solely on the patients' own "diagnoses," since, unlike nurses, they do not have the clinical decision-making skills that would allow them to assess the severity and urgency of problems. Using receptionists to triage patients threatens patient welfare and lays the organization open to unnecessary liability problems.

Administrators

Administrators must be concerned with the ways in which the telecommunications system is used to assist patients and communicate throughout the organization because of the potentially enormous cost of inefficiencies. It is easy, for example, to misuse clinical time with the telephone. An inadequate telecommunications system will tie up staff time and keep patients waiting or, in a worse-case scenario, will deny patients access altogether, resulting in patient dissatisfaction and lost revenues. Inappropriate telephone equipment solutions typically result in constant incremental changes, which add to the cost and confusion as staff members try to cope with new systems and procedures. Most costly of all are the potential liability problems that accompany the provision of inappropriate care and advice given over the telephone.

Nurses

Nurses contribute the largest labor force in ambulatory care and possess the basic clinical skills necessary to assess and triage the variety of callers and their problems. Forward-thinking organizations have incorporated the use of a professional telephone nursing service to solve problems ranging from increasing patient access to care to decreasing the inappropriate use of expensive medical and health care resources. Nurses are the key group for tackling the problem of how best to deal with patients over the phone. Within the framework of an organized telephone nursing service, many of the aforementioned telecommunications problems can be addressed.

TELEPHONE NURSING

Telephone nursing—the provision of health care information, assessment, triaging, and referral—is currently practiced either formally or informally by almost every nurse now working in an ambulatory care setting. Telephone nursing's new importance reflects the important changes occurring in the American health care system, especially those altering the structure of reimbursement and delivery systems. For example, patients are discharged "quicker and sicker," raising the level of acuity seen in ambulatory care environments as well as necessitating better home care support and information. These changes have created the need for highly skilled, specially trained telephone nurses and for organized telephone nursing systems. The formally recognized and supported telephone nursing program is appropriate in all ambulatory care settings and with all patient populations—in primary care as well as subspecialty areas. Studies have shown that telephone nursing services increase patient satisfaction levels (White 1989) and decrease utilization of inappropriate care ("Nurses on Call Reduce Emergency Room Visits" 1991), which is especially important in managed care settings and in organizations with a system similar to managed care, such as the Veterans Administration and the military.

Telephone nurses provide a vital link between the health care needs of people and the complex and often confusing system through which health care services are provided (see Figure 24-2). The appropriately trained telephone nurse knows the correct scope of practice (and can articulate that scope of practice); operates within well-defined organizational, professional, and nursing guidelines; can effectively assess and triage callers; and protects the organization by documenting pertinent aspects of the nurse–patient interaction.

Telephone nursing helps to address some of the biggest challenges facing providers in their attempts to provide high-quality, cost-effective care. Telephone nursing

- decreases the wasteful use of emergency settings for nonemergency care
- increases the accessibility of the health care system to all patients, regardless of their ability to pay or their familiarity with medical procedures, systems, and practitioners
- increases patient satisfaction, especially with after-hours care
- appropriately matches patients with physicians and services

Telephone nurses improve access to health care by identifying available resources. As both guides and interpreters within the health care "maze," they lower financial and informational barriers. They provide teaching to assist individuals and families in developing a broad range of health promoting behaviors. They encourage self-care by teaching health maintenance and illness prevention techniques. They are in a position to "sell" self-care and follow through with the medical regimen, which simultaneously serves the needs of patients, physicians, and an overburdened health care system.

The Multiple Functions of Telephone Nursing

Telephone nursing serves a number of important functions in a health care organization. As a patient care service, telephone nursing provides information to patients that allows them to gain access to appropriate care and make

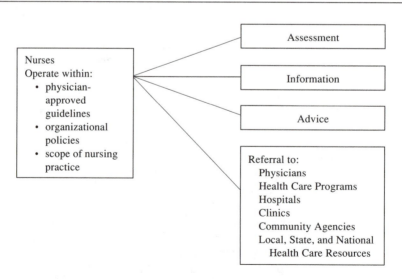

Figure 24-2 Telephone Nursing Linkages

informed decisions, while encouraging self-care and preventive measures for maintaining health. Those patients who are underinsured or uninsured obtain information that can help them to receive the right level of care at the least cost. Telephone nursing guidelines provide the nurse with a standard that, given an assessment of the caller's problem(s), identifies whether the patient needs to be seen in an emergency setting, needs to be seen in a physician's office within 24 hours, or can be self-managed at home, perhaps with further assistance from the telephone nurse or a physician. Telephone nurses may

- conduct phone interviews and assessments of callers with real or potential problems
- explain medical terms and procedures
- provide clarifying information regarding prescribed therapies and medications
- identify resources that may assist the caller such as those existing within the patient's home and family as well as physician, organizational, and community resources
- refer callers to appropriate health care providers and resources
- develop and implement caller follow-up programs
- document information to record continuity of care and protect the organization (risk management)

An important function of telephone nursing is triaging, which can help to ease the inappropriate use of emergency rooms and physician resources. Many emergency rooms not only are facing greater numbers of emergency patients (as more and more emergency rooms close their doors) but must also cope with increasing numbers of nonemergency patients who lack a primary care physician. Some of these patients can be referred to appropriate nonemergency care or can be given information on home care. One benefit of such referrals is that the patients would avoid the long waiting times faced by nonemergency patients who seek care in emergency rooms. Telephone nursing, in this scenario, is not only resource-efficient but also serves to increase patient satisfaction with access to care.

As a marketing tactic, telephone nursing matches consumer needs and wants with available health care services. The easy availability of free health care information is viewed very favorably by consumers. Telephone nursing represents an innovative way to provide convenient, fast, and potentially anonymous health care information and referral, benefiting many patient populations that find personal contact inconvenient (e.g., mothers with small children, elderly people, and working people). Some large, well-known HMO-based telephone nursing programs report that clients are consistently enthusiastic about the service. A health care organization can anticipate that its telephone nursing service will provide new patients and increase the loyalty of its current patient base.

Studies have shown that patients perceive nurses as being "safe" and "easier to talk to than physicians." Many patients "don't want to bother the doctor" when they are not sure of the import of their symptoms or problems.

As a means of managing scarce resources (e.g., physician time and emergency room space and personnel), telephone nursing assists organizations in cutting unnecessary utilization and in creating strategies to enhance patient flow and provider efficiency. Telephone nurses not only can refer patients, but can often schedule them, carry out follow-up activities for those already seen or hospitalized (helping to achieve continuity of care), and help them to gain access to the programs or providers best suited to their needs. Many organizations utilize telephone nurses in "gatekeeping" roles to minimize the use of scarce resources.

The Inevitability of Telephone Nursing

Telephone nursing is something that all ambulatory care nurses do at one time or another. The amount of time the typical nurse spends on the phone has gradually increased. For some, telephone nursing now takes up a significant portion of the day. Without an organized telephone nursing service, however, many nurses may have no formalized nursing guidelines for making assessments, no approved procedures to follow, no standardized methods of documenting calls, no structured education or training specific to nursing via the phone, no quality assurance process—in short, no means of providing consistent, high-quality care for their patients or of protecting their employers from the risks inherent in telephone nursing.

The emergency room nurse, for example, is frequently asked to speak to patients over the phone about their health problems. Nurses in private practice settings often offer advice and information to physicians' patients. Although many organizations have specific policies barring nurses from giving out information over the phone, it has been our experience that such activities do go on, even against policy. And without adequate training, many nurses do not realize the extent of the information they should and should not give out over the phone. Because many nurses are not operating under specific guidelines and policies, much of the information patients receive will lie outside the scope of telephone nursing. Without guidelines, a nurse might give out too little information (which does nothing to serve the patient or enhance cost savings); too much information (opening the organization and the nurse to liability problems); or inaccurate or outdated information.

Other programs, such as physician referral services, can end up operating as a sort of telephone nursing service in disguise. It is rare that calls to these services involve a simple referral; usually, the caller wants help with a specific illness or problem. But most physician referral services are not staffed by clinical personnel and do not have access to specific assessment guidelines. So they, too, can inadvertently place the patient and the organization at risk.

It is, therefore, in the organization's best interests to establish an organized program of telephone nursing that provides the appropriate nurses with the information, training, and resources necessary to do the job right, including the following:

- **Physician- and organization-sanctioned guidelines** for patient assessment, triaging, and referral. These assist the nurse in the assessment, problem definition, and planning phases of the call and are designed to maximize the level of information and assistance given the caller while minimizing the risk to the organization and the nurse.
- **Telephone nurse training and education,** which should focus on the nursing skills needed for assessment, triaging, resource identification, referral, documentation, and follow-up activities. Such training should emphasize the appropriate scope of nursing practice and ethical and legal issues as well as thoroughly familiarize the nurse with emergency, urgent, and nonurgent problems to facilitate correct patient triaging and information management.
- **Organizational support** such as systems for call documentation, staff selection and evaluation methods, communication equipment coordination, policies and procedures, and ongoing training and clinical consults.
- **Patient and physician information** to acquaint both consumers and affiliated physicians with the telephone nursing program's purpose, activities, and services.
- **Quality assurance policies and procedures** to monitor nursing activities and ensure that a proper standard of care is being consistently applied to all clients.
- **Adequate telephone equipment and systems.** The definition of "adequate" depends upon the organization's structure and the goals of the telephone nursing program. Considerations include the number of lines, the types of busy signals and call-holding devices, the use of call synthesizers, and linkages with computerized scheduling.

The Costs of Telephone Nursing

The additional costs of providing a fully staffed telephone nursing service can be recouped in a variety of ways. These services can both enhance revenues and decrease expenses. Revenues are affected by increases in overall market share (due to improved service and patient satisfaction levels) and by increases in referrals to affiliated specialists and programs. All areas of the organization are affected by improved patient service, increased patient satisfaction, and greater operational efficiency. Overall organizational expenses can be decreased as a result of the following:

- Increasing the efficiency of physician time (even those physicians who do not directly take calls have their time utilized by others who do).

- Redirecting many patient calls away from busy primary care areas, thus freeing those departments to concentrate more fully on patients who are actually present.

- Decreasing the number of patient complaints about access to care and information, which can result in decreased customer losses.

- Directing patients to the most appropriate level of care, which is especially important in managed care situations. For example, six months after instituting a telephone advisory nurse service, a large multispecialty clinic experienced a 15 percent decrease in visits to its emergency room, with accompanying savings to the HMO.

TELEPHONE NURSING IN DIFFERENT AMBULATORY CARE SETTINGS

Hospitals

Hospitals began to use telephone nursing to attract and retain patients. However, there are other important benefits of the service unique to the hospital environment but less apparent than marketing. These include the ability of telephone nursing to (1) support the medical staff on-call function; (2) provide discharge instructions and ongoing discharge follow-up for former inpatients; and (3) provide preadmission or preprocedure information and instructions. The telephone nursing service also provides patients with a means of dealing with the variety and complexity of services and programs offered by the hospital or medical center.

HMOs

In managed care environments, telephone nursing's ability to efficiently direct callers to the appropriate provider is an important means of reducing costs. Nurses in these organizations can serve in a "gatekeeper" role, helping to reduce nonessential visits and identifying the least costly provider appropriate for the patient's needs. Especially important is the goal of replacing the inappropriate use of the emergency room with access to other providers.

Military and Veterans Administration Ambulatory Care Centers

The benefits to these organizations are similar to those enjoyed by HMOs. In addition, the nurses can serve an important support function to those military families who may not have readily identified community or health care resources due to relocation or other dislocations resulting from active duty.

Corporate Settings

Between 1987 and 1990, the average cost of the corporate health care insurance bill rose 30 percent. Many corporations have attempted to seize control of their benefits expenses by changing the ways in which these benefits are delivered. Some have decided to self-insure; others have sought to keep costs low by cutting benefits or instituting copayment mechanisms to decrease utilization of services. Some, attempting to maintain employee benefits at their previous levels, have instituted wellness programs or provided limited medical services onsite to lessen employees' needs for expensive medical services. Whatever the mechanism used, such programs are here to stay: Most analysts believe little is being done that will slow or even control health care cost inflation in the foreseeable future.

A telephone nursing service is a creative alternative for a company facing substantial cost increases. The program can work in conjunction with the company's existing insurance and health care benefits, employee assistance programs (EAPs), and wellness and fitness programs. The telephone nursing service can be provided by an onsite nursing staff or can be contracted from local providers (hospitals, HMOs, etc.). Although it can help the company cut health care benefit costs, a telephone nursing program will not cut employees' benefits. It instead provides a new and better level of service: professional nursing advice and referral available around the clock. The limitations imposed by many insurance plans, combined with the complexity of procedures and the variety of providers available, leave many employees not knowing where to turn for information and guidance. With a telephone nursing service, employees are given one phone number to call for questions about their health and about health care options.

College Health Services

The young age of typical college students, combined with their distance from home and family and the stresses of academic life, can transform their health concerns into "emergencies." The availability of a telephone nurse to answer questions and address concerns is of real benefit to this population, who are often for the first time solely responsible for their own health care. Telephone nurses can teach preventive and self-care behaviors, match students to the right resources at the right time, and assist students in identifying their health care needs. Dissatisfaction with college health services, common among students, can fall dramatically when such a program is instituted. At one site where we helped to institute a telephone nursing service, complaints about lack of access to care dropped 90 percent.

Community Health Settings

Donation- or tax-supported community health organizations are typically strapped to the limit. Telephone nursing benefits them by creating ways of assisting callers who really don't need to be seen in person, by identifying other resources of use to their constituents, and by following up on constituents recently discharged from hospital programs.

CURRENT PROBLEMS IN TELEPHONE NURSING

Telephone nursing, while widely practiced, is often available only on an impromptu or informal basis. Although it has been estimated that over 95 percent of patient contacts with health care organizations and practitioners are through ambulatory care channels, only a small fraction of medical and nursing education focuses on ambulatory care areas. Without adequate familiarity and educational preparation, telephone contact with patients is difficult for all involved (receptionists, nurses, physicians, and administrators), and there is a heightened risk that inappropriate information or advice will be provided. The availability of nursing information without suitable guidelines and training leaves the nurses and the organization open to a host of liability questions and endangers the quality and consistency of patient care. In addition, such activities typically do not go far enough to truly enhance cost savings, as information and advice varies from nurse to nurse. Guidelines must be well thought out and then properly utilized by the nurses. Unfortunately, without good training, nurses can misuse the guidelines or not use them at all. For example, in one case a large pediatric group had prepared written guidelines that were given to each nurse in the department. In practice, however, the nurses typically consulted one another rather than the guidelines when confronted with a patient's concerns. So, even though there were guidelines, patients were still receiving personal opinions and inconsistent responses not approved by the physicians, who were all legally responsible for any information and advice given over the phone.

It has been our experience, in training dozens of telephone nurses, that many are ill informed about the appropriate scope of nursing practice. Several have expressed the opinion that nurses do offer medical diagnoses even if they aren't allowed to call them by that name. Such beliefs, and the actions that result from them, are dangerous to patients, nurses, and organizations. As was mentioned previously, orders to "not engage in telephone nursing" are met with resistance, especially in emergency settings. At one organization that we monitored, we found that even in the face of such a policy, telephone information and advice from the emergency department was regularly and frequently dispensed. During the one month we monitored this department, 500 calls were answered against stated organizational policy. When nurses are not educated in the concepts of telephone nursing, when issues like the scope of practice or the need for documentation are not addressed, nurses may not realize the importance of their telephone activities and may be inadvertently offering inappropriate or even dangerously incorrect information and opinions.

In addition, it has been our experience that many problems are being handled solely by receptionists, who are neither trained in nursing nor provided with "triaging guidelines." These individuals, who handle a high volume and great variety of calls, are only able to base triaging decisions on the callers' perceptions and their receptionists' own individual experiences and preferences. It is easy to see that many interactions with patients might be inappropriately handled by receptionists, who generally are not selected or trained to handle health care questions.

Change will only occur as organizations begin to recognize the inevitability of telephone nursing and take steps to control its provision by instituting an organized and planned service. When an organization formally decides to provide telephone nursing, it is critical that it do so completely, with adequate nurse selection and training activities, physician and administrative support, and resources designed to maximize the level of service and minimize liability risks.

SETTING UP A TELEPHONE NURSING PROGRAM

When we are charged with creating a telephone nursing program, we first begin with an assessment of the organization: its goals, strategic plan, personnel, philosophy, clientele, special patient populations, existing telephone systems, departmental organization, patient flow patterns, and the like. When we have a picture of the unique features of the organization, we then construct a program that builds on its existing strengths while ensuring that any weaknesses are counteracted by the nursing guidelines, the training program, the program policies and procedures, the program structure, and so on.

Several decisions that must be made by the organization prior to program initiation, ideally during the assessment process, are discussed below.

Populations Served. Is it the organization's desire to provide this service to all patients or to target selected groups (e.g., women, the elderly, or specialty medical populations)? Specially targeted services can be selectively marketed to a desired population, and telephone nurse training and protocols can zero in on that population's special problems, concerns, and needs.

Scheduling Considerations. Some organizations offer telephone nursing around the clock, others provide the service only when their normal office hours are over, and still others only on weekends. The decision as to the schedule should be based on considerations of physician on-call availability, patient needs, and the desired program budget (the direct cost of providing the service increases with the length of the schedule, although the actual savings may increase with the length of the schedule as well). The staff needed will depend on the anticipated volume of calls and the service's hours.

Nursing Staff. Typically, telephone nurses, who are responsible for clinical decisions, should be RNs who have had two or more years of clinical experience. LVNs have been used in certain settings, but if LVNs are used, there should be an RN in a supervisory role at all times. The RN is held accountable for judgments about whether standing orders are relevant for a particular patient and his or her particular circumstances. The telephone nurse must have the education and the expertise to decide which "path" to follow with regard to assessment. For example, a patient calling in with "indigestion" might in fact be experiencing a cardiac problem or the initial signs of appendicitis. If the nurse only goes down the indigestion path, he or she might miss a potentially critical problem. Often a caller will have predetermined how "serious" the problem is, but the nurse must do an appropriate assessment (utilizing resources and tools) of the severity and urgency of the problem if the service is to truly serve both the patient's and the organization's needs. Therefore, we recommend that the nurse's skills be viewed as a critical variable in the provision of advice. The guidelines and tools also need to be "state of the art" so as to provide the nurse with the most current information on which to base his or her assessments.

Scope of Advice. What are the boundaries set by professional nursing practice standards within which the telephone nurse can operate? State practice acts, professional nursing standards, and organizational policies and procedures should be reviewed prior to training. Some organizations initially provide very narrow guidelines regarding types of concerns that can be handled, but most often with time and experience organizations, physicians, and nurses expand into appropriate nursing practice. The decision regarding this issue, as well as decisions regarding other services issues, will determine the number and skill levels of nurses used to provide the service; the amount and level of education and training given to nurses prior to opening the program; the types of performance standards and evaluation methods used to assess the quality of the program; and the ways in which the telephone nursing guidelines are written and used.

EDUCATING THE TELEPHONE NURSING STAFF

Because there are risks inherent in giving health care information over the phone, even with the use of excellent tools and guidelines, education and training are key elements in setting up and managing a telephone nursing program. Nurses must quickly be able to engage in a number of steps that each involve clinical knowledge utilizing tools (such as computer guidelines), creative problem solving, and decision making. They must be able to ask the right questions of a caller to accurately determine the severity and urgency of the caller's problem(s). They must be able to identify risk factors within groups in the patient population and should be able to identify emergencies, "red flags," and urgent problems in all functional areas and systems—physical, psychosocial, and environmental. Most calls last less than five minutes, so telephone nurses must be able to demonstrate these skills in a fast-paced environment. Through his or her knowledge and the use of tools and systems, the nurse will be able to develop and suggest an appropriate plan of action (information, referrals, follow-up, etc.) during a successful interaction with the caller. Education in how to approach assessment and problem definition can give the nurse the skills to help the patient make the right decision.

The Training Program

The educational aspects of the program should include an explanation of the philosophy behind the program and clearly outline the scope of nursing practice. The telephone nurse must be able to define and articulate (both to callers and to other practitioners) exactly what it is that telephone nurses do as well as what they do *not* do. As previously mentioned, many nurses operate beyond the limits of what would be considered prudent or appropriate when answering patients' questions. Before the more detailed issues involved in clinical decision making can be dealt with, scope-of-nursing issues must be resolved so that all involved will be operating within the guidelines set by the organization.

Telephone nurses must be able to triage, provide health information, identify resources, and make appropriate referrals. The knowledge needed for these tasks must be integrated rather than simply "memorized." Nurses must be able to make assessments (regarding the urgency and severity of a caller's problem) quickly and accurately. Such a high level of skill and competence is a necessity from three perspectives: quality of care, cost-efficiency, and risk management. Effective telephone nursing is a difficult job, requiring specialized skills and tools. No nurse should be asked to shoulder the responsibility of this job without adequate education and supervised practice.

When we develop a program, we customize it by first determining the organization's needs and then working with physician and nurse project directors in order to create a curriculum that will meet the goals and objectives of the organization. Specific objectives, measurement criteria, and valuative processes should be established for the training program. Time should be allotted for reviewing or auditing simulated calls so that nurses can practice the concepts covered in the training and can obtain feedback on their communication and assessment skills.

Although our own training program is always customized to the specific needs of the organization and its nursing population, it inevitably includes the following elements:

- introduction to telephone nursing
- the nursing process applied to telephone nursing
- communication skills
- cultural differences influencing telephone contact
- the history: structure and process (chief complaint, present illness, past history, and review of systems) appropriate to the telephone
- coping with problem callers and problem calls
- documentation utilizing SOAP notes (in a manual or computerized format)
- practice standards
- consultation and referral
- legal issues: protecting your organization and yourself from liability problems
- the use of telephone nursing guidelines (computerized or manual)

We have found that the telephone nursing training program utilized by our firm is helpful to all ambulatory care nurses, as each one will continue to have telephone contact with patients even when centralized telephone nursing services are available. Such focused training aids an ambulatory care nurse in performing thorough assessment, problem definition, referral, and documentation activities.

Documenting Interactions

Documentation is the nurse's and the organization's *only* defense if litigation should arise. A standardized method for documenting each call should be used by the telephone nursing program. We recommend that information in the written record include

- information gathered during assessment (subjective history and objective findings obtained from listening to the caller), especially the information that leads to the problem definition and the nursing assessment of severity and urgency
- the nursing diagnosis or problem list and the nursing plan, as given to caller
- any advice, instruction, or other information given to caller
- the caller's response, including agreement or disagreement with the advice, instruction, or other information given by the nurse (if the nurse recommends that the caller go to the emergency room but the caller refuses, that refusal should be noted in the record)
- any consultation and recommendations made by other practitioners
- planned follow-up activities

FUTURE ALTERNATIVES IN TELEPHONE NURSING

Because telephone nursing has the ability to match patients with appropriate services, thereby decreasing unnecessary or inappropriate utilization, it will continue to grow in importance as health care resources become more scarce and valuable. The "linking nature" of telephone nursing also gives the service the ability to increase the accessibility of services, providers, departments, and programs within the health care setting.

We believe that, because of the growth in the number of telephone nurses and in clients' expectations, telephone nursing standards will be set and there will be a national certification in this important nursing specialty to standardize practice and ensure high-quality care and safe practices. Certification would also help answer the important question, What qualifies the nurse to give advice over the phone?

Beyond Marketing: Telephone Nursing As a New Patient Service

Although some organizations have visualized their telephone nursing program as a patient-oriented nursing service and have used it as a way of solving certain service delivery and service linkage problems, most organized programs are still driven by marketing concerns.

Telephone nursing programs were originally packaged as a means of attracting and retaining patients (for which purposes they are well suited), and they were advertised in such a way as to generate call volume and focus attention on the organization's providers and programs. But as resources become tighter, the need to offer real nursing services (e.g., preventive care information, self-management information, nursing advice, medical regimens clarification, etc.) becomes greater. This new focus requires improvements in the quality of nursing education and nursing guidelines so as to minimize risk. Some nationally marketed telephone nursing programs, for example, have nurses reporting to the marketing department, a situation that should not exist if any sort of true nursing practice is contemplated. The telephone nursing program of the future should be organized like an ambulatory care nursing service (with the appropriate level of physician guidance and administrative supervision), not simply as a means of attracting attention to the organization marketing the program. That said, it should be emphasized that, for the foreseeable future, such programs will continue to offer an attractive service for patients and will continue to differentiate organizations from their competitors.

Expanded Telephone Protocols

Innovative organizations are exploring ways to increase the level and types of services offered by telephone nurses to include the use of expanded telephone guidelines and linkages between telephone nursing and other areas of the organization. Expanding the guidelines used in telephone nursing utilizing expert systems approaches could include creating new protocols to fit common problems or patient populations encountered in the organization's specialty practice and creating some "higher-level" protocols containing more specific recommendations for care based on specific physician-approved information such as recommendations regarding commonly used over-the-counter drugs or self-care regimens. Computerized safeguards (clinical, professional, and legal) can be built into such systems. Protocol expansions such as these would carry the program a step further in its ability to decrease unnecessary utilization and provide new models of care delivery.

New Service Linkages

As previously mentioned, telephone nurses can serve a variety of functions in the health care setting. At the "front end" of the telephone interaction are the typical activities of the telephone nurse: assessing, triaging, giving health care information, and providing referrals. But it is easy to increase the range of activities to include programs for special patient populations, patient follow-up activities, special physician services, and marketing activities.

Special Patient Populations

Telephone nursing protocols and programs can be targeted to patient populations with unique and definable characteristics. Examples include oncology patients and their families, cardiac patients and their families, psychiatric and behavioral services patients, and patients utilizing home care services. Specialty telephone nursing programs would be especially attractive to organizations offering specialist services to a specific population.

Patient Follow-Up Activities

Telephone nursing can assist the organization in providing continuity of care for patients and in sharing patient information with subsequent providers. Patients can be called after telephone or in-person contact or after hospital discharge, and special guidelines can be developed to ensure that the follow-up activities are performed in accordance with departmental or organizational policies. The involvement of telephone nurses with follow-up frees other resources and is well within the legitimate purview of the service.

Special Physician Services

Because telephone nurses are specially trained to handle patient assessments via telephone, they can provide an increased level of service to on-call physicians. Some telephone nursing programs are being used as a more sophisticated version of the physician answering service, since a telephone nurse can more thoroughly apprise the physician of the caller's needs and problems. We have seen examples of other creative ways that telephone nurses are assisting physicians. For example, telephone nurses can provide "hassle-free" physician-to-physician referrals, eliminating the difficulties that often occur when physicians in outlying areas need to refer to medical center physicians or consultants.

Once physicians come to trust that the telephone nurses will only engage in appropriate practices (i.e., will not go beyond the scope of nursing practice), they often begin to utilize the nurses' services to improve the continuity of patient care and to mitigate communication problems between practitioners. In a group practice with rotating partners on call, for example, a telephone nurse can be used to relay information about patients who might contact a different physician each night because of an ongoing acute health problem. Rather than the physicians' having to repeatedly update their partners on the status of the patient, each physician can simply contact the nurse, who will provide this information to the next physician to come on call. We have found that many collaborative physician-nurse relationships develop once physicians are familiar with the strengths and limitations of the telephone nursing role.

Marketing Activities

To expand the effectiveness of a program's marketing function, the organization can work to thoroughly integrate information disseminated to the public through the telephone nursing service. The program should be sent departmental brochures, announcements, and information so that referrals can be coupled with up-to-date information. The ability of telephone nurses to "cross-sell" the organization's services is directly linked to the amount of information channeled to the telephone nursing program.

Computerized Guidelines and New Technologies

Changes in information systems technologies will have an impact on the kinds of decision-support tools that telephone nurses will have at their disposal. Currently, some telephone nursing programs utilize PC-based assessment tools. These tools can increase the quality of the telephone interaction by

- calling attention to possible "red flag" conditions necessitating further investigation by the nurse
- helping to eliminate avoidable errors such as the overlooking of important questions or conditions
- assisting in documentation efforts by providing "documentation menus" and other reminders and by performing redundant tasks
- improving the productivity of telephone nurses by making guidelines quickly accessible and easy to use
- providing the raw data needed to assess telephone nursing outcomes

With the advent of more powerful computing systems and more sophisticated software, telephone nurses could be linked into an organization's mainframe to follow up on what patients did and thus more accurately assess the real outcomes of telephone nursing interactions. Voice-activated information systems, new telecommunications technologies, and improved linkages between medical information systems will all influence the ways in which telephone nursing is delivered.

CONCLUSION

All ambulatory care practices are affected by the telephone, as are physicians, employees, and patients. The importance of the telephone to ambulatory care will continue to grow, as trends in health care delivery and reimbursement systems push organizations to offer better service while maintaining or reducing costs. The use of nurses to link patients to the variety of health care services available is just one of the ways the telephone can improve rather than detract from the delivery of patient care. Creative telephone nursing services can also serve the organization's financial, marketing, and physician-support goals; improve patient satisfaction and compliance; and position the organization to take advantage of coming improvements in communications and computer technologies that will lead to further efficiencies.

REFERENCES

"Nurses on Call Reduce Emergency Room Visits." *Wall Street Journal,* July 8, 1991.

White, Peggy. 1989. "Clients' Perceptions of the Quality of Advice by Registered Nurses in a Telephone Advisory Nurse Service." *Master's thesis,* University of Illinois.

Zylke, Jody. 1990. "Physicians Need Better Line on How, When To Respond to Patients via Telephone." *JAMA* 264.

BIBLIOGRAPHY

Brown, J.L. 1989. *Pediatric Telephone Medicine.* Philadelphia: J.B. Lippencott.

McGear, R., and Simms, J. 1988. *Telephone Triage and Management.* Philadelphia: Saunders.

Matherly, Sandra C., and Hodges, Shannon. 1990. *Telephone Nursing: The Process.* Denver: Center For Research in Ambulatory Health Care Administration.

Sinclair, Vaughn. 1991. "The Impact of Information Systems on Nursing Performance and Productivity." *Journal of Nursing Administration,* 21, no. 2.

"Telephone Nursing Can Increase Efficiency, Patient Satisfaction." 1991. *Physician's Marketing and Management,* February, p. 3.

25

Infection Control

Marjory A. O'Connor

In today's health care delivery system, many patients with infectious diseases previously treated in hospitals now receive their care in an ambulatory setting. Patients with infectious diseases of major severity, such as AIDS/HIV and hepatitis A and B, are now seen as outpatients as well as those with the more traditional outpatient diseases such as measles and flu. This increases the risk of acquiring these infections for ambulatory care personnel and other patients using the facility.

Compared to hospitals, ambulatory care has enjoyed a more permissive regulatory climate in regard to measures for the control of infectious diseases. In addition, the ambulatory sector has employed fewer professionals trained to deal with these problems. Physician outpatient practices are, therefore, frequently unprepared to cope in a consistent and effective manner with the problems and risks associated with communicable diseases. Ethical as well as legal considerations now mandate proper procedures in dealing with these conditions. This chapter presents a brief overview of factors affecting the transmission of communicable diseases, which is followed by the description of a methodology for reducing the risk of transmission of these diseases to staff and patients.

TRANSMISSION OF DISEASE

To reduce the likelihood of a communicable disease being transmitted in an outpatient setting, it is important to have an understanding of how infectious diseases sustain themselves. For a communicable disease to be transmitted, various elements must be present. Measures that afford control over one or more of these elements reduce the likelihood of transmission. These elements can be defined as follows:

- *Infectious agent.* Bacteria, virus, fungus, or parasite capable of causing disease.

334

- *Reservoir.* The milieu necessary for the survival of the infectious agent, including patients, staff, equipment, and the environment.
- *Portal of exit.* The path by which the infectious agent leaves the reservoir. Agents usually leave through body fluids such as blood, sputum, and wound drainage.
- *Means of transmission.* The means by which the agent enters the susceptible host. The entry might be by way of an inhalant such as air or water droplets or a contaminated needle or instrument.
- *Portal of entry.* The path through which the infectious agent enters the susceptible host. Common paths would include mucous membranes, breaks in the skin, and the gastrointestinal tract.
- *Susceptible host.* An individual incapable of resisting a specific infectious agent.

Not all diseases are equally infectious, nor are all people equally susceptible. Thus, of the above elements, the three most likely to affect disease transmission are the host (humans), the agent (organisms), and the reservoir (the environment).

Host susceptibility is affected by many factors, including age, sex, nutritional status, immune status, and the presence of underlying or secondary disease. Age is relevant in the case of infants and young children, since their immune systems are not fully developed, and the elderly, since their immune systems may be in decline. Gender can be a factor in urinary tract infections, for example, since their anatomical structure makes women more susceptible. Diet and nutrition can affect host susceptibility in the case of diabetics or anorexics.

Immune status is a function of the presence of antibodies in the host that can prevent or attenuate a particular infection. Individuals develop antibodies either by immunization with a specific vaccine or after recovering from an acute infection. Infection control in an outpatient setting can be enhanced by routinely providing suitable recommended vaccines to the patient population as well as keeping accurate records of immunizations and the past occurrence of contagious disease in the patients' medical records.

Underlying preexisting medical conditions can also have a dramatic effect on a patient's ability to resist infections. Diabetes, chronic obstructive pulmonary disease, and cancer are among the chronic conditions that increase susceptibility. Similarly, treatment modalities such as steroid medications, chemotherapy, and radiation therapy also adversely affect resistance. With less utilization of inpatient facilities, it is now much more common for patients with severely compromised health status to be seen in the ambulatory setting, thereby increasing the need for good infection control by the clinic.

The virulence of the agent or organism and the amount of infectious material absorbed by the host are other significant variables in disease transmission. Certain viruses such as the flu virus may vary in virulence or incidence from year to year. As a result of poor sterilization techniques, large numbers of bacteria can be transmitted to a host during a seemingly innocuous minor surgery.

The environment (reservoir) is also highly variable. Individuals in the "carrier state" of an infectious disease harbor the infectious agent (organism) but are not at the time clinically ill. Although a disease is communicable by individuals in the acute and carrier states, it is less readily identifiable in individuals in the carrier state, and therefore precautions are less likely to be taken to prevent transmission. As the number of cases and carriers in a population increases, so does the risk of transmission. Other variables affecting the environment include sanitation, crowding, seasons of the year, and the natural cycles of many of the disease entities.

Routes of Transmission

To develop a rationale for controlling the transmission of infectious diseases, the routes of transmission must be considered. Although there are four defined routes for an organism to travel from the portal of exit of the reservoir to the portal of entry of the host, more than one route may be operational at the same time. For example, chicken pox can be spread by both the contact and airborne routes. The four routes are commonly categorized as follows:

- Contact
- Airborne
- Vehicle
- Vectorborne

Contact Route

Contact transmission can occur as a result of direct physical contact between an infected person and a susceptible host. An example would be direct contact of the skin of a susceptible staff member with drainage from a patient's chicken pox vesicles. It can also occur indirectly by the transfer of organisms to a susceptible host through contaminated equipment or soiled dressings. A common example of this is the transmission of hepatitis B following a needle puncture with a contaminated needle. Another method of contact transmission involves close contact with small droplets of saliva or mucous produced by coughing, sneezing, or laughing. These droplets generally do not travel beyond a three-foot radius. Influenza and the common cold are spread in this fashion.

Airborne Route

Unlike droplet contact, which involves large particles that travel only a few feet before falling to the ground, airborne transmission involves the inhalation of very small particles that may stay suspended in the air for long periods of time. Chicken pox and measles are spread through this route. There have been several reports of measles and chicken pox being transmitted to susceptible hosts as long as 90 minutes after the patient has left the area. Exhibit 25-1 presents a list of diseases that are usually transmitted by this route.

Vehicle Route

The vehicle route transmission occurs through contaminated media such as food, water, blood, drugs, or intravenous fluid. Multiple cases of infection are often the result of vehicle transmission such as food poisoning after a picnic. Hepatitis B or AIDS contracted through contaminated blood would be another example of transmission by the vehicle route.

Vectorborne Route

Vectorborne transmission occurs when a living intermediary, such as a mosquito or tick, is the carrier of infection. Malaria, Rocky Mountain spotted fever and Lyme disease are transmitted through the vectorborne route. This route would rarely occur in a medical office.

Exhibit 25-1 Diseases Spread through the Airborne Route

- Anthrax
- Chicken pox
- Diphtheria
- Epiglottitis
- Measles
- Meningitis (H-flu, meningococcal)
- Mumps
- Pertussis
- Pneumonia (H-flu, in children)
- Rubella
- Respiratory syncytial virus
- Smallpox
- Tuberculosis (pulmonary, bronchial, laryngeal)

PREVENTION OF TRANSMISSION

Universal Precautions

Many methods are available to reduce the risk of transmitting diseases in the medical office. One preventive system, a carryover from hospital practice, is titled "universal precautions." The Centers for Disease Control (CDC) recommends implementing universal precautions to prevent the spread of pathogens such as HIV and Hepatitis B to patients and health care workers. These precautions were originally designed to protect against blood, semen, vaginal secretions, and other fluids that could act as a vehicle for transmission of these pathogens. Today, universal precautions encompass measures designed to protect against body fluid transmission of any bacteria or virus disease. Consequently, universal precautions should be observed any time there is the potential for contact with blood or body fluids, mucus membranes, or nonintact skin.

Although universal precautions will protect against many diseases, infections spread through the airborne route need special consideration. Patients with known or suspected airborne diseases should not wait in a common reception area but be placed in an exam room immediately. The door to the exam room should be kept closed, and only immune personnel should care for the patient. If the patient needs to leave the room for any reason, the patient should wear a mask. Because organisms spread through the airborne route, such as measles and chicken pox, stay suspended in the air for long periods of time, the exam room ideally should not be used by any susceptible persons for 60–90 minutes.

The following is a summary of the fundamentals of universal precautions.

1. Gloves should be put on before touching blood or body fluids, mucous membranes, or nonintact skin. They should also be used for handling items or surfaces contaminated with blood or body fluids and for performing invasive procedures.

2. Gowns or aprons should be used during any procedure where soiling with blood or body fluids is likely to occur.

3. Masks and protective eyewear or face shields should be worn during any procedures that are likely to generate droplets of blood or body fluids in order to prevent exposure of the mucous membranes of the mouth, eyes, or nose.

4. To minimize the need for emergency mouth-to-mouth resuscitation, mouthpieces and resuscitation devices should be readily available.

5. Hands should be washed before any patient contact and after removing gloves. Hands and other skin surfaces should be washed immediately and

thoroughly if contaminated with blood or body fluids. Handwashing still remains the most effective means of preventing disease transmission. Gloves do not take the place of handwashing.

Environmental Cleaning

Cleaning is the mechanical removal of all visible dirt, dust, or foreign material from both environmental surfaces and patient care equipment. Any hospital-grade, EPA-approved disinfectant detergent can be used. Products are available premixed or in concentrated form requiring dilution. Premixed products can be used until the container is empty, but products that are diluted from concentrate must be discarded weekly. It is essential to comply with the manufacturer's instructions regarding dilution and use. Solutions that have been overly diluted may be ineffective, whereas solutions that contain too much chemical can damage the surfaces and equipment. Phenols and quaternary ammonium products are generally available and acceptable disinfectants.

Cleaning schedules will vary depending on the type of surface and the amount of soil present, but of course all spills of blood and body fluids must be cleaned immediately. Exam tables, for example, should be cleaned after each patient, and the paper should be changed. Floors and horizontal surfaces should be cleaned on a regular basis—at least daily. Walls, curtains, blinds, and windows need only be cleaned when visibly soiled.

Sterilization and Disinfection

Sterilization is a process that destroys all microorganisms, including spores. Sterilization can be achieved by using heat (autoclave) or chemicals. In order for a chemical sterilant to achieve sterilization, the item must be soaked at least 6 to 10 hours. It is essential to follow the label instructions concerning temperature, time activation, and reuse. Chemical sterilants may be useful in the ambulatory environment for equipment and parts that are not disposable and that might be damaged by autoclaving.

Items requiring sterilization include those that enter sterile tissue or the vascular system such as surgical instruments, needles, scalpels, and catheters, and that, because of complexity and expense, are not disposable.

The same chemical used to sterilize can be used as a high-level disinfectant for semicritical items. Disinfection kills or destroys most disease-producing organisms except spores. When high-level disinfection is required, the item is soaked a minimum of 20 minutes. Again, it is essential to comply with the label instructions. Semicritical items include those that come into contact with mucous membranes or nonintact skin such as endoscopes, anesthesia equipment, and respiratory therapy equipment.

Before any item can be sterilized or disinfected, it must first be thoroughly cleaned. Instrument cleaners that help remove protein soils are commercially available. Noncritical items such as stethoscopes and blood pressure cuffs can be disinfected from time to time with a hospital grade, EPA-approved disinfectant.

Sterilization Process Monitoring

All autoclaves should be monitored weekly with a biological indicator (spore test). If the spore test is positive, indicating that spores are not killed, the sterilizer should be checked for proper use and function and another spore test be performed. If the second test is positive, the autoclave should be taken out of service.

The Association of Operating Room Nurses (AORN) recommends that all items processed in a suspect load be reprocessed and resterilized. However, the CDC does not require reprocessing after a single positive test.

Each load autoclaved should contain a chemical indicator that will change color to indicate that the item has been through a sterilization process, although the indicator alone does not guarantee sterility. Each load should also be checked to ensure that the proper temperature has been achieved for the appropriate length of time.

Reportable Diseases

State laws usually require physicians, dentists, and clinics to report specific diseases to the local health officer. The local health department can furnish a current list of reportable diseases and the mechanism for reporting them. Once a report is made, the date and disease being reported should be documented in the patient's medical record.

Infectious Waste

State laws define and regulate the labeling, handling, storage, and disposal of infectious waste. Local ordinances generally control waste disposal in landfills. All such regulations need to be considered when developing policies and procedures for handling infectious waste. Although individual laws vary, generally infectious waste is considered to include

- laboratory waste such as specimens, cultures, and surgery specimens or tissues removed during surgery
- blood, blood products, and equipment containing blood such as vials, dialysis equipment, and transfusion packs and tubing
- "sharps," including syringes, needles, pipettes, slides, suture needles, scalpels, and disposable instruments

Infectious waste usually does not include containers that have been emptied, gauze, bandages, dressings with dried blood, or paper products such as hand towels, gowns, or table liners.

Infectious waste must be contained in impervious bags and stored separately from other waste. These bags must be of a specific strength and color and must be appropriately labeled. Sharps must be contained in containers that are rigid and puncture- and leak-resistant. Once sealed, infectious waste and sharps must be stored in appropriately labeled rigid containers for handling and transport. Sharps containers should be sealed when three-quarters full and replaced. State laws also usually regulate the length of time infectious waste can be stored before removal. Often infectious waste can be removed from the facility only by a registered infectious waste handler. The local health department can detail the area's specific requirements.

Surveillance

Surveillance ensures compliance with infection control policies and procedures. It will vary with the scope of services being offered. Attempts should be made to identify and track infections associated with medical treatment such as surgery or invasive procedures. A urology clinic, GI lab, or ambulatory surgery center could develop monitors to identify urinary tract infections after instrumentation and gastroenteritis after endoscopy and surgical wound infections. Several simple methods may be utilized. A phone call to the patient several days after an invasive procedure could include questions concerning signs of infection. Some facilities use a postcard system. The card is sent to the physician one month after the procedure by the infection control office. The physician records any signs of infection or cultures taken and returns the card to the infection control office. Infections identified are recorded in the nosocomial statistics in the month they are identified. New infections identified within 14 days of the procedure are considered nosocomial. This tabulated information can then be reported to physicians, nurses, and administrators for any appropriate action.

Quality Assurance

Once an infection control program has been implemented, it is important to monitor the compliance and effectiveness of the program. Monitoring should be an ongoing process, and the results of the monitoring should be used to educate staff and develop or modify policies. Exhibit 25-2 is a sample of a surveillance report employed by a large group practice to monitor infection control.

EMPLOYEE HEALTH PROGRAM

With so many serious diseases treated in outpatient settings, health care workers who are employed in such settings have the potential for exposure to a variety of infectious diseases. Every new employee should have a health assessment examination. This might range from a health history or inventory to a physical examination. Emphasis should be placed on the employee's immunization status and history of preexisting conditions. The health inventory could be used to determine if a physical examination is necessary. A PPD (tuberculin skin test) should be done. Employees with a history of a positive PPD should have a chest x-ray if signs of TB are present.

Consideration should be given to immunizing susceptible employees. The current CDC recommendation for health care workers at risk of exposure to measles is at least one dose of MMR vaccine. Persons born since 1957 should have evidence of two MMR vaccinations. Flu vaccine should be offered to employees annually. Employees who might transmit rubella to pregnant patients or coworkers should be tested to ascertain immunity to rubella. OSHA regulations require health care facilities to offer Hepatitis B vaccine to all employees who have potential for exposure to blood (effective 12/1/91). OSHA regulations apply to any company with 11 or more employees.

Postexposure Care

The CDC has developed recommendations for postexposure prophylaxis for health care workers. The local health department or hospital's infection control department can provide current information on appropriate treatment.

Employee Education

All new employees should receive an orientation specific to their job assignment. In addition, principles of disease transmission, universal precautions,

Exhibit 25-2 Infection Control Surveillance Report

Location: _____ Date: _____

CRITERIA	YES	NO	COMMENTS
1. Handwashing facilities available	____	____	_____
2. Environmental	____	____	
a. Disinfectant available and labeled if required	____	____	_____
b. Walk area clean	____	____	_____
c. Tables cleaned between points	____	____	_____
d. Patient bathroom clean/facilities available	____	____	_____
e. Trash contained	____	____	_____
f. Area free of food	____	____	_____
g. Refrigerators clean, temp checked, no food present	____	____	_____
3. Universal precautions			
a. Equipment available (used for all patients; used appropriately)	____	____	_____
b. Goggles available	____	____	_____
c. Needles and sharps discarded appropriately	____	____	_____
1) Containers 3/4 full	____	____	_____
d. Staff aware of isolation	____	____	_____
1) Rooms available	____	____	_____
2) Signs available	____	____	_____
4. Disposable equipment discarded appropriately	____	____	_____
5. Reusable equipment disinfected appropriately	____	____	_____
6. Scopes disinfected/autoclaved	____	____	_____
7. Multidose vials dated when opened, discarded per policy	____	____	_____
8. Communicable disease reported to County	____	____	_____
9. Medical history includes immunization, exposure to infectious disease	____	____	_____
10. Needle sticks/exposures reported to EHS	____	____	_____
11. Infectious waste handled appropriately	____	____	_____

isolation, and employee safety should be included. Ongoing education should be encouraged. Employees requiring additional education should be identified and the appropriate information given either one on one or in a formal class setting. Pamphlets describing universal precautions and various safety issues are commercially available.

BIBLIOGRAPHY

Benensom, A. 1985. "Control of Communicable Diseases in Man." In *The American Public Health Association.* 14th ed.

Berg, R. 1988. *The APIC Curriculum for Infection Control Practices.* Vol. 3. Dubuque, Ia: Kendall/Hunt Publishing Company.

Bradford, M., and Flynn, N., 1988. "Ambulatory Care Infection Control Quality Assurance Monitoring." *American Journal of Infection Control* 16: 21A–28A.

Flanders, E., and Hinnant, J. 1990. "Ambulatory Surgery Postoperative Wound Surveillance." *American Journal of Infection Control* 18: 336–339.

Garner, J., and Favero, M. 1985. "Guidelines for Handwashing and Hospital Environmental Control, 1985." *Hospital Infections Program,* Centers for Disease Control, U.S. Public Health and Human Resources, Atlanta, Ga.

Garner, J., and Simmons, B. 1983. "CDC Guidelines for Isolation Precautions in Hospitals." *Hospitals Infections Program,* Centers for Disease Control, Atlanta, Ga.

"Guidelines for Prevention of Transmission of HIV Virus and Hepatitis B Virus to Health Care and Public Safety Workers." 1989. *Morbidity and Mortality Weekly Report,* June 23.

"Head Lice and Scabies Infestation, Update on Control Measures." 1990. *California Morbidity,* November 30.

"Measles Prevention: Recommendations of the Immunization Practices Advisory Committee." 1989. *Morbidity and Mortality Weekly Report,* December 29.

Principle of Epidemiology. 1980. Atlanta, Ga.: Centers for Disease Control.

"Protection against Viral Hepatitis: Recommendations of the Immunization Practices Advisory Committee." 1990. *Morbidity and Mortality Weekly Report,* February 9.

"Recommendations for Prevention of HIV Transmission in Healthcare Settings." *Morbidity and Mortality Weekly Report,* August 21.

"Report of the Committee on Infectious Diseases." 1988. In *American Academy of Pediatrics.* 21st ed. Elk Grove Village, IL.

"Rubella Prevention: Recommendations of the Immunization Practices Advisory Committee." 1990. *Morbidity and Mortality Weekly Report,* November 23.

Rutala, William A. 1990. "APIC Guidelines for Selection and Use of Disinfectants." *American Journal of Infection Control,* Vol. 18, no. 2, (April 1990), pp. 99–177.

Schuman, L. 1980. *Principles of Epidemiology.* Atlanta, Ga.: Centers for Disease Control, Bureau of Training.

Soule, B. 1983. *The APIC Curriculum for Infection Control Practice,* Vol. I & II. Dubuque, Ia.: Kendall/Hunt Publishing Company.

26

Patient Classification in Ambulatory Care

Judith Moore Johnson

Patient classification is a general term and may refer to many types of categorization such as diagnosis, reason for visit, and so on. This chapter uses the term *patient classification system* to refer to the methodology that categorizes patients for the amount of nursing care required. The reader who is unfamiliar with the basic concepts of patient classification as it relates to nursing workload is referred to the classical article by Phyllis Giovannetti (1979), "Understanding Patient Classification Systems."

PATIENT CLASSIFICATION SYSTEM COMPONENTS

A patient classification system comprises five components:

1. patient classification instruments
2. quantification of nursing care hours per class
3. validity and reliability measurements
4. system reports
5. ongoing system maintenance mechanisms

Patient Classification Instruments

A patient classification instrument is a physical document used by a nurse to determine a patient's class or category. There are dozens of patient classification instruments in use, most of them modifications or versions of two basic types of instruments: prototype evaluation and factor evaluation instruments. A *prototype evaluation instrument* uses broad descriptive categories to classify patients. A *factor evaluation instrument* uses specific elements of care for which the patient is rated independently; the ratings on each element are combined to place the patient in the overall category.

345

In determining classes or categories of patient care, the instruments attempt to establish groups that are mutually exclusive. *Critical indicators of care* are the indicators that are most crucial to the correct identification of a patient's category of care.

Quantification of Nursing Hours per Class

Quantification is the process of determining the hours of care for each category or class. The hours of care per class are predetermined in some systems, whereas others are site-specific and determined through observational sampling. *Observational sampling* is the onsite tracking of all nursing caregivers' activities on a representative sample of shifts to determine the amount of time nurses spend in direct and indirect care as well as unit-related and personal activities. *Direct patient care* is care delivered in the presence of the patient and/or family. It includes activities such as education, psychosocial support, administering medications, and monitoring vital signs. *Indirect patient care* includes activities done for the benefit of an individual patient but not in his or her presence such as preparing medications, arranging referrals, ordering tests, and calling the physician. Also tracked are unit-related time and personal time. *Unit-related activities* are those activities not directed at individual patients but performed for the good of all patients such as meetings and phone calls to or from patients not on the unit. *Personal activities* includes breaks, lunches, and socialization among staff. The data from an observational sampling study are used to determine the hours of care per class and to determine the number of staff required to deliver the care.

Validity and Reliability Measurements

Validity and reliability are generally established during the installation of a patient classification system. Without evidence of validity and reliability, the manager using the patient classification system data has no way of knowing how accurate or representative the data are.

Validity is the degree to which an instrument measures what it purports to measure. Several types of validity are important in patient classification. *Content validity,* which is based on the judgment of nurse experts, is the ability of the instrument to represent the area it is meant to measure. *Face validity,* a version of content validity, specifies the degree of agreement among users that the instrument seems reasonable and representative. *Criterion-related validity* includes *predictive validity,* which is determined by comparing the nurses' classifications with observational sampling data.

Reliability is the consistency or repeatability of an instrument. Usually this means that two nurses classifying the same patients will arrive at the same class. This form of reliability is known as *interrater reliability*.

System Reports

System reports are those reports that are compiled by using data associated with patient classifications, corresponding workloads, and available staff. In recent years, with the onset of inexpensive and timely computer options, rich data bases and user-defined reports have enhanced the usefulness of patient classification system data.

Ongoing System Maintenance Mechanisms

Ongoing system maintenance includes educating nursing staff and managers to use the instruments and reports, monitoring validity and reliability, and modifying the instruments and/or hours of care as the need arises.

REVIEW OF THE LITERATURE

Until recently, patient classification has been primarily associated with inpatient acute care settings. Today, developments in reimbursement practices mandate that increasingly complex care be provided in outpatient settings. This movement of care to ambulatory practices brings with it the need for more sophisticated nursing and nursing information systems. Staff and patient scheduling, budget planning and tracking, productivity monitoring, and the gathering of costing and charging data must become standard activities in the management of the nursing service (see Exhibit 26-1).

A major step forward in categorizing ambulatory patients occurred in an innovative practice setting at Nokomis Clinic in Minneapolis. As part of the University of Minnesota Medical School's Department of Family Practice and Community Health, Nokomis Clinic was a site for testing practice systems (Solberg and Johnson 1981). The amount of time and the types of providers (physician, physician's assistant, medical assistant, or family nurse) to be seen were determined by several patient categories: new or returning patient, age, and type of visit (acute minor illness, chronic condition, follow-up, complete physical). The amount of time for which the patient was scheduled was based on experienced estimates of the staff providing the services. This categorization of patients for time and providers worked well in that middle-class practice.

Exhibit 26-1 Objectives of Patient Classification Systems in Ambulatory Care

---

- Budget planning and tracking
- Budget justification of needed positions
- Description of clinic activities
- Staffing utilization data (productivity and efficiency)
- Staffing trending and planning
- Costing of care
- Charging for care
- Nursing research links with:
  —Ambulatory visit groups
  —ICD-9 codes
  —Procedure codes
  —Nursing minimum data sets
  —Nursing diagnoses
- Quality assurance:
  —Tracking of primary nurse care delivery
  —Assessment of appropriate use of skill levels
  —Quality of care delivered using site-specific definitions
  —Evaluation of equity of nursing assignments
  —Costing of research protocols

The daily schedule became the (manual) data initiation point for tracking patient and staff information such as staff productivity, charges, and patterns of appointments.

While categorizing patients for types of visit has gone on for almost two decades (Schneider and Appleton 1977; Hastings 1987), the specific use of patient classification systems to measure nursing workloads is fairly new. Most of the literature that describes efforts to develop a patient classification system or study ambulatory care nursing can be found in the nursing literature of the last decade, with the exception of a reference manual developed in the late 1950s (Adams 1957) and published by the Department of Health, Education, and Welfare. This manual suggests several methods for studying ambulatory care and highlights many of the difficulties in conducting studies, including the episodic nature of care, the large volume of patients, and the costliness of conducting research. Adams's study areas focus on supportive care, continuity of patient care, and patient education. Hastings (1987) echoes Adams and also describes the problems arising from the large volume of phone calls and the coordination of care activities for patients who are not presently in the clinic.

Several patient classification or nursing workload studies have been conducted in ambulatory care, all with limitations. Self-report studies have been the most common. Henninger and Daily (1983) described a self-report study conducted at the Johns Hopkins Oncology Center. In this study, nurses used a checklist of direct care activities and a tally sheet for reporting indirect and unit-related activities. One of the strengths of this study was its effort to account for the time spent in meetings, care conferences, and other unit-related tasks. The time spent on a procedure was converted to a relative value index standard. To this standard, a component of fixed time (unit-related care) was added. The results of the study were used to plan future staffing.

Another self-report study was conducted at Henry Ford Hospital in six internal medicine clinics (Genovich-Richards and Tracy 1984). The nursing staff listed their nursing tasks and estimated the time required to perform the tasks and the frequency with which the tasks occurred during the shift. Average times for activities were derived by applying a multiple regression model to the tasks and times data. Only direct patient care activities were assessed in this study, which took place in a private office group practice and utilized nonprofessional nursing staff. The study did not take into account the range of activities performed by professional nurses, which include education and case management.

None of the self-report methods appear to be used on an ongoing basis. Rather, the studies were done for specific, immediate purposes. Other research-ers have developed systems or suggested methodologies for ongoing use. Hoffman and Wakefield (1986) describe an approach for developing an ambu-latory system using the familiar inpatient factor evaluation model. The steps they propose for developing an instrument include identifying relevant patient care factors, estimating times for the activities, and conducting a self-report or observational study. No mention is made of the daily use of the instrument once it has been developed, how validity would be maintained, how reliability would be monitored, or how the instrument would be kept current.

Smith and Elesha-Adams (1989) describe the development of an instrument for the student health service at East Carolina University. They extend their criteria to include, in addition to those listed above, a monitoring mechanism and a method for modification of the instrument if required. No discussion of these additional components or developments appears in the article.

Verran's (1986a) work at the University of Arizona focuses on the develop-ment of a taxonomy of nursing care activities rated by experts for complexity. The original purpose of the data was not to quantify workload, though some ambulatory settings have used modifications of the Verran taxonomy for classi-fication purposes (Giovannetti and Burkhalter 1988). The author of this chapter also spoke informally to managers in two ambulatory care settings who have applied average care times to nursing care descriptions. In these settings, the instruments are used on an ongoing basis.

The Verran taxonomy was employed at Tulane Medical Center as one of three sources of data used to plan staffing (Miller and Folse 1989). Average times were assigned to the nursing care activities for direct patient care. Unit-based activities were identified, and the frequency and times of these activities were determined through self-reporting. These two components, together with

average-census-by-day-of-week data, were used to develop staffing requirements and adjust daily staffing. In this setting, the system is not used on a daily
basis to collect patient-specific data but only used once annually to identify
changes in care delivery.

At Strong Memorial Hospital (University of Rochester), an inpatient instrument was modified for use in the ambulatory surgery center (Parrinello 1987).
Ambulatory surgical indicators were used and nursing care hours established
through a self-report mechanism. The article reports on the study process; it is
not clear if the instrument was used on an ongoing basis.

A recent study conducted at the National Institutes of Health (NIH) in the
Ambulatory Care Research Facility (ACRF) evaluated Verran's taxonomy and
three established inpatient instruments modified for ambulatory care
(Giovannetti and Burkhalter 1988; Johnson 1989). The four instruments (Verran,
Saskatchewan, San Joaquin, and ARIC) were used by 10 of the ACRF clinics.
Each instrument was used for five consecutive clinic days. The professional
nurse who cared for the patients classified them and completed several additional questions about the patients and the instrument. Reliability was monitored using the method described by Verran (1986b), in which the nurse
classifier tapes an account of the patient and the expert classifier then classifies
the patient. The two classifications were then compared for agreement. At the
end of four weeks the nurses in the study clinics were asked to rate each
instrument using the selection criteria established earlier in the study. The
Verran and ARIC instruments scored favorably and higher than the other
instruments. As this component of the study only evaluated user acceptability
and face validity, additional factors such as adaptability to the research setting,
onsite development of clinic-specific critical indicators, onsite validation, and a
computerized data base structure prompted the selection of ARIC, as ARIC
provides for these considerations.*

Implementing a patient classification system in ambulatory care is difficult.
Exhibit 26-2 summarizes some of the problems encountered in developing
ambulatory care systems.

FUTURE USES OF PATIENT CLASSIFICATION SYSTEMS

The future uses of patient classification data will depend to a large extent on
the accuracy of the data. If ambulatory patient classification systems can be
developed that are valid, reliable, and easy to modify as case mix changes, the

---

* ARIC (Allocation, Resource Identification and Costing) is a nursing information system developed by James
Bahr Associates of Plymouth, Michigan. The ARIC system software and documentation are protected under U.S.
copyright laws and trade secret laws. Patents covering many of ARIC's unique features are pending.

Exhibit 26-2 Problems in Developing a Patient Classification Instrument for Ambulatory Care

- New critical indicators reflecting the nature of ambulatory care need to be developed.
- Ambulatory nursing and inpatient nursing use different nursing technologies.
- There is no existing national data base for ambulatory nursing.
- Workload and staffing requirements must be retrospective.
- There is little time available to classify patients.
- The patient populations change over time.
- The specialization of nursing functions often makes reallocation of staff impractical.
- The scheduling of patients is difficult, because of overbooking, walk-ins, emergencies in and out of the clinic, and missed appointments.
- The patients may be in clinic or on the phone.
- Ambulatory care is episodic rather than continuous.
- The treatment period is unclear—treatment continues after the patient leaves the facility.
- The workload capacity is surpassed as a result of walk-ins, phone calls, and emergencies to which physicians must respond.
- The patients are in control of their arrival time.

information can be used for "productivity monitoring, long range planning, budgeted staff tracking, trend analysis, costing, charging, and the linking of patient classification data to a wide range of pertinent data such as quality data, nursing diagnosis, and medical diagnosis . . . negotiating contracts with HMO's, evaluating trends in patient care demands, and generally minimizing risks" (Giovannetti and Johnson 1990).

As the patient classification system becomes more integrated with other data bases, the data can be linked almost endlessly for purposes of management analysis. For example, a grievance filed by a staff member alleging unfair patient assignments can be viewed more objectively when assignments, patient visit types, and the patient classifications of the complaining staff member are compared with other staff of the same rank.

NURSING INFORMATION SYSTEM REQUIREMENTS

A nursing information system has several requirements if it is going to be useful as a management tool in ambulatory care:

1. The system needs an *accurate patient classification* component that reflects the nursing workload. The patient classification system needs to be responsive to changing populations of patients, have demonstrable reliability and validity, and be simple to use on an ongoing basis.
2. The information system needs to be *staff-specific* to enable the manager to determine which staff are caring for which patients.

3. The information needs to be *patient-specific* so that age, sex, reason for visit, procedures, research protocols, primary nurse, nursing diagnoses, and medical diagnoses may be linked for research, quality assurance, costing, and charging purposes.

4. The system must use *computer hardware that allows for growth.* The hardware must be affordable.

5. The computer software must be written with a data base development system that allows for *site-specific tables and values* that can be maintained and modified by the user.

6. The software must include an *ad hoc report design and development capability.*

7. The software must provide for *ease in dealing with large patient volumes.*

8. The software must have *built-in accuracy checks.*

ARIC-A SYSTEM

ARIC-A (Allocation, Resource Identification and Costing—Ambulatory) is an ambulatory care patient classification system that appears to meet the above requirements. ARIC-A has a well-defined methodology for implementation, which is outlined in the following steps:

1. Identification of clinical areas with unique sets of dependent orders.
2. Identification of clinic-specific dependent orders and times.
3. Identification of clinic-specific critical indicators.
4. Definition of independent nursing functions.
5. Development of clinic-specific instruments.
6. Instruction in the use of instruments.
7. Establishment of reliable use of instruments.
8. Validation of instruments.
9. Ongoing use of the system.
10. Implementation of system maintenance mechanisms.

The time needed to implement this system is about 18 weeks. An example of a clinic-specific ARIC-A classification instrument appears in Exhibit 26-3.

Daily Use of the System

The day-to-day use of the instrument involves a plan to use patient and staff data from preexisting systems as well as daily classification of patients. The

Exhibit 26-3 ARIC Classification Instrument—Oncology Clinic

DEPENDENT DESCRIPTION (Range)	INDEPENDENT NEEDS	CODE	CLASS
Type S (0–10 min)	Very Low (0–15 min)	V	1
Type A (11–29 min)			
Blood Pressure and Heart Rate	Very Low (0–15 min)	V	1
Height, Weight, Temperature	Low (16–30 min)	L	2
Oral or Topical Meds	Moderate (31–60 min)	M	2
Assist with Physical Exam	High (1–2 hrs)	H	3
	Extremely High (>2 hrs)	X	3
Type B (0.50–1.49 hrs)			
Blood Pressure and Heart Rate	Very Low (0–15 min)	V	3
Height, Weight, Temperature	Low (16–30 min)	L	3
Oral, IM, Sub Q, Topical Meds	Moderate (31–60 min)	M	3
Venous Blood Draw-Single	High (1–2 hrs)	H	4
Assist with Physical Exam	Extremely High (<2 hrs)	X	4
Urinalysis			
Type C (1.50–2.49 hrs)			
Blood Pressure and Heart Rate	Very Low (0–15 min)	V	4
Height, Weight, Temperature	Low (16–30 min)	L	4
Chemotherapy	Moderate (31–60 min)	M	4
Venous Blood Draw	High (1–2 hrs)	H	4
	Extremely High (2 hrs)	X	4
Type D (2.50–3.49 hrs)			
Blood Pressure and Heart Rate	Very Low (0–15 min)	V	4
Height, Weight, Temperature	Low (16–30 min)	L	4
Chemotherapy	Moderate (31–60 min)	M	4
Standard Protocol Instructions	High (1–2 hrs)	H	5
Bone Marrow Biopsy	Extremely High (>2 hrs)	X	5
Venous Blood Draws-Serial			
Type E (3.50–4.49 hrs)			
Blood Pressure and Heart Rate	Very Low (0–15 min)	V	5
Height, Weight, Temperature	Low (16–30 min)	L	5
Standard Protocol Instructions	Moderate (31–60 min)	M	5
Chemotherapy, Complex	High (1–2 hrs)	H	5
Venous Blood Draws-Serial	Extremely High (>2 hrs)	X	5
IV Fluids			
Type F (4.50 hrs & over)			
Blood Pressure and Heart Rate	Very Low (0–15 min)	V	6
Chemotherapy, Complex	Low (16–30 min)	L	6
Blood/Blood Products	Moderate (31–60 min)	M	6
Venous Blood Draw-Serial	High (1–2 hrs)	H	6
Standard Protocol Instructions	Extremely High (>2 hrs)	X	6
IV Fluids			
Transfusion, Blood, Blood Products			

Source: ARIC Patient Classification Instrument. Copyright James Bahr Associates, 1988.

method used in a given site will depend on the availability of preexisting systems such as a patient scheduling system and a nurse scheduling system. For example, an appointment document could be designed that obtains the patients' names and the times they are scheduled from the patient scheduling system. Nurse staffing data may be preprinted on the data entry form in one of two ways. If the staffing is stable and constant, it can be printed as default data. That is, the system assumes that all staff are on all schedules for a certain number of hours. Entries then are needed only to change the default data: The nurse called in sick, left one hour early, went to a conference, and so on. If there is a nurse scheduling system, that data can be downloaded to the classification form. This staff schedule again is modified by exception from what was planned.

Items required by the patient classification system as well as additional site-specific data elements are identified and placed on the patient classification form (Exhibit 26-4). If no automation is available for staff or patients, the information can be manually placed on the form. Data in the ARIC-A system are patient- and staff-specific. Patient and staff data are stored in the system's data base, and the system retrieves the data by name or identification number.

Patient-specific data include caregiver identifications and patient classifications. Additional data are user-defined and can be set as optional or required. One site identified the following additional data elements: research division, physician, visit type (screening, active treatment, follow-up, consult, emergency, other), procedures performed, and research protocol. All of these data elements are built into tables in the software to facilitate data entry. Other types of data that might be useful include CPT codes, ICD-9 codes, supplies and medications used, Ambulatory Visit Group, and other billing data. The combination of these data might be used at least for costing purposes and possibly for charging. When entering data into the computer, built-in accuracy checks are performed by the software to prevent data entry errors.

Patients are classified immediately after being seen in the clinic by the nurse who provided the care. For example, a cancer patient coming into the oncology clinic for chemotherapy would be rated at the time of departure after all care had been delivered.

The following case study may help to illustrate the process.

Case Study

Barbara Burton is a 47-year-old woman receiving a course of I.V. chemotherapy. In this oncology clinic, the nurse takes the patient's blood pressure and weight, assesses her physical and emotional status, provides psychological support, and instructs her on the possible side effects of the medication. The nurse draws blood for a CBC and chemistry profile and starts an I.V. When the blood analysis is completed, the physician reviews the results, meets with the

Exhibit 26-4 Daily Clinic Census and Staffing Report

Date: _____ Cost Center: _____

	Staff Information							Patient Information									
No.	ID	Name	Func.	Begin	End	Hours Worked	No.	ID	Name	Time	Type	Dep.	Ind.	Class	Nurse No.	Proc.	Other
1	5288	Olson J	RN	8:00	17:00	8.0	1	47140	Burton B	9:15	3	C	M	4	1	04	
2																	
3																	
4																	
5																	
6																	
7																	
8																	
9																	
10																	
11																	
12																	
13																	
14																	
15																	
16																	
17																	
18																	
19																	
20																	

Visit Types: 1. Initial Visit 2. Follow-up (routine) 3. Chemotherapy 4. Follow-up (long-term) 5. Emergency 6. Other
Source: Courtesy of Wellcare Ambulatory Care Services, Minneapolis, MN.

patient briefly, and orders the I.V. chemotherapy. (On this visit, because Ms. Burton is an established patient, the physician time is only about 10 minutes.) The nurse gives the I.V. medication over an hour, monitoring the patient intermittently. At the conclusion of the visit, Ms. Burton asks the nurse to assist her with arranging transportation for future visits. This takes an additional 10 minutes of nursing time. A future appointment is also arranged, as ordered by the physician.

The nurse goes to the daily clinic census and staffing report (Exhibit 26-4) at the nurses' station and classifies the patient, using the classification instrument (Exhibit 26-3) as a guide. As required in the case of all patient classification instruments, the nurse uses professional judgment in classifying the patient.

The nurse first identifies the dependent description that best fits the doctor-driven care (in this example, Type C). Then the independent needs category (education, psychosocial support, and coordination of care) that is most appropriate is selected (in this example, M for moderate). The dependent and independent categories are combined to determine the care category or class: 4. The nurse enters six data elements into the daily clinic census and staffing report: visit type (see the user-defined legend printed at the bottom of the form), dependent category, independent category, patient classification, nurse number, and procedure code. The procedure code is optional; in this example, 04 is entered for "Chemo I.V. complex." The classification process takes about 20 seconds per patient.

The following day, the data are entered into the computer. The system may already contain the patient schedule and nurse staffing data, which are only modified if changed. Thus, only the six data elements the nurse marked are entered. Data entry may be done directly into the computer by the caregiver, bypassing the manual step if there are clinic-based terminals.

ARIC-A System Reports

One of the benefits of any patient classification system is the financial and productivity information generated. The ARIC-A system produces nursing workload reports as well as other reports, depending on the types of data entered. Reports may be generated for any time intervals (daily, weekly, monthly, quarterly). The most common reports are listed below and described briefly by recommended frequency.

Daily Reports

Visits by Visit Type and Care Required. This report (Exhibit 26-5) gives the total number of visits in each user-defined category, summarizes the total care

Exhibit 26-5 Visit by Visit Type and Care Required and Delivered

Visit Type	Visit Description	No. of Visits	Care Hours Required	Care Hours Available
1	Screening	163	346.46	
2	Active treatment	550	1991.49	
3	Follow-up	261	451.81	
4	Consult	13	19.37	
5	Other	4	33.92	
Totals		991	2843.05	1818.75

For Dates: 8/1/90–8/31/90   Cost Center: ONC   Department: OPD

Source: Courtesy of Wellcare Ambulatory Services, Minneapolis, MN.

hours required using patient classification data, and compares required care hours with available care hours using staff hours worked data.

Visits by Patient Classification. This report lists the number of patients in each classification group and the total care hours for each group. Total required hours is compared with available work force. (Required hours include both variable and fixed time.) This report assists the administrator in evaluating the mix of visit types and its implications.

Weekly Reports

Visits by Day of Week. Each clinic is reported separately by day of week, with totals for the department by day of week. This report helps analyze whether the patient schedules are efficient.

Census and Classification by Day of Week. Each clinic is reported separately, with the number of visits for each patient classification shown for each day of the week. Total visits for each day and totals for each classification for the week are provided. This report will assist the administrator in evaluating not only patient volume but patient complexity.

Procedures Performed by Day of Week. Procedures codes (up to 99) may be defined for each clinic. The codes are listed along with the frequency of each procedure by day of the week as well as daily and weekly totals. This report (Exhibit 26-6) will assist the administrator in evaluating productivity and utilization of special equipment and staff.

Caregiver Summary. This report (Exhibit 26-7) provides a daily or weekly summary (or a summary for a longer period) of the number of patients in each

Exhibit 26-6 Procedures Performed by Day of Week

For Dates: 8/1/90–8/31/90   Cost Center: ONC   Department: OPD   Clinic: Oncology

Procedure Code	Description	Sun	Mon	Tues	Wed	Thu	Fri	Sat
01	Adm chem IV/IM simple		8	3	5	3	9	
02	Chemo premed IV/IM		50	59	89	58	29	3
03	Adm chemo IV interm		46	44	74	44	44	6
04	Adm chemo IV complex		54	75	69	59	34	
05	Adm chemo pump refill		8	5	6	11	8	
06	Intra-arterial chemo		1					
07	Adm medication IM/SQ/IV		17	9	22	12	15	1
08	Adm antibiotics		2	1	2	1	1	
09	IV hydration		84	73	84	66	74	1
10	Amphotericin infusion		1		1			
11	Platelets transfusion		2	2	4	2	4	1
12	RBC transfusions 1st unit		5	6	12	7	10	2
Totals			278	277	368	253	219	14

Total Procedures: 1419

Source: Courtesy of Wellcare Ambulatory Services, Minneapolis, MN.

clinic by caregiver. RN-only visits and the RNs' workload requirements are compared with the RNs' available hours. This report provides the clinic manager with a tool for evaluating equity and appropriateness of assignments.

Workload and Service Level by Day of Week. This report lists number of visits, required workload, and available work time by day of week. A service level (productivity) percentage is calculated by dividing the available work time by the required workload. This report assists the administrator in evaluating productivity.

Monthly Reports

Trend Report by Cost Center. This report lists the required workload, available work time, visits, and percentage change in required workload and visits. It provides trending information for planning as well as a method for judging growth predictions.

Trend Report by Protocol. An example of a user-designed report by clinic and research protocol, it depicts the monthly required workload and percentage change from the previous month by research protocol.

Exhibit 26-7 Caregiver Summary

For Dates: 8/1/90–8/31/90		Cost Center: ONC	Department: OPD			
Name	# Patient Visits	RN Visits	Available Work Time (hrs)	Dependent Workload (hrs)	Independent Workload (hrs)	Total Workload (hrs)
Johnson, J	2	0	3.0	11.96	1.54	13.80
Olson, O	217	10	400.0	22.53	19.58	41.50
Peterson, P	181	20	410.0	31.30	23.47	55.00
Swanson, S	2	0	8.0	4.09	5.57	9.75
Nelson, N	3	0	24.0	22.57	9.72	32.38
Totals	405	30	106.0	92.45	59.88	152.33

Source: Courtesy of Wellcare Ambulatory Services, Minneapolis, MN.

Total Patients by Cost Center. This report depicts the number of visits by patient classification and associated required workload.

WHO NEEDS A PATIENT CLASSIFICATION SYSTEM?

Ambulatory care settings all have a need to track and analyze patient visit data. At what point is the *nursing workload* data sufficiently important in terms of costs to justify close monitoring of resources? No single dollar or FTE amount serves as a guide. Certainly an ambulatory care setting that is large enough to have a nursing director, head nurses, and staff nurses with its own budget and cost centers will benefit from patient classification data.

The primary cost of a nursing division is labor. Tracking productivity and providing the budget justification that can reduce or more appropriately allocate staffing by even a single FTE is worthwhile. It is important that nursing management in large facilities be able to respond by cross-training and cross-staffing whenever possible. In certain areas where reimbursement may be modified by documenting exceptions (for example, chronic hemodialysis) patient classification data will provide accurate nursing care evidence of patient needs.

The ARIC-A system was first installed in a large ambulatory care facility with 13 major outpatient care areas, approximately 100 nursing staff, and 70,000 visits per year. Facilities of this complexity and patient volume certainly will benefit from patient classification data. Other types of settings that would benefit from a patient classification system in addition to research and university/tertiary care centers include large HMO outpatient settings such as Group Health, Inc. and Kaiser Permanente. The ability to track nursing activities accurately may be crucial in determining budgets, negotiating contracts, and monitoring staff utilization.

REFERENCES

Adams A. 1957. "How To Study the Nursing Service of an Outpatient Department." Washington, DC: U.S. Government Printing Office.

Genovich-Richards, J., and Tracy, R. 1984. "An Assessment Process for Nursing Staff Patterns in Ambulatory Care." *Ambulatory Care Management* 5: 69–79.

Giovannetti, P. 1979. "Understanding Patient Classification Systems." *Journal of Nursing Administration* 9, no. 2: 4–9.

Giovannetti, P., and Burkhalter, B. 1988. "Test and Monitor Patient Classification Systems." Final Report. Contract NO-CL-7-2101. Bethesda, MD.: National Institutes of Health.

Giovannetti, P., and Johnson, J. 1990. "A New Generation Patient Classification System for Nursing." *Journal of Nursing Administration* 20, no. 5: 33–40.

Hastings, C. 1987. "Classification Issues in Ambulatory Care Nursing." *Ambulatory Care Management* 10, no. 3: 50–64.

Henninger, D., and Daily. 1983. "Measuring Workload in an Outpatient Department." *Journal of Nursing Administration* 13, no. 9: 23–33.

Hoffman, F., and Wakefield, D. 1986. "Ambulatory Care Patient Classification." *Journal of Nursing Administration* 16, no. 4: 23–30.

Johnson, J. 1989. "Quantifying an Ambulatory Care Patient Classification Instrument." *Journal of Nursing Administration* 19, no. 11: 36–42.

Miller, P., and Folse, G. 1989. "Patient Classification and Staffing in Ambulatory Care." *Nursing Economics* 5, no. 4: 167–72.

Parrinello, K. 1987. "Accounting for Patient Acuity in an Ambulatory Surgery Center." *Nursing Economics* 5, no. 4: 167–72.

Schneider D., and Appleton, L. 1977. "Reason for Unit Classification System for Patient Records in the Ambulatory Care Setting." *Quality Review Bulletin* (January): 20–26.

Smith, S., and Elesha-Adams, M. 1989. "Allocating Nursing Resources in Ambulatory Care." *Nursing Management* 20, no. 1: 61–64.

Solberg, L., and Johnson, J. 1981. "Physician and Nurse." In *A Manual for Collaboration*. Minneapolis, MN: University of Minnesota Medical School.

Verran, J. 1986a. "Patient Classification in Ambulatory Care." *Nursing Economics* 4, no. 5: 247–61.

Verran, J. 1986b. "Testing a Patient Classification Instrument for the Ambulatory Care Setting." *Research in Nursing and Health* 9: 279–87.

Part IV

Support Services

27

Case Management

Nancy Parliman Brown, Gloria Gilbert Mayer, and
Linda K. Jackson

Providing health care to the frail elderly, chronically ill, high-risk perinatal, or high-risk adult patient in the ambulatory setting provides new and exciting challenges for health care providers. Traditional health care delivery systems must be operationally restructured to meet the needs of these patients. An interdisciplinary case management model provides an exemplary framework for the restructuring process. The effective configuration and consequential application of an interdisciplinary case management model entails the collaborative involvement of administrators, physicians, nurses, and all levels of the professional and support staff who will be accountable for the implementation, utilization, and continued development of the model. This chapter presents case management as an innovative system for managing complex health-related problems in the ambulatory setting.

WHY CASE MANAGEMENT?

Shifts in population demographics, accompanied by changing consumer expectations, will continue to force operational restructuring of health care delivery systems as the year 2000 approaches. One example of a population shift is described by Ken Dychtwald (1989) in his book *Age Wave*. Dychtwald predicts a massive demographic shift to an older population with an average age of 65 and a potential life expectancy of 80 years. He suggests that America will need to be redesigned to meet the changing needs of this maturing marketplace. Will health care, a special concern to the older adult, have systems ready to meet the demands of a mature marketplace? One of the answers to this question may be found in a case management approach to patient care.

Case management provides a *known* strategy for dealing positively with the health, economic, and human perspectives of health care and offers a framework for operationally restructuring health care systems. The phrase "balancing cost and quality" abounds in current health care literature, indicating that many recognize the need to accomplish this balance. How can this be done? Case management, a model where the pathways of business, client, and health professionals intersect to provide an integrated approach to the delivery of health care, has surfaced as a viable solution.

TOWARD A DEFINITION

The challenge confronting the health care industry today is to provide more effective health care to patients in settings that differ vastly from the hospital and physician office settings of the past. Historically, patients with varying degrees of illnesses have been cared for in institutions that provided an environment in which the patients were constantly visible, requisite services were instantly available, physicians were immediately accessible, patient care was planned, and nurses were continually present. Additionally, patient care was provided in a physical environment that was conducive to meeting the needs of patients—an environment that had, for example, special beds, wide hallways, and handrails. Patients were nearing the end of their convalescence upon discharge from this institutional setting. National attention continues to focus on the spiraling costs of the delivery of health care within this model, driving the need for the development of health care delivery systems that reduce cost while simultaneously providing patient-focused care (Lathrop 1991).

Case management models have been used in public health and community settings for a number of years. These models generally comprised a set of logical steps and a process of interaction within a service network that ensured that patients would receive needed services in a supportive, effective, efficient, and cost-effective manner (Conti 1989). Within institutional health care environments, case management has been operationalized as a systematic approach to

- identifying high-risk, high-cost patients
- assessing opportunities to coordinate care
- assessing and choosing treatment options
- developing treatment plans to improve quality and efficacy
- controlling costs
- managing a patient's total care to ensure optimum outcome (Desimone 1988)

The nursing case management model, in which the RN is held accountable for financial and clinical patient outcomes, is currently winning wide acceptance in acute care delivery systems (Zander 1988). Within this model, nursing case management activities have centered on redesigning work, enhancing clinical management skills, and developing concurrent monitoring and feedback. In inpatient settings, the loci of control are critical paths or multidisciplinary action plans (MAPs). Such plans cover an episode of illness and specify interventions that must occur in a timely manner to achieve discharge within a set length of stay. In some health care delivery settings, application of the nursing case management model has extended services from hospital care into the community to provide comprehensive nursing services, including acute care, preventive care, and health promotion and education as well as ambulatory, home health, and long-term care (Lamb and Huggins 1990).

The main differences between the various case management models are the level of authority directly controlling service utilization, the type and systems of service provision, and the method of service payment (Schraeder et al. 1990). Application of case management in the ambulatory setting is the counterpart of bedside managed care that provides care to patients on a continuum. "While cost containment is clearly one objective of a case management program, its prime focus is the organization and sequence of services and resources needed to respond to an individual's health care problem" (Merrill 1985, 5). In the coming years, effective case management models will need to utilize the expertise of all health care professionals and be carefully structured to meet the health needs of targeted patient populations.

THE CASE MANAGER ROLE

Generally, the roles of all health care professionals within all categories have remained relatively constant during the 1970s and early 1980s. Currently, national fiscal and quality challenges are forcing reexamination and consequent expansion, redefinition, cross-training, and creation of definitive performance standards for all job categories within medical organizations. Although health care providers in discharge planning, social service, utilization review, and therapy positions are adapting to "case management" roles, it is felt by many experts that RNs are best suited for the title role of case manager. Three factors make RNs the most likely candidates for this position: (1) Their range of professional duties can be summarized as "the diagnosis and treatment of human responses to actual or potential health problems" (American Nurses' Association [ANA] 1980, 9); (2) the educational role of nurses prepares them to focus on a total approach to the patient's body, mind, and spirit; and (3) they have an orientation toward a scientific problem-solving approach, which is termed "the nursing process."

Case management models familiar to other professionals (e.g., medical, social, and primary care models) should not be depreciated. Rather, these models need to be strengthened and integrated into an interdisciplinary case management model. This is accomplished by fostering the expertise of RNs in collaboration and coordination while simultaneously providing an organizational structure that facilitates the integration of all models.

Specific roles for the RN as case manager emerge within the case management concept: assessor, planner, coordinator, collaborator, advocate, counselor, educator, and evaluator. In addition to these management and professional roles, the RN must possess clinical expertise in the care of patients targeted for case management. Current literature supports the view that the case manager role places the RN in an advanced practice arena requiring knowledge obtained through both education and clinical experience. The American Nurses' Association recommends a baccalaureate in nursing and three years of appropriate clinical experience (ANA 1988). At lease one university is offering a master's degree program to prepare nurses as case managers (Graham 1989).

THE CASE MANAGEMENT PROCESS

Case management models serve as the hub for the delivery of multilevels of patient care within the ambulatory setting. For example, a patient experiences a health crisis and, at his or her residence or during a visit to the health care provider, is placed in one of the following categories:

Level I: Defined treatment on a short-term basis.

Level II: Intensive care via visits, followed by telephone management until discharge.

Level III: Continuous long-term care management via coordination with other services and monthly visits.

Level IV: Home health services with minimal dependence on external services.

Level V: Coordination of care, which provides a linkage between the health care facility and client's residence.

The process of case management begins with the referral of a patient. The need for referral is usually determined by means of a screening process. The screening takes into account factors present in the patient's situation that are indicators for continued health care. These indicators may include, for example, prescribed intake of four or more medications, living arrangements with environmental hazards, absence of social support systems, cognitive disorders, multiple illnesses, hospital readmissions, and difficulty accomplishing activities of daily living.

Once the referral has been transmitted, comprehensive and in-depth assessments are performed to establish baseline data for developing a plan for managing patient care on a continuum. Major components of the assessment process include

- demographics
- functional status
- legal issues
- financial issues
- cognitive status
- assessor's impressions
- medical history
- living arrangements
- support systems
- medication profile

This assessment is then summarized, and a written case management plan for the client is established, triggering the case management process. Case management activities may include physical assessments, referrals, arranging for needed services, health teaching, home visits, resource identification, follow-ups, recordkeeping, family counseling, and periodic reassessments. Through formal interdisciplinary collaboration, the case manager, physician, social worker, caregiver, and all other disciplines involved in the care of the patient, are continually engaged in the planning of care, the evaluation of the patient's progress, and problem-solving activities. The case manager is at the hub of all services provided to the patient and is directly accountable and indirectly responsible for the services.

OPERATIONALIZING CASE MANAGEMENT

Getting started is readily accomplished by holding a meeting of all interested individuals and using a brainstorming methodology to pool ideas regarding the creation of a case management service model. A steering committee can be established to guide the continued development, implementation, and evaluation of the model. Work groups accountable to the steering committee can then tackle various aspects to make the model practicable. The model should enable the users to visualize, and subsequently efficiently achieve, concrete and specifically delineated goals (Egan 1985).

Initial attention should focus on the structure, process, and planned outcomes of the model. Cooperation of all services within the organization should be obtained, and physician support must exist. Strategic planning should include the mission, goals, objectives, case-finding methodology, and demographics of patient populations that could benefit from case management. Additional topics might include policies and procedures; tools; determination of available services; internal and external marketing; financial planning; staffing determinations, including clerical support; clinical competencies for case managers; physician direction; and plans for utilization review of services. One planning requirement is to decide on a methodology for evaluation of the impact of the proposed model. Aspects that will need to be addressed following implementation of the model include transportation, consolidation of services, caseloads per manager, cost of services, reimbursement, and patient satisfaction in relationship to improved quality of life.

Once consensus has been obtained on the initial plans, a pilot program should be launched to test the suitability of the model. During the initial starting phase, adjustments to the plan may be made based on surfacing problems, continuous evaluation of the dynamics of the organizational structure, and the patient outcomes that are achieved.

FUTURE CONSIDERATIONS

As the various health care delivery systems struggle to enhance service while controlling costs, modifications of case management systems will occur. During this evolutionary period, several questions will be answered, including these: Are case management systems a cost-efficient method for delivering quality health care to diverse patient populations? Will patient satisfaction be evident? How will reimbursement systems be redesigned to cover noninstitutionalized postacute health care? What is the job description for the health care professional who is a direct provider of services within a case management system? Opportunities are unlimited for service providers in this exciting area.

BRIDGING SYSTEMS AT FRIENDLY HILLS

Friendly Hills HealthCare Network (FHHN) is an integrated managed care provider—a medical group practice and a hospital medical center combined into one entity. With its satellite offices, the campus stretches over a 12-mile radius. The primary mission of FHHN is to be a high-quality, comprehensive health care system that continues to be fully integrated and financially responsible. Health care is provided to over 100,000 subscribers of health maintenance organizations on a capitated basis. A full range of services is available either on campus or through contracted tertiary care centers for the 600,000 patient visits that physicians, professionals, and support staff deal with yearly.

The philosophy of managed care at FHHN is embodied in the organization and functioning of all departments and service areas. Services to patients have been restructured to fit with FHHN's integrated model of managed care, which combines acute and ambulatory settings.

The census at the medical center averages approximately 100 patients daily. An in-house team of physicians are responsible for the medical care of patients during their stay at the medical center. MAPs provide the means of control for managing care during patient stays. A screening process identifies patients for referral to the continuing care center, which is structured as an interdisciplinary case management system.

The case management model at FHHN bridges systems and services to ensure that care of each patient is managed on a continuum and that rapport with and support of the patient continue past the initial contact. Patients are referred to the continuing care center from the FHHN's medical center, physician offices, and tertiary care settings. The following are indicators for referral:

- functional deficit
- patient education required
- continuing medication management required
- history of readmissions to the medical center
- further diagnostic testing required
- lack of social support system
- lack of patient compliance due to decreased mental capacity
- chronic illness

Under the umbrella of the continuing care center, patients are provided varying levels of services directed toward posthospital stabilization of their medical condition through emphasis on compliance with medications and treatment regimens, management of medical conditions through counseling, medical condition rechecks, health education, and orchestration of biopsychosocial aspects. Within the continuing care center, patient care is managed for short to indefinite periods of time. When the services of the continuing care center are no longer required, patients are transferred to the service areas that can best maintain their health status (some patients remain within the continuing care center for indefinite periods of time).

The continuing care center provides a formal interdisciplinary managed care process that significantly impacts the ability of patients to self-manage their care, remain autonomous, and receive required health care services. Quality of life is enhanced and the direct cost of readmissions and overutilization of health care services is simultaneously reduced.

CONCLUSION

Application of case management in the ambulatory setting offers a strategy for significantly impacting patient care in a positive manner by simultaneously addressing the concerns of patients, families, physicians, health care professionals, paraprofessionals, and administrators in the accomplishment of individual and common goals. A functional case management system can be developed through the cooperative actions of a team headed by an RN and consisting of administrators, physicians, and other professionals. Future adaptations of the case management model will allow for the management of a wide range of health, social, and economic problems in the ambulatory arena.

REFERENCES

American Nurses' Association. 1980. *Nursing: A Social Policy Statement.* Kansas City, MO.: American Nurses' Association.

————. 1988. *Nursing Case Management.* Kansas City, MO.: American Nurses' Association.

Conti, Roberta. 1989. "The Nurse as Case Manager." *Nursing Connections* 1, no. 1: 55–58.

Desimone, Betsy S. 1988. "The Case for Case Management." *Continuing Care* (July): 22–23.

Dychtwald, Ken. 1989. *Age Wave.* New York: St. Martin's Press.

Egan, Gerard. 1985. *Change Agent Skills in Helping and Human Service Professions.* Monterey, CA.: Brooks/Cole.

Graham, Barbara. 1989. "Preparing Case Managers." *Caring* (February): 22–23.

Lamb, Gerri S., and Huggins, Delma. 1990. "The Professional Nursing Network." In *Patient Care Delivery Models,* edited by Gloria Gilbert Mayer, Mary Jane Madden, and Eunice Lawrenz. Gaithersburg, MD.: Aspen Publishers, Inc.

Lathrop, J. Philip. 1991. "The Patient-focused Hospital." *Healthcare Forum Journal* (July–August): 17–21.

Merill, J.C. 1985. "Defining Case Management." *Business and Health* 2: 5–9.

Schraeder, Cheryl, Fraser, Cindy, Bruno, Candy, and Dworak, Donna. 1990. *Case Management in Primary Care: A Manual.* Englewood, CO.: Center for Research in Ambulatory Care.

Zander, Karen. 1988. "Nursing Case Management: Strategic Management of Cost and Quality Outcomes." *Journal of Nursing Administration* 18, no. 5: 23–30.

28

Ancillary Services

David R. Morgan

INTRODUCTION

Not long ago, the only tools a physician commonly used to diagnose and treat patients were a tongue depressor and thermometer. Often these were all that were needed. Frequently, however, serious illnesses that can be easily detected today went unnoticed. Only within the past 50 years have we seen the development of diagnostic testing procedures and equipment that significantly assist physicians in the care of patients. At first, many of these tests could only be performed in a hospital, and the patient had to be admitted for one to several days. Now, however, physicians are armed with a large number of highly technical diagnostic tests and procedures that can be performed in the doctor's office or an outpatient setting.

Ancillary services (or clinical services, as they are sometimes called) typically encompass the following diagnostic and treatment modalities:

- pharmacy services
- inhalation therapy
- pulmonary function testing
- electrocardiography
- electroencephalography
- electromyography
- echocardiography
- diagnostic ultrasonography
- diagnostic radiography
- nuclear medicine
- clinical laboratory services
- dialysis

- physical therapy
- occupational therapy

As more instruments and procedures are developed, there will be a continued expansion of the role of these services in the provision of ambulatory care.

THE ROLE OF ANCILLARY SERVICES

As diagnostic and treatment tools, ancillary services play an integral role in the determination of both the diagnosis and treatment. They also extend into the actual treatment and care of patients, as in the case of rehabilitation services. For example, a patient with suspected coronary artery disease may have a cardiac catheterization performed for diagnosis. After the procedure, a cardiac rehabilitation program might be prescribed involving physical therapy and possibly respiratory therapy.

Although the function of ancillary services is the same in both fee-for-service and managed care settings, their role is quite different. In a multispecialty group practice under fee-for-service reimbursement, ancillary services are viewed as potential revenue generators or profit centers. By providing ancillary services, a medical group is able to maintain a continuum of health care services and thus capture most, if not all, potential revenue. The more ancillary services utilized, the more revenue.

In a prepaid managed care setting, ancillary services are viewed very differently. Rather than being treated as profit centers, they are considered to be cost centers or cost-saving centers. Instead of capturing revenue, a prepaid managed care system strives to contain actual and potential costs. This goal is achieved by creating a health care delivery system that includes many ancillary services but effectively manages the costs.

DEVELOPING ANCILLARY SERVICES

Ancillary services can be as simple as a single laboratory or as complex as multiservice diagnostic and rehabilitation centers. Typically, the two most widely utilized ancillary services are laboratory and radiology services. From these services, magnetic resonance imaging (MRI), computerized tomography (CT), ultrasonography, dialysis, neurological testing, and many other services have emerged. The benefits of ancillary services are both medical and financial. Although startup costs can range from hundreds of dollars to several million dollars, the incremental costs of operating these services is minimal in comparison with other more labor-intensive areas of the health care delivery system. Therefore, return on investment (ROI) is typically very high for most ancillary services.

When considering which ancillary services to establish, it is necessary to define (1) the needs of the population to be served, and (2) the needs of the physicians who will be utilizing services. This step is crucial, since there is usually significant capital investment for equipment and materials. Choosing anciallary services that wind up being underused can be disastrous.

COMMON ANCILLARY SERVICES

Radiology Services

For many years the primary utilizer of radiological services were large general practice and orthopedic medical groups. However, with reductions in some equipment and installation costs, it is not uncommon today for solo practice physicians to have radiographic suites. Interestingly, the largest percentage of radiographic suites, in recent years, have been installed in chiropractic offices.

Because radiology services include ultrasonography, echocardiography, MRI, CT, and angiography (invasive radiology) as well as roentgenography, a more accurate term would be *imaging services*. Technological advancements in imaging services are allowing physicians to examine the fetus before it is born, study the flow of blood through the heart and vessels, and pinpoint blood clots and remove them (sometimes even on an ambulatory basis). The nature of imaging services allows them to operate optimally in an ambulatory setting. The main problem is to figure out which services should be offered by a particular provider.

Service Mix

In determining service mix, patient need is the first concern. Although the patient is the person actually receiving the service, it is the physician who utilizes the information provided by imaging services in the care of the patient. Therefore, in determining which services to provide, one must look at the requirements of the physicians who will be ordering the services as well as the demographics of the patient population (see Figure 28-1). For instance, a multispecialty group would probably consist of family practice, OB/GYN, internal medicine, pediatrics, ENT, orthopedics, and radiology departments. Typical imaging services for this type of practice mix would include standard radiography, fluoroscopy, ultrasonography, and mammography. Breaking down

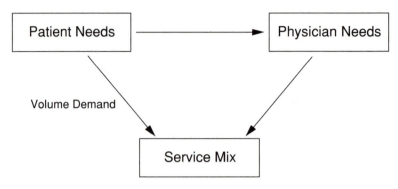

Figure 28-1 Service Mix Development

the individual imaging services by physician utilization, the following pattern is typical:

	Primary	*Secondary*
Ultrasonography	OB/GYN	Family practice
Fluoroscopy	GI/internal medicine	Family practice
Radiography	Orthopedics	Family practice
MRI	Orthopedics	Family practice, neurology, chiropractic
CT	FP/internal medicine	Orthopedics/chiropractic
Echocardiography	Cardiology	Internal medicine

Utilization may vary from group to group, but as a general rule these utilization patterns hold true and can be used to determine the appropriate imaging services mix.

Since a patient's illness generates a need for imaging services, knowing the patient demographics of a service area is helpful in predicting future service demand. For example, a multispecialty group practice in an older community may provide OB/GYN services. However, because the community does not have a large number of young families and pregnant women, the OB/GYN department may not be a significant utilizer of ultrasonography (unlike mammography, which will be subject to heavy demand).

Department Design

The actual design or layout of the ancillary services departments will be dictated by the type of services to be offered. For example, "women's centers" are very common today and rely heavily on diagnostic imaging services. A typical imaging department for a women's center would comprise ultrasonography, mammography, and radiography. These services often require easy access to restroom facilities that may double as dressing rooms. Both ultrasonography and mammography services require only one-third the space of the usual radiographic suite. Mammography needs only minimal lead shielding and ultrasonography does not require any special shielding.

The elderly are the greatest users of health care resources today, and they will increase their utilization rate over the next two decades. Successful imaging departments should be designed around the needs and types of illness afflicting the elderly. Elderly patients typically suffer from pulmonary, bowel, and cardiac illnesses. Therefore, the design of an imaging service mix should be specific to these types of illnesses. An example of a department that would meet the needs of the elderly would have echocardiography, ultrasonography (specifically carotid scan capabilities), fluoroscopy, and standard x-ray services.

Besides diagnostic equipment, minimal space must also be allocated for film developing. For example, it is necessary to have a processor, which will require a four-by-four-foot plumbed area attached to the darkroom. Depending on the type of equipment and the number of procedures performed, an additional processor may be obligatory. This should be taken into consideration when purchasing equipment and in the departmental design. It is often economical to locate processors near bathrooms, which allows utilization of available plumbing.

Capital and Cash Flow

Developing and operating imaging services is very capital-intensive. The initial capital outlay can be as low as twenty thousand dollars for a simple single-phase radiographic suite to over a million dollars for an MRI center. Therefore, once the type of imaging services mix is determined (but prior to any capital expenditure), a profit and loss analysis should be done. This analysis will determine the return on investment (ROI), the payback period, and the monthly cash flow needed for operations. It should include startup costs (e.g., equipment and construction costs) and operational costs (e.g., supply, service contract, maintenance, and labor costs) (see Table 28-1). Most financial institutions will require a profit and loss analysis prior to approving loans.

Staffing

Salaries constitute the largest percentage of the costs associated with imaging services. Like other health care services, radiology is labor-intensive and requires a high degree of technical expertise. All states require personnel to

Table 28-1 Financial Analysis

		1991	1992	1993	1994	1995
	0	1	2	3	4	5
Initial Costs						
Equipment	307,223					
Remodel	41,140					
Training	1,200					
Total	349,573					
Additional Costs						
Staff		263,606	276,786	290,626	305,157	320,415
Service Agreement		6,276	6,276	6,276	6,276	6,276
Supplies		50,000	53,000	54,000	55,900	57,000
Total Cost	349,573	319,882	336,062	350,902	367,333	383,691
Projected Revenue						
Patient Revenue	0	360,000	425,250	464,625	511,875	559,125
Total Profit	(349,573)	40,118	89,188	113,723	144,542	175,434
Payback	(349,573)	(309,455)	(220,267)	(106,544)	37,998	213,432

have some form of training in an approved program. Such programs are often two years in duration and require the student to pass a rigid state examination. Because the demand for radiographic technologists has risen sharply over the last few years and the number of training programs is limited, the law of supply and demand has increased the salaries of technologists, making labor costs even greater in comparison to other direct costs.

Laboratory Services

Laboratory services, by volume, are responsible for the largest number of diagnostic tests and the bulk of ancillary service operations. It is not uncommon for an average-size lab to perform between twenty and thirty thousand tests per month. For many years, physician offices have performed various laboratory tests and have enjoyed large returns on investment due to low incremental operating costs. However, in recent years the new regulations from Medicare and state agencies have made it unlawful to perform most lab tests without proper licensing. Because of these barriers, more and more physicians have entered into partnerships and joint ventures to establish offsite licensed laboratories. This partnership route has enabled many physicians to meet government agency regulations and limit their financial liability.

Within the HMO provider environment, ownership and operation of a lab has the additional benefit of controlling costs. Under a capitated contract, the burden of laboratory and other diagnostic tests costs are born by the medical provider. Compared to sending specimens outside, operation of a lab can greatly reduce costs and, with varying degrees of success, control excess utilization.

Developing Laboratory Services

As with radiology, the first step is to determine which physicians will be utilizing lab services and project the expected volume. The utilization rates will be based on the physicians' specialties and the patient populations served. For example, an OB/GYN physician will order a high percentage of pregnancy, blood typing, and hormone or fertility tests. On the other hand, a pediatrician may rely more heavily on microbiologic tests, strep screens, CBCs, and so on.

Once the needs of the physicians and the patient populations are determined, the next step is to select a laboratory director. Federal regulations and the regulations of most states require that each licensed lab have a medical director who is either a pathologist or has a doctorate in chemistry or microbiology or an equivalent degree. The primary role of the laboratory director is to review and ensure the quality (validity and reliability) of the reported tests. Additionally, the laboratory director will guide the development of new testing procedures.

When physically designing a laboratory, it is important to remember that the two primary functions of a lab are specimen collection and specimen processing or analysis. The specimen collection area must include a patient waiting area and private specimen-drawing areas. The collection area should also include a place for patients to lay down if they feel faint. A centrifuge and refrigerator should be located near the collection area for storage and specimen preparation. Lastly, a bathroom should be located adjacent to the lab so that a specimen pass-through box can be used for urine or stool samples. The processing or analysis section of the lab is typically divided into areas for urine analysis, hematology, chemistry, and microbiology. Usually one main analyzer per area will handle most of the tests, with a few smaller analyzers for more specialized testing. Each area should have ample electrical outlets providing appropriate power.

Purchasing Equipment

A laboratory analyzer can cost tens of thousands of dollars and yet only have a useful technological life span of five to seven years due to technological advances. Because of the high capital cost, some financing arrangements are frequently needed. At present, there are four basic methods of acquiring equipment: lease to purchase, operating lease, reagent lease, and straight purchase. Each of these methods is generally available through the manufacturer or the local representative, and each has its own advantages and disadvantages.

Lease to Purchase. In this kind of arrangement, the health care organization agrees to lease a piece of equipment (laboratory analyzer) for a specific monthly payment over a fixed period of time. At the end of the lease period, the organization is given the option of purchasing the equipment, usually for a minimal amount of money.

Operating Lease. This is a straight lease, and at the end of the contracted lease period the organization has the option of continuing the lease at a reduced rate or trading in the old analyzer for a new one.

Reagent Lease. This kind of lease is available only through the manufacturer and requires the organization to purchase a minimum amount of reagents. In turn the laboratory analyzer is leased to the organization at no cost, and the lease usually includes a buyout option that comes into force at the end of the contract period. A potential negative in this arrangement is that the organization is locked into a particular reagent supplier and is therefore unable to benefit from competitive pricing by other vendors.

Purchase. The organization can always simply purchase the equipment outright.

When considering a particular option, an organization must consider its current cash position, access to capital, and asset management philosophy. Lease options are the most common, because lab equipment has a short technological life span, no capital outlay is required, and the monthly payments are minimal. As with radiology equipment, lessors will require a copy of the organization's current financial statement and a profit and loss projection analysis.

The downside to leasing, in most cases, is that the organization does not own the equipment and makes lease payments at a hefty interest rate. Reagent lease agreements on the surface seem very appealing, since there is no capital outlay and no lease payment. Although reagents must be bought whatever the equipment, in fact the organization pays "rent" on the equipment through higher reagent costs.

Staff

In a large lab, the two main functions, collection and analysis, are performed by phlebotomists and medical technologists, respectively. The collection function, especially in the case of smaller providers, may be performed by properly trained nursing personnel or medical assistants. Training programs for phlebotomy can take four to six months and can be taught in house by a medical technologist. Many community or junior colleges offer phlebotomy training programs.

Among the most educated health care professionals are medical technologists, who often have more than six years of formal and clinical training. Typical medical technology programs require a four-year degree in chemistry, microbiology, or a related field. This is then followed by one or two years of clinical rotation. The supply of graduates of these programs has not generally kept up with the demand.

Cardiopulmonary and Neurological Testing

In general, cardiopulmonary and neurological testing include the following services:

- electrocardiography
- electroencephalography
- electromyography
- pulmonary function testing
- cardiac testing (treadmill testing)

Most of these services can be used by both primary care physicians and specialists. Since cardiopulmonary and neurological testing require minimal operating costs and relatively modest capital expense, these ancillary services have proven to be reliable profit centers for fee-for-service physician practices.

Developing Services

As with other diagnostic services, the mix of cardiac and neurological tests should be based on physician demand. For example, cardiologists will utilize cardiac testing, stress or treadmill testing, cardiac rehabilitation, and electrocardiography. Neurologists will typically utilize electroencephalography and electromyography, and pulmonologists will use pulmonary function testing and pulmonary rehabilitation. Multispeciality groups or free-standing diagnostic centers that are utilized by cardiologists, neurologists, and pulmonologists will find it advantageous to provide a full range of tests.

Staff

Of all the diagnostic services, cardiopulmonary and neurological testing services are the least difficult to staff, since personnel typically are not required to be licensed. Most states, however, require that individuals performing the tests have some type of certification as proof of training. Nursing personnel can also be cross-trained to perform some of these tests. An additional advantage of these services is that the bulk of the testing is done on the day shift and can often be scheduled in advance.

Rehabilitation Services

The three rehabilitation services are physical therapy, occupational therapy, and speech therapy. Rehab services have long been excellent revenue generators due to the fact that treatment is often for an extended period of time and requires minimal startup and equipment costs as compared with other ancillary services. Primarily associated with orthopedic and industrial medicine, rehab services have found their niche in both ambulatory sports medicine centers and long-term rehab facilities.

As stated earlier, the primary utilizer of physical therapy services are orthopedists. The nature of orthopedic medicine lends itself to a symbiotic relationship with physical therapy. On the other hand, occupational therapy is more closely associated with geriatric medicine and neurology (e.g., the rehabilitation of stroke patients). Speech therapy for communicative disorders is utilized by a wide variety of medical disciplines such as primary care; ears, nose, and throat; pediatrics; and neurology.

Developing Services

"Space" is key for a successful rehab department. Like radiology services, physical therapy can be very space-intensive. A typical department in a large group practice will contain

- five to ten individual treatment tables
- one or two treatment mats
- two or three whirlpools (various heights)
- paraffin baths
- hot and cold pack units
- ultrasound units
- neuromuscular stimulant units
- assorted wall pulleys
- parallel bars

The department should be designed to accommodate patients who have locomotive and neuromuscular problems by providing ample siderails, wide corridors, and, of course, restrooms suitable for the handicapped.

Staff

Rehabilitation services staff comprise registered physical, occupational, and speech therapists. All of these staff members require degrees from accredited university programs. Employment of aids and students can be a cost-effective way to supplement department staff.

MEASURING OPERATIONS

Should an additional piece of equipment be purchased? Is expansion of a department necessary? How productive are operations? What is the projection for future service demand? What is the cost of performing a particular test? What should the charge be? At some point, all of these questions will be asked. Having the answers or knowing how to get them will mean the difference between profitability and unprofitability. Continuing measurement of operations is essential for determining pricing, projecting future operational resource demands, and pinpointing operational inefficiencies quickly. By obtaining and utilizing operational data such as cost per procedure, man-hours per procedure, procedure mix, and procedure volume, effective decision making can occur.

Productivity and Volume Analysis

Because health care services are labor-intensive, procedural volumes influence the type and amount of labor needed for operations. By tracking daily service volumes, it is possible to use personnel more efficiently. The following are typical volume units of measure:

	Primary	*Secondary*
Radiology	Relative value units (RVUs)	Procedures
Laboratory	College of American Pathologists (CAP) units	Procedures
Cardiopulmonary and neurological testing	Relative value units (RVUs)	Procedures
Rehabilitation	Modalities	Procedures

The primary units of measurement, RVUs, CAPs and modalities, are based on the time utilized to perform a specific procedure or test. In other words, the units are time weighted to allow for more time-consuming procedures. Although counting procedures is a simpler method of tracking service activity, it is less accurate than measuring RVUs, CAP units, and modalities because each procedure is treated equally thus ignoring the actual length of an exam (see Figure 28-2).

Knowing a department's productivity will allow optimization of staffing. Ideally, staffing should be volume-driven, with staffing maximized at those hours when the peak number of procedures are performed. With this system, the productivity graph would be close to a straight line. This is because staff hours would efficiently flex or vary as procedural volumes varied and thus productivity in terms of man-hours per procedure would remain constant. Widely fluctuating productivity values on this scale of measurement signal an inefficient or nonvolume-driven use of staff (Figure 28-3). Of course, the ideal straight line can never be reached because minimal staffing is usually always necessary and because governmental regulatory agencies may impose their own staffing requirements.

Procedure Mix

Different tests or procedures vary with respect to use of space, type of equipment required, and length of time required for completion. Because each of these elements will affect profitability or cost and future operational plans, it becomes advantageous to track and analyze the procedure mix of ancillary services. For example, a mammogram costs less and takes less time to perform than an upper G.I. series. But although a mammogram commands a lower price, its low incre-

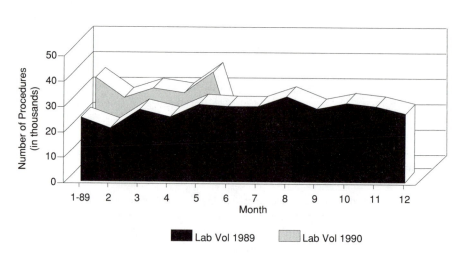

Figure 28-2 Laboratory Procedure Volume Analysis

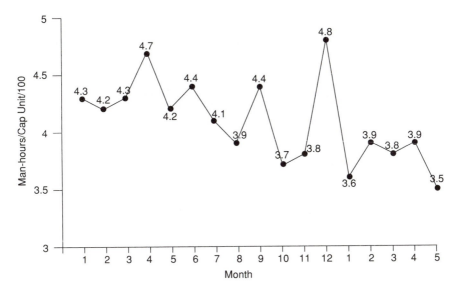

Figure 28-3 Laboratory Productivity

mental cost (direct variable costs), coupled with its high throughput, gives it a greater potential for contributing to the profitability of a fee-for-service practice.

Additionally, the startup costs for mammography are significantly less than for G.I. procedures, and mammography requires much less operating space. The demand for a diagnostic service and the service's throughput and contribution margin are directly related to its profit potential. Careful analysis of these elements will assist in developing a procedure mix or product line that has a positive financial impact. In a fee-for-service practice, knowledge of these factors can help create a beneficial marketing strategy (see Figure 28-4).

THE FUTURE OF ANCILLARY SERVICES

Ancillary services will continue to expand their role in diagnosis and treatment as a result of new technology, increased automation, and improved clinical information systems.

The rapid development of new technologies over the past 20 years has enabled the diagnostic services to provide physicians with more than test results. As in the case of MRI, the ability to view the actual internal structure of a patient without invasive procedures has led to rapid diagnosis and treatment of many illnesses that in the past would have gone undetected or required

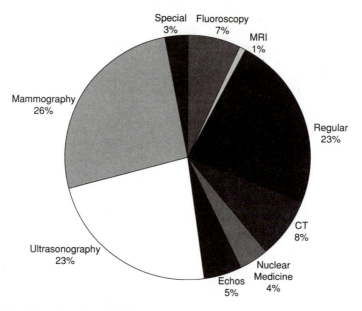

Figure 28-4 Radiology Procedure Mix

invasive procedures or even surgery. The capabilities of ancillary services will continue to develop and expand in parallel with technological advancements.

The ability to do it faster, better, and cheaper has been a longstanding goal of business, and this also applies to ancillary services. Economic pressures, especially high labor costs, will continue to be the driving force in the development of more automated systems. All ancillary services, by the nature of their production processes, lend themselves to the application of automation. Laboratories, especially in recent years, have seen an enormous application of automation technology.

The revolution that is taking place in the transmission and processing of information is just beginning to touch the health care industry. Information systems are emerging and evolving in all ancillary service areas, enabling diagnostic information to be processed faster and be available to physicians more rapidly than ever before. For example, computerized laboratory results systems allow multiple "caregivers" to view test result information simultaneously from local and remote locations. Radiology information systems are available that allow a radiologist to read x-rays from a remote location through computer transmitted images, eliminating the need for the actual x-ray film. The application of information systems to ancillary services seems limitless and will play a significant role in the future.

29

Marketing Techniques

Mary Jo Littlefield and Steve Daily

MARKETING AND MEDICINE

"Marketing . . . sales . . . advertising." As little as one generation ago, these words would have struck any physician as discordant. But today, few observers dispute the importance of competition in health care or the key role marketing plays in building and maintaining a viable medical practice. This is especially true for the large-scale multispecialty medical group, an organizational model whose main advantages lie in the economies of scale that come with expansion.

How did all of this marketing talk begin? A few clues can be found in the terms used in health care today: *affordable, contract, third-party payment, cost containment*. These are the terms of the marketplace, not the operating theater. In the new lexicon of health care, *competition* and *market share* are no longer foreign phrases but key concepts vital to long-term survival.

In a free economy, marketing is intrinsic to the act of buying and selling any product or service, including health care. Today, patients (and third-party players in the reimbursement game such as employers and insurance carriers) are truly consumers of health care, with the same discretionary powers as any other group of consumers. This means that health care organizations are now subject to the same economic laws as other commercial enterprises.

THE WAY WE WERE

In a discreet and limited way, marketing has always been part of medicine. In the past, marketing simply took the form of networking and maintaining cordial relations with other physicians, especially referral sources. Examples are the holiday parties thrown by the local cardiologist or orthopedic surgeon and the flattering "thank you for allowing me to see your patient" letters sent by consulting physicians to referring physicians.

Marketing in those days was a subtle, back room affair conducted by the members of an exclusive professional club. Fee-for-service was the rule of the day. Physicians routinely did their financial planning from the bottom up, arriving at a desired income level by raising fees, providing more services to each patient, or scheduling more patients from a virtually inexhaustible supply. Physicians were paid on a cost-plus basis, with no questions asked. There were not enough physicians to meet the demand for health care, so there was no need to court the public directly. It was a classic example of a seller's market.

THE WAY WE ARE NOW

In those days, even placing a Yellow Pages advertisement with the practice's name in bold print was considered unethical. Newspaper advertising was for quacks and charlatans. Yet today, outright and unabashed promotion is considered normal in many competitive areas. Why?

There is no simple answer, but the seeds of change were sown in a complex series of events during the seventies and eighties:

- Following the inexorable laws of the marketplace, prices rose to meet the surging demand for health care services.
- More young people, attracted by high incomes, trained to become physicians.
- Relaxed immigration laws allowed an influx of foreign-trained physicians.
- Physicians passed on the costs of increasingly expensive technologies and the malpractice crisis in the form of higher fees.
- Patients and insurers became increasingly knowledgeable about health care.
- The economywide cycle of inflation and recession resulted in increased employer demands for cost containment in health care and spurred the move toward alternative systems of reimbursement.

The new result of these developments was a complete transformation: The seller's market became a buyer's market. Medicine hit the wall of fiscal reality. The same economic laws that always applied to Procter & Gamble and General Motors now suddenly applied equally to Dr. Smith around the corner.

The seventies and eighties removed the insulation that once surrounded health care providers. After having it all their own way for many years, they now must learn to live with the realities of the marketplace.

MARKETING TERMINOLOGY

Marketing, according to Webster, is "an aggregate of functions involved in moving goods from producer to consumer." In a health care environment, marketing encompasses all the functions that relate to protecting and increasing *market share*—the portion of a service area's patient population that comes to a provider for health care. Marketing goals include retaining current patients, attracting new patients, establishing a positive image for the organization, and promoting the interests of the group to the public, potential business partners, and government agencies. Components of marketing include strategic planning of services, market research, and the various forms of advertising. *Market research* is the process of quantitatively measuring the various factors that determine an organization's survival in the market, especially the opinions of consumers. *Positioning* is the art of staking out unique territory from which to sell, then establishing a brand preference in the minds of consumers. *Advertising* is the pointed end of the marketing stick: the outward projection of image that aims to increase top-of-mind awareness and thus market share.

SMALL VERSUS LARGE

The need for marketing is not size-dependent. Large or small, all health care providers need to include some component of marketing in their plans for long-term stability.

The marketing plan for a small primary care practice may focus on sending out reminder postcards for routine checkups, letters containing a postappointment patient satisfaction survey, or holiday and birthday cards for all current patients. An area hospital may be willing to help a small practice with marketing. It needs referrals, which the practice can supply. Therefore, what is good for the practice is also good for the hospital.

In the case of a specialty practice, marketing may take the form of seeking and maintaining strong links with primary care physicians, backed up by the cultivation in-house of a customer service mentality. In the case of a large multispecialty practice, marketing will have many facets, including aggressive advertising and promotion of programs.

The time to address marketing issues is now. If the organization is already prosperous, marketing will enable it to remain that way. If it is facing difficult times in its service area, the stakes are even higher. Indeed, an effective marketing program can be the difference between survival and extinction.

MANAGED CARE VERSUS FEE-FOR-SERVICE

Just as small size does not excuse a practice from marketing, neither does the patient mix or reimbursement method. There are differences, but both major types of practice must still market.

For a multispecialty medical group or health care network dealing primarily with prepaid managed care patients, the principal marketing goal is to increase and sustain patient enrollment, which in turn increases the level of capitated funds entering the financial stream. Therefore, it is a common practice to time marketing efforts to coincide with seasonal open enrollment periods. Heavy emphasis is also placed on patient education and retention, both of which contribute to long-term stability and efficient use of health care services.

For organizations still based on fees for service, marketing assumes an added dimension of urgency. Managed care patients typically can only change providers during an annual open enrollment period, so once they are drawn in, the main task is retention. Fee-for-service patients can at any time go elsewhere—and often do. Therefore, they need to be marketed more aggressively. Also, in the fee-for-service marketplace, profit margins per visit and per procedure are higher, making more elaborate and costly marketing efforts feasible.

LOOKING FOR AN EDGE

Uniqueness provides an edge in marketing. As part of building an effective marketing plan, an organization needs to create a unique appeal. The key here is to establish in the public's mind a difference between the organization and the competition. The organization can offer longer office hours than the competition, have office hours on Saturdays, offer a free van service for cataract surgery patients, or have nurses make next-day follow-up calls to all surgery patients. It's up to the organization to find or create new marketing wrinkles, but the possibilities are endless.

THE PATIENT FACTOR

Keep in mind that patients are the cheapest and most effective means of marketing. If listened to, they will describe what they want. The extent to which the organization gives it to them will determine its marketing edge.

Staff should start "marketing" the minute a patient enters the waiting room. A satisfied patient will tell two people; an unhappy patient will tell ten.

A THREE-PHASE PLAN FOR EFFECTIVE MARKETING

Marketing does not mean just shotgun-style advertising. It requires a measured, valuative, strategic program. It is best approached in these three distinct but overlapping phases:

1. *Assessment of position.* Make an honest appraisal of the organization's current situation, both internally (through dialogue among physicians and other personnel) and externally (through objective market research).
2. *Internal reinforcement.* The organization's image and unique selling points must be understood and made part of the corporate culture. The organization must cultivate a shared sense of purpose and a customer service orientation.
3. *External projection.* To increase top-of-mind awareness in its service area, the organization must broadcast its message and identity. This phase can be truly effective only after the first two have been addressed.

Phase 1: Assessment of Position

If positioning is the art of staking out territory from which to sell, then assessment is the science of surveying the ground. It means evaluating one's current place in the market area, determining what unique services can be offered to consumers, and making educated guesses about what the competition is going to do, then taking steps to establish a unique niche.

This first and all-important phase of the marketing process encompasses three subphases.

The Internal Audit

The first step in assessment is to take a long, hard look at just what the organization has to offer. What kind of business is it in? Who comes to it and why? Where do the people in the organization think it is going? Where do they want it to go?

The internal audit is best approached using a series of offsite retreats where physicians, management personnel, and other staff members can engage in dialogue about topics relating to marketing such as quality of service, quality of care, and so on. The actual discussion topics will vary, but the goal is to understand what is special, and thus marketable, about the organization. Retreat participants should focus on uncovering strengths and weaknesses and analyzing the root causes. It is a time for clear thinking and complete honesty.

The final result of the internal audit is a complete picture of what the organization now has to offer, which areas need improvement, and what opportunities may exist for future marketing.

The Market Survey

This subphase can be conducted simultaneously with the internal audit. The purpose of the market survey is to ascertain the current state of public recognition and perception. To build an effective marketing plan, the organization needs to know who its current patients are, what patients and nonpatients think, what the public knows about it, what they think about it, what the current share of market is, who the competition is, what they are doing, what the demographics of the market area are, and what the success rate of any current marketing effort is.

Methods used in market research include written questionnaires, random telephone surveys, and formal focus group studies using paid respondents from the community. Besides talking directly with the public, the organization might also interview insurance carriers, benefits administrators, and other representatives of area employers.

The internal audit incurs little cost, since it requires only the participation of employees. But external market research is a different matter, since it involves going directly to a representative sample of the public and asking direct questions about the organization. There is no way to do this objectively without the services of an outside firm. An operational assessment by an outside professional is also the best way to ascertain the effectiveness of current marketing. Costs for a comprehensive market survey will run from $10,000 to $50,000, depending on the size of the area surveyed, the methods used, and the fee structure of the individual research company. Obtaining referrals from other similar organizations before choosing a marketing firm is always recommended.

The Marketing Plan

The net result of the internal and external audits is a comprehensive, objective picture of both internal and external marketing issues. Once the organization has a good grasp of the current situation in its market area, it is ready to build a realistic marketing plan, targeting specific goals for business development.

The overall marketing plan will include marketing goals, the means to achieve them, and the costs and timeframes involved. Many companies assign a percentage of their net income for marketing, typically between 5 and 10 percent. In managed care situations, the HMOs, insurance companies, and other payers usually devote a substantial portion of their income to marketing. Therefore, the individual group's percentage may be lower. However, whatever the percentage, the group should have a detailed written budget for each year. The linchpin of successful marketing is an overall marketing plan that addresses both current and future needs and forms an integral part of the group's strategic plan for long-term, stable growth.

To increase effectiveness, it is standard practice to segment the market and develop programs specifically tailored to the needs of each segment—the so-called rifle approach. For example, weight reduction programs, senior discount programs, industrial medicine, and perinatal services all target fairly well-defined market segments that can be reached through mailing lists.

Phase 2: Internal Reinforcement

The second major phase of marketing involves putting one's own house in order. Health care is a service business—service is the product. In order to sell something, an organization has to have something to sell. Therefore, it must develop the capability to offer consistently high-quality service before it can realistically hope to gain market share. This ensures that when it sells, it can live up to the promises made in its advertising.

This phase centers around developing an organizational personality or corporate culture—a positive team spirit among staffers, personal rapport between staff and patients, and an overall orientation toward serving patient needs and solving patient concerns.

Strategies that help to solidify the product include developing staff training programs, holding special events and parties, devising motivational programs and providing incentives, bringing in outside motivational speakers, establishing standards for customer service, and setting up a patient relations committee and a formal grievance process.

In a field where service is the product, consumers will measure the organization by the kind of service they get from its staff and physicians.

Phase 3: External Projection

The final and most visible phase of marketing involves going into the community and projecting the organization's image and message. Like all parts of the marketing process, getting the image out into the community is a long-term building process, not a one-time shot.

The goal of this final phase of marketing is to increase top-of-mind awareness among consumers (or, in the case of specialty groups, referring physicians). The emphasis on top-of-mind awareness (the reflexive association of the organization's name and its line of services) is based on the direct relationship between this kind of awareness and market share. If 5 percent of respondents in a survey of the local population associate the organization's name with health care, it probably serves about 5 percent of the population in that area. Therefore, it can theoretically increase market share by increasing top-of-mind awareness.

The drive for awareness can take the form of promoting individual services targeted at specific audiences (such as weight control programs) or more general approaches (e.g., a newsletter that promotes all facets of a large group on a regular, rotating basis).

Increasing top-of-mind awareness is basically accomplished in two ways: (1) through the efforts of staff within the community and (2) through professionally produced advertising that promotes the unique appeal of the organization.

In-house efforts that can be effective in building awareness include

- marketing directly to area employers
- having staff physicians speak to organizations and get involved in the community
- developing a scholarship program with local schools
- providing health education and other community outreach programs
- participating in health-related events in the community
- building strong relations with local newspapers and other media
- finding ways to encourage referrals from satisfied patients

All of these efforts are valuable in the context of an overall marketing plan, but they are essentially passive. The aggressive portion of this phase is best accomplished by working with outside professional resources. The effective marketing plan will have some of the following components. (Obviously, the larger the advertiser, the larger the budget and the more can be done.) The major facets of external marketing are as follows.

Corporate Identity. The organization should develop a graphic identity expressed through the design of its stationery, signage, and uniforms and even apparent on company vehicles. The graphic identity includes the logo and logotype, the company colors, the names of special programs, and the way the logo is used on ID badges. The organization should have a set of comprehensive graphic standards so that all communications have a polished, professional family look.

Direct Mail (Direct Response) Advertising. Direct mail is the most targetable of all media. It includes any printed material the organization sends by mail directly to its audience—brochures, newsletters, and the like. In most situations faced by health care organizations, the bulk of the advertising budget will go toward some form of direct response advertising. There are hundreds of lists available, and the organization can send a mailing to every household in the service area, only to families with two or more children under 18 and an annual household income of over $50,000, or to numerous other groups of similar or lesser specificity. Direct mail provides an opportunity for the organization to put its message where it cannot be ignored by recipients. To rise above the background clutter of junk mail, direct mail materials should be carefully thought out, visually attractive, and of high quality.

Collateral. This broad category covers brochures and other informational materials that give patients information of value wrapped inside the organization's image. Collateral includes brochures explaining the benefits of specific lines of service, general patient information materials, and health education materials.

Mass Media Advertising. The mass media include radio, television, newspapers, magazines, billboards, bus benches and bus placards, and even the Yellow Pages. The mass media are glamorous but often prohibitively expensive. If the organization's service area encompasses all or most of the surrounding metropolitan area, then using television, radio, and newspaper advertising can be effective.

For example, in a city of 200,000 with its own broadcast outlets, advertising through radio and television may be cost-effective for an organization with satellite offices throughout the city; after all, the media audience and target market are the same. But for a group of the same size in a city of five million, the ad rates will be much higher and only a small fraction of the media audience will be potential patients, which makes use of the broadcast media questionable at best. In this scenario, the group would be paying for useless media coverage, and it would do better to concentrate on targeted media like direct mail.

SELECTING A CREATIVE RESOURCE

Marketing is, by its very nature, a creative field. And nowhere is that creativity more crucial than in the actual messages broadcast to the world. For its marketing efforts to succeed, the organization will need to retain the services of an advertising agency or creative design group to help develop the message and present it in ways that get results. The extent to which it uses advertising professionals will depend on its marketing goals, budget, and service area.

Creative advertising agencies provide services like graphic design, advertising copyrighting, print and broadcast production services, management of printings and mailings, and media buying. These capabilities can also be developed in-house, but generally it is feasible to do so only if the organization is large enough to support the intrinsic costs of personnel and facilities and if at least one person high up in the organization has the necessary skills and contacts to build an in-house advertising department.

From a long-term perspective, generally the best results are achieved by assigning the implementation of these services to a single source. It is preferable not to use a mixed bag of free-lancers. In general, the more services one firm can provide, the greater the accountability and cost-effectiveness. Also, these creative services are provided by people, and people need to get to know their clients in order to do their best work.

A creative resource should be chosen in much the same way as a market research firm is—by asking for referrals from other health care organizations and collecting effective advertisements, then finding out who created them.

Once the organization has begun implementing its marketing plan, it should review the results on a periodic basis. It should also hold a review of its account in order to measure the performance of its advertising firm.

BENEFITS AND RISKS OF MARKETING

The goal of advertising is the same in health care as it is at Procter & Gamble—to create a positive image in the consumer's mind and to establish a brand preference. For an organization that becomes the brand of choice, the benefits are obvious.

But marketing effectively to a mass audience, whether by print, mail, or electronic media, is not cheap. Typical rates of response on direct mail run between .5 and 4 percent, and with 2 percent being considered very good. A long-term view is also required: Health care is generally a "slow-burn" environment, since it usually takes time for patients to switch providers. Therefore, a serious commitment is required if a marketing plan is to have any chance of success.

CONCLUSION

Marketing is part of the new reality of health care. In order for health care organizations to prosper, they must take their cues from the professionals who have sold things for generations. *Marketing* is no longer a dirty word in medical circles. Indeed, the success of privately funded health care will partly depend of the marketing skills of health care providers.

30

Marketing in the Managed Care Setting: Patient Survey Techniques and Other Factors in Assessing Patient Satisfaction

Kevin W. Sullivan and Meryl D. Luallin

In health care, as in all other service industries, the ultimate measure of success is customer satisfaction.

In the 1980s, as managed care prepayments represented greater portions of monthly revenue for multispecialty groups, many physicians and managers interpreted "locked in market share" as suggesting that patients, once enrolled at the lower premiums, were unlikely to leave the health plans or switch providers. In theory, the prepaid plans would ensure that member solicitation, enrollment, and continuing "relations" would be services of the HMOs, thereby enabling professionals in the delivery system to focus on operating efficiencies and utilization review.

In practice, however, the marketing promises of managed care plans are rarely kept. Instead, many plans focus almost exclusively on enrollment, leaving members uneducated or even misinformed regarding health coverage and rules of access. As a consequence, significant numbers of patients remain willing to switch providers for "service" reasons, even in managed care settings. The table excerpt below is from Sullivan/Luallin patient surveys conducted from 1989 to 1991 for multispecialty groups with HMO members constituting 50 to 95 percent of their total patient bases.

Have you ever switched doctors in order to obtain a better medical service?

	Yes	No	No Reply
Clinic "A"	31.3	58.6	10.1
Clinic "B"	44.5	53.4	2.2
Clinic "C"	35.1	57.4	7.2
Clinic "D"	35.8	60.8	3.4
Clinic "E"	34.9	60.4	4.8
Clinic "F"	37.6	54.8	7.6
Clinic "G"	49.4	44.4	6.2
Clinic "H"	36.1	60.4	3.6
Average responses	38.1	56.3	5.6

Despite the claims of HMOs, the responsibility for "patient relations" remains with the business offices and clinical departments of the provider groups. In this context, the thought is often expressed that, for providers and staff members functioning in a high-volume managed care setting, the ability to maintain patient satisfaction has been buried under staggering workloads and mounting levels of job stress. This feeling is reinforced by feedback from patients that "the doctor rushed me through the visit," or "the clinic receptionist was surly," or "I felt like a number instead of a person."

THE MARKETING PROCESS

At one time, the process of delivering products to Americans was dominated by a *selling* process in which companies decided what products they wanted to offer and how they wished to structure their operations. Henry Ford's attitude that "our customers can have any color they want, as long as it's black" was echoed in many other industries. Customers, knowing no better, accepted the status quo.

Following World War II, as competition grew and profit margins narrowed, many U.S. companies began to offer new options to consumers (e.g., Marshall Field built his retailing empire on the slogan, "Give the lady what she wants"). In the new era, businesses took the trouble to learn what consumers wanted, and they enhanced their products with features reflecting what they had learned. The marketplace quickly responded to companies that showed sensitivity to customer preferences.

The advent of the service economy in the past 20 years has intensified a nationwide transition to a customer-sensitive philosophy of doing business. At present the health care industry is in the latter stages of the evolution from selling—"hanging out the shingle" and expecting that patient volume will result without further effort—to a three-step marketing process that reflects the realities of an environment in which consumers and payers have the power of choice and have demonstrated their willingness to use it.

In a service industry like health care, the three steps of the marketing process are as follows:

1. Study the needs, perceptions, and expectations of patients, referral sources, and other target audiences.
2. Involve providers and employees in a cooperative effort to meet patient or referrer expectations (including the elimination of operational barriers that impede clinic staff when they attempt to fulfill patients' desires for caring and efficient service).

3. Develop a "recovery" system for dealing effectively with patients and referrers when service lapses occur.

This chapter focuses on the three steps of the marketing process: surveying the needs of patients and referring physicians, building an internal service marketing program, and installing a service recovery program.

Step 1: Surveying Patients and Referring Physicians

Surveys of customer audiences give practice marketers the most reliable measure of the group's strong points and weak points in terms of its ability to protect the existing revenue base and attract new capitated members. Survey findings identify specific areas where maintaining or increasing responsiveness to consumers not only reinforces the loyalty of current patients and referrers but also generates new managed care membership through word-of-mouth referrals during enrollment periods in the workplace.

Patient Surveys

Appendix 30-A to this chapter contains a recommended patient survey that has been used successfully by many group practices committed to the managed care model. The issues addressed in the survey include

- sources of referrals
- satisfaction with the managed care plan
- selection criteria
- provider or department visited
- experience when making the appointment
- satisfaction with specific performance areas
- overall rating
- willingness to recommend the practice
- past utilization patterns
- current utilization of clinic services

Patient surveys should be conducted at least semiannually so that practice leaders can stay abreast of changes in patient perceptions. In cases where "trouble spots" have been identified, more frequent surveys will provide current data on the effects of management attempts to improve clinic services or performance.

Survey Distribution. Patient surveys can be conducted in several ways, which differ in the results obtained and the amount of time and money spent. For example, a telephone survey, although relatively expensive, allows interviewers to probe beyond the basic questions and elicit specific information regarding the patients' perceptions of clinic systems and performance. A written-response survey, like the example in Appendix 30-A, is much less costly but limits interpretation to the actual items circled and comments made.

Surveying is a "sampling" technique in which responses from the sample population are projected over the clinic's total patient base. From a statistical standpoint, a sample of 385 qualified respondents can be said to represent the thinking of the entire patient base, particularly if the majority of the respondents give the same answers. Statisticians refer to the "95 percent confidence level," in terms of which a population of 385 respondents represents an error tolerance of plus or minus 7 percent.

However, if the total sample is further divided into subcategories (e.g., satellite location, department, etc.), the smaller populations are less likely to warrant a high level of confidence in the findings. For example, if the intent is to measure patient satisfaction at each of six locations, *each* location would need 385 respondents to keep the error tolerance within 7 percent.

The reliability of survey findings is also affected by the number of possible responses to each question. In the sample survey, Q8 and Q9 are yes–no questions to which there are only two possible responses, whereas Q1 and Q2 not only offer multiple possibilities but also permit more than one response. Answers to the yes–no questions are much more reliable than responses to Q1 and Q2.

Distribution of the survey can be by mail or over the counter during the patient visits. With some exceptions, neither method is superior in terms of producing valid results; however, direct distribution by clinic employees has certain advantages. Not only does this method personalize the survey and increase the probability of returns, it also focuses the attention of providers and staff on the surveying process and reinforces management's insistence on service as a measurement of job performance.

What Survey Results Should Be Expected? No medical practice would be satisfied with a 10 percent error rate in diagnosis or a similar lack of accuracy in laboratory test procedures. For the purpose of maintaining patient loyalty and generating new referrals, the service issues contained in patient and referrer surveys are at least as important as the quality of the medical care provided. In 12 years of surveying patients for single-specialty and multispecialty groups, our firm has reviewed many thousands of comments, very few of which were unrelated to some aspect of service. In marketing the practice, therefore, no less should be expected in the area of service than is demanded in the clinical and ancillary departments.

In Q6 of the patient survey (Appendix 30-A), an overall rating of 90 percent (good plus excellent) would mean that one in ten patients was not satisfied with the encounter. If, as discovered in research by Humana Corporation and others, a dissatisfied patient will tell nine other people of the experience, the downside risk of failing to meet patient expectations has a ninefold effect on public perceptions of the group. If the service lapses of a medical practice were to antagonize ten patients per week—not unlikely in some high-volume groups—in one year's time a total of 4,680 persons will know about it (ten unhappy patients per week times nine family members or friends times 52 weeks).

To meet the growth requirements of most marketing plans, the overall patient satisfaction rating (Q6) should be at least 93 percent. Further, in nearly all the patient surveys done by our firm, there is a correlation of less than 2 percent between the overall rating (good plus excellent in Q6) and the patient's willingness to refer others to the practice (Q7).

In analyzing the survey findings, the overall rating (Q6) comprises the individual satisfaction ratings in the preceding question (Q5), which give a reliable indication of specific areas for management attention. By addressing the Q5 issues quickly and effectively, practice managers can arrest downtrends and recapture marketing momentum.

One such example is provided by a multispecialty group in Southern California, more than 80 percent of whose nonMedicare patients belong to managed care plans. A 1989 patient survey had indicated slippage in several performance areas (Q5) and a loss of 4 percentage points in the overall rating (Q6).

Management began an immediate effort to involve its providers, supervisors, and staff members in identifying the barriers that interfered with patient-centered service and correcting the deficiencies. A formal "service marketing" program was instituted, featuring a revised appraisal system to ensure that service concepts would be converted into on-the-job performance. In a subsequent survey one year later, Q6 "excellent" ratings had increased more than nine percentage points, overall satisfaction (good plus excellent) had grown from 89.7% to 93.4% in less than 12 months, and dramatic improvements had been achieved in several areas of patient satisfaction, as illustrated in Exhibit 30-1.

Surveying Primary Care Providers

Critical for the satisfaction of members of prepaid health plans is the process by which specialist physicians meet patient expectations when referred by the gatekeeper providers. For this reason, marketers need reliable feedback from primary care physicians to ensure that the referral process is smooth and patient-centered.

Appendix 30-B contains a recommended referring physician survey for measuring the effectiveness of the referral process. Key issues in the survey include

Exhibit 30-1 Patient Survey Results for a Multispecialty Group

Q5. How satisfied are you with:
(1990 findings in italics; 1989 findings on second line of each pair.)

	Very Satis	Somewhat Satis	Somewhat Dissat	Very Dissat	N/R
Appointments scheduled at times	67.9	20.2	3.1	1.1	7.3
that are convenient for you?	13.0	59.2	22.3	4.2	1.4
Normal waiting times acceptable to you?					
In the registration area?	66.0	24.2	2.2	0.6	6.7
	57.3	22.8	4.8	2.4	12.7
In the reception area?	53.8	29.5	5.7	1.2	9.5
	46.7	28.4	8.0	3.7	13.3
In the exam room?	52.0	27.4	5.4	1.1	13.8
	49.9	26.5	6.1	1.1	16.4
In the lab?	41.8	25.9	4.8	1.0	26.5
	39.5	24.4	8.2	2.9	24.9
Being informed of test results	52.6	25.9	6.1	2.0	13.1
in a reasonable amount of time?	51.2	24.7	4.8	2.9	16.2
Phone calls handled in a prompt	61.8	23.1	7.1	4.2	3.5
and courteous manner?	57.3	26.0	4.8	3.4	8.5
Our after-hours answering service	42.6	15.3	2.3	0.7	38.7
prompt and courteous?	34.5	19.9	1.3	0.8	43.5
Receptionists friendly and	83.7	12.5	0.8	0.7	1.9
courteous?	77.7	16.4	1.1	0.5	4.2
Nurses sympathetic to problems and	78.3	15.1	2.2	0.6	3.5
concerned about you as a person?	70.6	17.8	1.9	0.8	9.0
The people in our business office	63.8	20.6	4.2	1.4	9.6
concerned about helping you?	58.9	21.8	4.5	0.8	14.1
Our answers to your questions about	58.0	18.9	4.1	1.6	17.1
insurance forms and payment?	51.7	22.5	5.0	1.9	18.8
Our staff members' willingness to	72.2	15.8	1.3	0.7	9.6
to go out of their way for you?	64.5	19.1	1.9	0.5	14.1
Our ability to solve your problems	56.3	25.6	4.2	1.6	12.0
in a timely manner?	50.4	28.1	3.2	1.9	16.4
Provider seeing you in reasonable	62.5	26.8	5.7	2.0	2.5
amount of time after you arrive?	55.7	26.5	5.8	3.7	8.2
Provider taking time to answer	75.6	17.4	1.8	1.6	3.4
your questions?	67.9	19.1	4.0	1.6	7.4
Provider's interest in you as a	74.6	15.7	3.4	1.7	4.3
person?	65.5	22.3	4.5	0.8	6.9
Provider returning your calls	56.0	20.6	2.5	2.2	18.3
within a reasonable amount of time?	51.5	21.2	4.0	0.5	22.8

continued

Exhibit 30-1 continued

	Very Satis	Somewhat Satis	Somewhat Dissat	Very Dissat	N/R
The comfort of our facilities?	79.2	13.2	0.8	0.5	6.0
	61.0	24.4	3.2	0.8	10.6
Adequate parking?	51.3	29.0	12.0	3.7	3.7
	25.2	29.7	22.8	14.9	7.4
Reasonable charges?	58.1	22.3	2.8	0.8	15.7
	47.7	26.5	3.4	1.6	20.7
Our billing and payment procedures clear?	61.9	17.6	4.0	1.9	14.3
	50.4	23.3	4.0	1.9	20.4
Our hours convenient for you?	74.7	17.4	1.9	0.2	5.4
	67.9	21.5	1.6	0.3	8.8
Our office convenient to your home or work?	68.1	20.5	2.9	2.6	5.5
	60.2	23.1	4.2	1.9	10.6

Q6. What is your overall rating of our clinic?

	1989	1990
Excellent	49.6%	58.8%
Good	40.1	34.6
Fair	5.6	2.9
Poor	0.8	0.1
Did not answer	4.0	3.2
	100.0%	100.0%

- volume of referrals to the department
- criteria for making referrals
- referral patterns outside the provider network
- ratings of department responsiveness
- ratings of individual physicians
- patient feedback regarding specialists
- suggestions for improving the referral process

In effect, primary care providers are "clients" of the specialist departments. As managers of the health care team, they deserve full and timely communication regarding diagnosis and treatment. Indeed, the need for adequate communication is heightened by the fact that, in most group models, a patient may be seen by several primary care providers, all of whom need up-to-date information when the patient returns from the specialist's care.

A corollary issue involves "curbside consults." A key objective of the survey is to measure both the specialist's willingness to be available to primary care providers and the specialist's ability to recognize when *not* to insist on seeing the patient for diagnosis.

What To Do with Survey Results

Results of the patient survey measure the performance of primary care providers (Q3 asks the respondent to name the physician or department visited); results of the referring physician survey measure the performance of specialist physicians or departments. Since nonphysician marketers are usually outranked by the providers, the practical question is how to use the survey results.

Providers, even those in salaried positions with large groups, resist the concept of measurement and only in recent years have submitted to outside review of their clinical decisions. It can be added with confidence that few physicians and midlevel providers are ready to accept constructive criticism of their "bedside manner."

This problem is particularly acute in academic practices, where the performance of residents is a major determinant of patient satisfaction. Despite indications that patient loyalty is necessary for survival, faculty physicians rarely see their teaching roles as including supervision in nonclinical areas.

The quality assurance program can function as the mechanism for conveying survey findings to providers and counseling them in behavioral areas. The process involves expanding the role of medical directors, who, in concert with department heads, are already responsible for monitoring clinical performance and correcting practice patterns as appropriate. Using patient and referrer surveys, the annual evaluations of physicians and other providers can be extended to include the service standards described later in this chapter.

Step 2: Service Marketing Program

The second step in the service marketing process is to institutionalize the concept of patient satisfaction and convey the message that service is everyone's job. This process is as critical for managed care practices as for those groups marketing to fee-for-service patients. In one survey conducted among HMO members enrolled at a large multispecialty group, 37.6 percent said that they had asked a fellow employee about the clinic before choosing a provider from the managed care plan's network. Further, much research by the plans themselves indicates that, although cost may be a major factor in the selection of a plan, patient perceptions of service are a primary determinant in selecting and staying with a particular provider.

The case for service marketing is well made, but there is an additional benefit in focusing on service performance as a means of maintaining patient loyalty and building market share: This marketing strategy utilizes resources that are already paid for (i.e., the providers and those who support them) and avoids the added expense of external marketing techniques such as premium offers and advertising campaigns.

Anatomy of a Service Marketing Program

The schematic diagram in Figure 30-1 is a typical implementation plan for a service marketing program. The aim is to involve all clinic professionals—both those on the front line and those working behind the scenes—in a common effort to align the "corporate culture" with the perceived needs of patients. The program has three objectives:

1. To describe in criteria-based terms the specific performance standards expected of providers, employees whose jobs bring them into contact with patients, and support staff whose efforts are essential to the patient-centered performance of clinical and ancillary departments and the business office.
2. To deliver the service message in a clear and unambiguous manner so that everyone recognizes service standards as measurements of job performance.
3. To maintain the momentum of the program by involving providers and staff on an ongoing basis and by integrating service standards into the clinic's system for performance appraisal.

In the following sections, each of the major phases of implementation is discussed using the experience of the Southern California clinic whose dramatic improvements were noted earlier in this chapter.

Management Issues and Objectives

In meetings with the board of directors, clinic management proposed general objectives for the service marketing program. Although no specific goals were set for overall patient satisfaction (Q6), it was noted that a significant improvement would be required to counter the moves of area competitors and continue the clinic's growth pattern as stipulated in the business plan.

Specific patient satisfaction issues (Q5) were singled out for priority attention during the coming year, notably telephone procedures, appointment scheduling, waiting times in the clinic, business office performance, and the quality of provider time spent with patients.

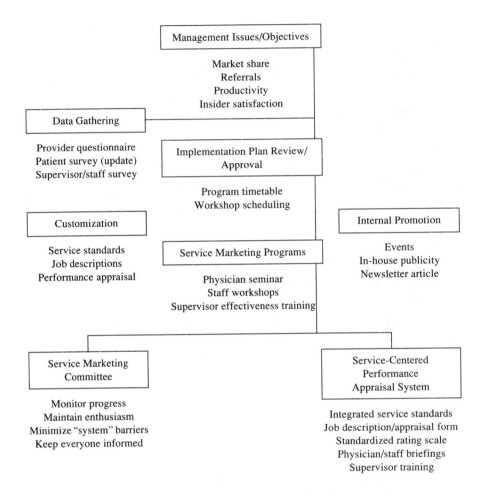

Figure 30-1 Typical Service Marketing Program Implementation Schematic. *Source:* Copyright © 1991 Sullivan/Luallin. All rights reserved.

The program and its goals were formally announced to the entire practice at the outset so as to focus attention on the importance of the service issues and the commitment of clinic leadership to effecting improvements.

Data Gathering

Once the objectives were established and publicized, an introductory meeting was scheduled in which the disappointing results of the 1989 patient survey were discussed with providers and supervisors, along with the results of questionnaires sent to providers, supervisors, and staff asking for input regarding the "pinch points" and other obstacles to fulfilling the service mission. The administration and the board emphasized that, since available capital was committed to other growth purposes, the performance problems would need to be solved without increasing current staffing levels. A timetable for program activities was presented, and a special call for cooperative effort was made.

Service Marketing Workshops

There followed a series of "patient relations" workshops designed to communicate the standards to be met by each of the clinic's professionals in order to achieve the desired turnaround in patient satisfaction.

Physicians and other providers participated in a seminar that reviewed the market forces affecting managed care providers and presented a set of recommended practice protocols (Exhibit 30-2).

Supervisor training programs presented proven techniques for motivating and managing employees, including situational concepts for diagnosing employee performance, applying effective management techniques, dealing with problem employees, dealing with job stress, and managing time.

In-service workshops for staff members included group exercises that focused attention on patient needs and practice sessions to improve performance in using the telephone, handling patient flow, resolving complaints, cooperating with other clinic departments, and other areas.

Performance Appraisal

Recognizing that service "sermons" are short-lived, a major priority was to develop a system for communicating to employees what is expected of them (job descriptions) and an objective means to evaluate their performance (appraisal system).

The Service-Centered Performance Appraisal System met these needs by developing criteria-based job descriptions for each position in the practice, including department-specific job descriptions for registered nurses, licensed practical nurses, and medical assistants. A new rating scale was developed to make the appraisal process more objective and consistent throughout the organization. The program was extended for use in new employee interviews and orientation as well as formal evaluations. (A sample job description from the Service-Centered Performance Appraisal System is provided in Appendix 30-C.)

Once the new job descriptions were completed, a series of employee briefings were scheduled to explain the program and answer questions about the appraisal process. It should be added that, owing to careful preparation by the

Exhibit 30-2 Service Guidelines for Physicians

---

1. Begin each appointment no more than 15 minutes late (and always with an apology when running behind).
2. Greet patients with a smile and a handshake.
3. Sit at eye level with patient; use eye contact.
4. Use patient's last name.
5. Use layperson's language whenever possible.
6. Ask if patients understand answers and instructions.
7. Return telephone calls to patients and referring physicians as promptly as possible.
8. Praise good staff performance frequently; don't criticize staff in front of patients.
9. Take leave of patients with a handshake or a pat on the shoulder.
10. Be available for consults with primary care providers as appropriate.
11. Provide dictation for patient charts within 24 hours of encounter.
12. Use standard forms to communicate diagnosis and/or treatment to primary care physician within 72 hours of encounter.
13. Return patients to primary care providers at the earliest appropriate time.

---

administration and the inclusion of supervisors in customizing the job descriptions, employees were nearly unanimous in accepting the new standards.

Service Marketing Committee

A final strategy for maintaining the momentum of the service program was to establish a committee comprising selected providers, supervisors, and staff members, aided by department heads from marketing, human resources, data processing, and operations.

The committee's charge was to monitor patient surveys and other information, to identify and remove operating system barriers and other barriers, and to keep everyone informed of progress.

Step 3: Service Recovery Program

Even in the most carefully constructed service program, mistakes are inevitable. In medical practices, where the services are performed in the patients' presence, there is little opportunity to correct errors before they are noticed. This is particularly the case in clinics where cost-cutting measures have thinned out the staff and placed major burdens on people and operating systems in the business office and clinical departments. Further, the medical delivery system is represented primarily by people whose performance will vary according to workloads, job stresses, and the personal baggage that every employee brings to the job.

Since service lapses will occur occasionally, the marketing program must develop procedures for responding to and recovering from problems. (In fact, patient complaints have been shown to be excellent marketing opportunities, since many patients become more loyal to the provider organization when problems are solved quickly and with concern for the patients' feelings.)

A systematic and effective approach to identifying and dealing with service lapses involves the ability of front-line employees to take responsibility for fixing problems. When management trusts its employees to this extent—after giving them adequate training and attentive supervision, to be sure—the employees nearly always become enthusiastic about the challenges of their expanded roles.

Unfortunately, most clinic protocols have the opposite effect, instructing employees to send complaints up the chain of communication for resolution at a higher level. Too often, these problems get lost in the shuffle, suppressed by insecure managers or simply ignored in the clutter of more pressing deadlines. In these cases, missed opportunities are quickly converted into lost market share.

A service recovery system is simple to set up and operate. It involves the following steps:

1. *Set up a "performance watch."* Establish effective tracking mechanisms that enable front-line employees to notify management immediately of problems occurring at their station. This ad hoc system, which complements the more general approach of regular patient surveys, is aimed at providing immediate solutions rather than programmatic solutions, which involve a longer, more formal process.

For example, clerks in the billing department can coordinate the immediate correction of data in the clinic computer system if they have the cooperation of the data processing staff. No doubt, interrupting the work schedules of data entry clerks is inefficient and may delay posting of other data; but the benefits to patient relations (and, concurrently, the marketing effort) far outweigh the disadvantages of interrupting workflow in the data processing department.

2. *Get the service marketing committee involved in finding solutions to recurring problems.* Every clinic has trouble spots where avoidable problems occur with regularity. For these service lapses, the more formal committee approach can be used to analyze problems and suggest solutions for use in departments throughout the organization.

For example, while physicians in obstetric departments are frequently called away to deliver babies, some doctors are more skilled than others in dealing with patients whose appointments were canceled without notice because of these emergencies. The committee might institute a special protocol in which a "green card" is inserted in the chart of a canceled patient so that the physician can make a special effort to apologize and explain during the next visit.

3. *Train front-line employees.* Since patient problems and complaints are best resolved at the point of service, staff members need special training in protocols for dealing with specific situations—both those in which solutions can be found and those where the employees are not able to provide an immediate resolution.

Staff training, although concentrating on procedural rules for dealing with specific problems, should include the following advice:

- If a problem exists, the involved staff member should be willing to recognize that it does. Taking the patient to a private place, if possible, the staff member should practice "active" listening techniques, dealing with the problem (not the patient's personality) and focusing on possible solutions.
- Staff members should demonstrate a willingness to empathize with patients, apologizing for a service lapse without being defensive or denying or minimizing the problem.
- Staff members should be adept at analyzing a problem situation, asking questions, and proposing alternatives without blaming the patient or another department.
- In cases where problems can be resolved, staff members should know the specific procedures, focusing on what can be done and following through on promises made to patients.

It should be noted that resolving patient problems does not always mean giving patients exactly what they want. When an alternative solution is the only practical course, the staff member might need to be persuasive in satisfying the patient that the clinic is doing its best to be accommodating. For example, the attendant at a clogged clinic parking lot may not be able to manufacture an empty space for an arriving patient but may be able to direct the patient to an alternate parking facility.

For employees to perform effectively in service recovery programs, extensive training is needed to explain and discuss all the recommended protocols. Further, nonmonetary incentives can be employed to recognize and reward employees whose performance in this area is exemplary.

4. *Communicate with patients.* Since patients value timely communication almost as much as getting their problems solved, a quick-response system can be implemented in which front-line employees can notify a designated individual (probably in the patient services department) of a problem and its resolution without going through regular line management. In this manner, the patient can be contacted by telephone to communicate the clinic's concern that the problem happened, the solution that has been implemented, and an invitation to call the patient services representative directly if future problems occur.

Other communication strategies include letters (with "real" signatures) and a special column in the clinic's patient newsletter reviewing problems solved in the preceding period.

A program for recovering from mistakes is as important as the basic system for preventing service lapses in the first place. Such a program is not without risk, for at its heart is a commitment by management to trust in the dedication and judgment of its lowest paid employees. Once implemented, the program requires continuing support by the administration, the board of directors, and the physicians and other providers. However, the magnitude of the investment is more than offset by the marketing benefits that can result.

CONCLUSION

In marketing, as with other medical management activities, there is no single formula for success. Strategies that work well in one situation may not be effective in another. Some providers or policies may receive positive reactions from some patients and negative responses from others.

Because marketing is neither art nor science, there are no ironclad rules. Patient and referrer surveys can help identify performance issues; "performance marketing" committees can solve them. Patient relations workshops can communicate service standards to employees; supervisors can monitor performance to see that the standards are met. Criteria-based job descriptions can define expectations; service-centered appraisals can reward employees for meeting them.

In the final analysis, marketing is a willingness to place a premium on patient satisfaction, a commitment to focus on marketing issues as part of the decision-making process, and the good fortune to consistently do the right thing at the right time.

Sample Patient Survey

Dear Patient:

Would you take a few minutes of your time to help us? Our goal is to provide comfort, convenience, and satisfaction as well as the very best medical care to all our patients.

We'd like to know how you feel about our medical services, our patient-handling systems, and our physicians and staff members.

Please return the completed survey as quickly as possible, either in the survey boxes in the lobby or using the return envelope. Your comments will help us evaluate our operations to ensure that we are truly responsive to your needs.

Thanks in advance for your help.

PLEASE CIRCLE THE NUMBER NEXT TO YOUR ANSWER.

Q1. How were you referred for this visit?
(please circle all that apply)

Friend/family member	1
Physician referral	2
Member of prepaid health plan (HMO)	3
Member of preferred provider organization (PPO)	4
Yellow Pages	5
Company medical plan	6
Saw your advertising	7
Recommended by the hospital	8
Other:_____	9

Q2. If you are a member of a prepaid health plan (HMO), why did you join that plan? (please circle all that apply)

Liked the plan benefits (coverage of services)	1
Liked the low cost	2
Liked the provider panel	3
Other:_____	4

Source: Portions of the survey are reprinted from the *Medical Marketer's Guide* by Sullivan/Luallin, with permission of Medical Group Management Association, 104 Inverness Terrace East, Englewood, CO 80112-5306, 1991.

Q3. What was it about our practice that attracted you? (please circle all that apply)

Your reputation for quality medical care	1
I've been to your doctors before	2
You're convenient to my home or work	3
You have convenient hours	4
Your cost is low	5
I like all health care services under one roof	6
Other:_____	7

Q3. Which physician/department did you visit?

_____

Q4. If you had any difficulty making this appointment, please tell us what happened:

_____
_____

Q5. Do you agree or disagree with the following:

	Strongly Agree	Agree Somewhat	Disagree Somewhat	Strongly Disagree
Your waiting time in the reception area was reasonable.	1	2	3	4
Your waiting time in the exam room was reasonable.	1	2	3	4
The waiting time for lab results was reasoanble.	1	2	3	4
You were informed of your test results within a reasonable amount of time.	1	2	3	4
Your phone calls were handled in a prompt and courteous manner.	1	2	3	4
Our after-hours answering service was prompt and courteous.	1	2	3	4
Our receptionists were friendly and courteous.	1	2	3	4
Our nurses were sympathetic to your problems and concerned about you as a person.	1	2	3	4
The people in our business office were concerned about helping you.	1	2	3	4

	Strongly Agree	Agree Somewhat	Disagree Somewhat	Strongly Disagree
We were able to solve your problems in a timely manner.	1	2	3	4
Your provider saw you within a reasonable amount of time after you arrived.	1	2	3	4
Your provider took time to answer your questions.	1	2	3	4
Your provider was interested in you as a person.	1	2	3	4
Your provider returned your calls within a reasonable amount of time.	1	2	3	4
Our facilities are clean and comfortable.	1	2	3	4
Our parking is adequate.	1	2	3	4
Our charges are reasonable.	1	2	3	4
Our hours are convenient for you.	1	2	3	4
Our office is convenient to your home or work.	1	2	3	4

Q6. What is your overall rating of our practice?

Excellent 1
Good 2
Fair 3
Poor 4

If *fair* or *poor*, please tell us why:

_____

_____

Q7. Would you recommend our practice to a family member or friend?

Yes 1
No 2

If *no*, please tell us why not:

_____

_____

Q8. Have you ever switched doctors in order to obtain better service?

Yes 1
No 2

Q9. Do you receive all of your medical care at our clinic?
    Yes   1
    No   2
    If *no*, please tell us what services you receive elsewhere:

_____

_____

Q10. Other comments:

_____

_____

_____

_____

Thank you for helping with this survey.

Appendix 30-B

Sample Referring Physician Survey

Dear Doctor:

Your opinions are valuable in helping our specialist departments serve your patients and maintain a high degree of responsiveness to your needs. Would you take a few minutes to respond to this survey and return it in the enclosed envelope. We will keep your responses strictly confidential. Thank you.

DEPARTMENT:_____

Q1. Approximately how many patients do you refer to specialists in this department each month?

0–5	1
6–10	2
11–15	3
16–25	4
26 and over	5

Q2. What criteria are most important to you when making referrals? (rate each factor on a scale of 1 [least important] to 5 [most important])

	Least Important			Most Important	
Personal relationship with physician	1	2	3	4	5
Physician sends patients back to you	1	2	3	4	5
Patient's request	1	2	3	4	5
Severity of illness	1	2	3	4	5
Physician's communication about patient	1	2	3	4	5
Feedback from patients after consults	1	2	3	4	5
Quick appointment scheduling	1	2	3	4	5
Competence of physician	1	2	3	4	5
Alumnus of a particular medical school	1	2	3	4	5
Other: _____	1	2	3	4	5

Source: Portions of the survey are reprinted from the *Medical Marketer's Guide* by Sullivan/Luallin, with permission of Medical Group Management Association, 104 Inverness Terrace East, Englewood, CO 80112-5306, 1991.

Q3. Do you ever refer patients outside our system?

Yes   1
No   2

If *yes,* please indicate your reasons for preferring the services of other providers:

_____

_____

Q4. How would you rate the ability of this department to serve your patients and your practice?

	Excellent	Good	Fair	Poor
Ease of getting an appointment	1	2	3	4
Friendly/courteous staff	1	2	3	4
Timely return of phone calls	1	2	3	4
Consult information	1	2	3	4
Answering patient questions	1	2	3	4
Concern for patient feelings	1	2	3	4
Timely return of patient	1	2	3	4
Overall quality of service	1	2	3	4

Q5. Please describe the response of physicians in this department when you ask for consultations or other information:

	Excellent	Good	Fair	Poor
Interest in the patient	1	2	3	4
Responsiveness to my request	1	2	3	4
Willingness to make time for me	1	2	3	4
Sensitivity to my needs	1	2	3	4
Ability to communicate	1	2	3	4
Concerned about my problem	1	2	3	4

Q6. How would you rate the written communication from this department regarding your patients?

	Excellent	Good	Fair	Poor
Timeliness of communication	1	2	3	4
Accuracy of information	1	2	3	4
Completeness of information	1	2	3	4
Other:_____	1	2	3	4

Q7. If your patients make any positive or negative comments about this department when they return to your care, please describe:

_____

_____

Q8. What suggestion(s) would you make to help this department improve its ability to serve the needs of patients and referring physicians?

_____

_____

Thank you for your time. Your input will be of help to us in structuring our practice to be more responsive to you and your patients.

Appendix 30-C

Job Description/Appraisal Form

Name: _____

Title: Receptionist **Department:** General **Reports to:** Office Manager

Summary:

The Satellite Receptionist performs various procedures associated with routine patient encounters; and maintains positive relationships with patients, family members and other visitors, and fellow employees.

Qualifications:

Minimum requirements include experience working with the public; ability to maintain composure when confronted with fast-paced and stressful situations; pleasant attitude; neat appearance; excellent communication skills; excellent telephone communication skills.

Note:

This document is intended to describe the general nature and level of work performed. It is not intended to serve as an exhaustive list of all duties, skills, and responsibilities required of personnel so classified.

A. DEPARTMENT STANDARD

Rating

Perform Department Duties in a Timely and Efficient Manner.

(1)   Manage all phases of the patient encounter; verify patient's name, address, phone number, and health coverage; direct patients to appropriate clinic locations as indicated by the schedule.

(2)   Open the department on time according to the checklist.

(3)   Give departing patients an appointment card with appropriate information; repeat the date and time of the next appointment, physician's name, and location of appointment.

(4)   Each afternoon, call patients with next-day appointments and verify time and place.

(5)   Monitor the outside front lobby area and be ready to assist if patients or visitors encounter difficulties.

(6)   Maintain a fresh coffee supply in the reception area and keep the coffee area clean and tidy.

(7)   Perform other tasks as assigned.

EVALUATOR COMMENTS:

( ) _____

( ) _____

(Use reverse side for additional comments.)

B. SERVICE STANDARD

Rating

Demonstrate Courtesy and Helpfulness toward Patients, Family Members, and Others.

(1) Acknowledge patients/others immediately; use eye contact and smile (when appropriate).

(2) Let patients know if delays are expected; keep patients/others informed of their status.

(3) Use the patient's last name until you sense that a less formal approach is appropriate.

(4) Use layperson's language whenever possible.

(5) Be an "active" listener; pay attention to what the person is saying.

(6) Make sure the information you give is accurate and complete.

(7) Be helpful to patients/others who need assistance in finding their way around the facility.

(8) Give clear, understandable directions; repeat your remarks and answer all questions with patience and concern.

(9) Reassure anxious patients/others; ask what you can do to make the situation easier for them.

(10) Conclude every encounter with a friendly "thank you" when appropriate.

EVALUATOR COMMENTS:

( ) _____
_____
( ) _____
_____

(Use reverse side for additional comments.)

C. SERVICE STANDARD

**Ensure Smooth and Efficient Telephone
Communication.**

Rating

(1) Answer the telephone within three rings when possible; say "(Department), (your name), may I help you?"

(2) Speak to callers in a friendly, helpful tone of voice.

(3) When putting callers on hold, ask "Can you hold, please?" and wait for a response.

(4) Keep "on hold" callers apprised of their status.

(5) When returning to the line, thank the caller for holding.

(6) If you cannot help the caller within a reasonable time, take name/number and promise a call-back; follow through on all promises made to callers.

(7) When taking messages, repeat the information to ensure accuracy; use the appropriate form and distribute messages in a timely manner.

EVALUATOR COMMENTS:

(   ) _____
_____

(   ) _____
_____

(Use reverse side for additional comments.)

D. SERVICE STANDARD

Handle Complaints in a Responsive and Professional Manner.

(1) Stay calm; don't take complaints personally.

(2) Listen for the facts; let the patient tell the whole story and make sure you understand the source of the problem.

(3) Don't respond to complaints with arguments or excuses; apologize if errors have been made.

(4) Refer abusive patients immediately to the appropriate supervisor or Administration.

(5) Let the complainer know that you're interested in solving the problem.

(6) Describe what you plan to do to solve the problem; never make promises you can't keep.

(7) Follow through on whatever promises you make to solve the problem.

(8) Monitor feedback and let your supervisor know how you handled the problem.

EVALUATOR COMMENTS:

( ) _____

( ) _____

(Use reverse side for additional comments.)

E. TEAMWORK STANDARD

Be Cooperative and Helpful with Co-Workers and Employees in Other Departments.

Rating

(1) In dealing with fellow employees, recognize that everyone's job is important to the success of the organization.

(2) Take the initiative in offering your help to co-workers in overload situations (when possible).

(3) Respond to requests from other departments in a timely, positive, and pleasant manner.

(4) Keep your promises to co-workers and employees in other departments.

(5) Approach all disagreements with fellow employees as problems to be solved; attempt to solve problems yourself before taking them to your supervisor.

(6) Avoid criticizing other members of the clinic in front of patients or fellow employees.

(7) Assist your supervisor by suggesting methods for avoiding problems in the future.

EVALUATOR COMMENTS:

( ) _____

_____

( ) _____

_____

(Use reverse side for additional comments.)

F. PROFESSIONAL STANDARD

Ensure That Your Appearance and Personal Conduct Are Professional at All Times.

Rating

(1) Arrive at your work station and be ready to begin work at the appropriate time.

(2) Follow the dress code; wear your name badge correctly.

(3) Be courteous with physicians and fellow staff members.

(4) Limit personal phone calls and side-talk.

(5) Observe department rules for food and drink at your work station.

(6) Adhere to established policies as contained in the Personnel Manual.

(7) In the community, represent the organization in a positive and professional manner.

(8) Maintain patient confidentiality at all times.

(9) Respond calmly and professionally in emergency situations.

EVALUATOR COMMENTS:

( ) _____

( ) _____

(Use reverse side for additional comments.)

Final Rating Worksheet

Job Standards	Rating ×	Level of Importance =	Total Points
A. Perform department duties in an efficient and timely manner.	_____ ×	_____%	= _____
B. Demonstrate courtesy and helpfulness.	_____ ×	_____%	= _____
C. Ensure smooth and efficient telephone communication.	_____ ×	_____%	= _____
D. Handle complaints in a professional manner.	_____ ×	_____%	= _____
E. Be cooperative and helpful with fellow employees.	_____ ×	_____%	= _____
F. Ensure that your appearance and personal conduct are professional at all times.	_____ ×	_____%	= _____

100%

Total Points _____

Divided by   *100*

Final Rating _____

31

Human Resources

Judy M. Marsh

What are human resources? Is there a difference between human resources and personnel? And why should ambulatory care administrators be concerned about human resources? This chapter will answer these questions and provide a guide for companies considering the establishment of a professional human resources function. It will also provide basic guidelines and suggest caveats for organizations that do not have a human resources department.

HISTORY

The personnel department experienced a metamorphosis during the last ten years: It became the human resources department. This metamorphosis was not simply a change in terminology. It was a change in function. The old personnel department evolved as an adjunct of the payroll department, handling routine functions primarily associated with recordkeeping (e.g., personnel files) and "hiring and firing." Beginning in the mid-1960s with the enactment of civil rights legislation, especially antidiscrimination laws, the role of the personnel department began to change, since its recordkeeping functions had to be modified and enlarged to accommodate the new laws. The personnel manager's job expanded to include expertise in the various antidiscrimination statutes and their application in the employment setting, particularly in hiring and terminating employees. The goal was to keep the organization from encountering difficulties with the Equal Employment Opportunity Commission (EEOC) and the various individual state agencies set up to monitor state antidiscrimination laws.

Organizations that failed to comply with the new employment laws discovered that their employees were frequently quite knowledgeable about civil rights issues and applicable statutes. This resulted in the filing of many well-publicized lawsuits and complaints with the EEOC and the state agencies. These in turn frequently generated high awards for applicants and employees who were victims of discrimination.

During the 1970s, even more laws protecting employees and restricting employers were passed, for example, the Employee Retirement Income Security Act (ERISA), which affects benefits administration. As more and more laws and regulations affecting the employer-employee relationship were enacted, a demand arose for professional personnel managers who were trained, educated, and skilled in the practical application of employment law. In the early years, personnel professionals were primarily trained on the job. But with the passage of time, formal university education in personnel management and administration became the rule.

The 1980s continued the trend of restrictive employment laws with the passage of laws such as the Consolidated Omnibus Budget Reconciliation Act (COBRA), which required employers to offer group insurance at group rates to terminated employees. Judicial decisions that clarified existing statutes such as the court decisions regarding wrongful terminations resulted in multi-million-dollar awards granted to employees who had been "wrongfully discharged." The term "human resources department" emerged during the 1980s as a more generally descriptive term for a department that was engaged not only in hiring and firing but also in providing the many services necessary to maintain the employer-employee relationship. These services include functions mandated by law as well as procedures designed to protect employers from inadvertently violating existing regulations and statutes. This shift in emphasis was enhanced as employers realized that employees were not simply a cost item on balance sheets but had become their most important resource.

GENERAL FUNCTIONS

Passage of the Americans with Disabilities Act (ADA), signed by President Bush on July 26, 1990, indicates that the trend toward employer restrictions will continue into the 1990s. As employers or representatives of employers, ambulatory care administrators must be aware of the limitations imposed by governmental agencies and the courts. Ignorance could result in significant financial loss to the organization through litigation fees, mandated fines, or negotiated settlements. Recent court decisions in wrongful termination, sexual harassment, and other employment-related lawsuits have resulted in hundreds of thousands of dollars in settlements. The human resources department serves the organization as a clearinghouse for information relevant to the ever-changing laws dealing with the employer-employee relationship. Ambulatory care administrators should view an effective human resources department as a form of insurance against litigious applicants and employees as well as an information source about employee relations issues for the entire organization.

However, human resources is not only a preventive function. Today's enlightened manager realizes that an organization's most valuable resource is its employees. In a service industry such as health care, labor is the most costly expenditure. It stands to reason that a manager should care for an organization's employees just as he or she cares for an expensive piece of equipment. The human resources department assists ambulatory care administrators in caring for the organization's employees.

Because of the acute shortage of skilled health care professionals in the current job market, the human resources department can contribute to an organization's profitability through professional administration of its recruiting, selecting, and retention procedures.

Although today's health care is highly technical, it cannot be delivered by machine. Patients need and demand the attention and warmth of human caregivers. Unfortunately, good skilled employees are difficult to find. Human resources personnel can assist ambulatory care administrators by locating and hiring qualified employees at minimal cost. In addition, by reducing turnover through positive employee relations techniques and equitable enforcement of policies, human resources personnel can improve an organization's financial position. They can accomplish this by reducing employment costs while at the same time ensuring consistently good patient care through the retention of skilled employees.

ESTABLISHING A HUMAN RESOURCES DEPARTMENT

When should an organization establish a separate human resources department? Generally, an organization of 50 or more employees should have some part-time professional assistance (e.g., a consultant or an onsite human resources representative). An organization with 100 or more employees should establish a human resources department with one full-time human resources professional. Part-time clerical assistance may also be needed to help with the recordkeeping. However, it is important to note that federal antidiscrimination laws apply to employers of as few as 15 employees. In California, one of the states with the most stringent laws dealing with the employer-employee relationship, the antidiscrimination laws can cover employers with as few as one to four employees (e.g., the laws governing the employment of pregnant women). Therefore, the astute ambulatory care administrator must have a working knowledge of state and federal civil rights laws.

Managers of even the smallest organization should begin reviewing its business practices for compliance with antidiscrimination laws. It is important to note that an employee is defined as a person who receives money in the form of wages, salary, or commission in return for services performed. Nonowner physicians and managers are also employees and are therefore protected by the various laws. Ambulatory care managers should not make the mistake of presuming a physician or high-level manager will not seek recourse for a grievance through the courts. In fact, professionals are more likely to file a complaint against an organization than are blue- or pink-collar workers.

In addition to civil rights laws, ambulatory care administrators must be familiar with the wage and hour laws of the jurisdiction in which they work. Wage and hour laws govern such things as compensation and the working environment. All employers are governed by the Fair Labor Standards Act, which covers areas such as overtime payments, breaks, and working conditions. In addition, many states and some local governments also enact wage and hour laws. How does one determine which of the various laws to follow? The safest course to follow when federal and state wage and hour laws conflict is to abide by the most stringent. The courts do not recognize ignorance of the wage and hour laws as an excuse for failure to comply. An employer is seldom viewed favorably by a judge or jury for failing to observe published or general knowledge laws dealing with the employer-employee relationship. The employer is considered the superior in the alliance and therefore the controlling force in the employee's life. Therefore, the employer has the responsibility to understand and abide by the wage and hour laws.

It is difficult and time consuming for an ambulatory care administrator to stay abreast of and comply with the complex and changing employment laws and regulations. Human resources professionals can assist the employer in observing the laws. (Many payroll specialists are also knowledgeable about wage and hour laws, especially those dealing with compensation.) Sources for information regarding employment laws include organizations that market reference book series, professional human resources organizations such as the Society for Human Resource Management and the Healthcare Human Resources Management Association, law firms that specialize in personnel or labor law, and human resources practitioners working as consultants (see Suggested Resources at end of chapter).

Establishment Procedure

How should an ambulatory care administrator proceed in establishing a human resources department? First, choose a seasoned human resources practitioner. Suggested minimum qualifications for the position include at least three years of professional human resources experience, preferably in a health care environment, and some college work in personnel administration, with the optimum being a degree. Health care human resources experience is important because of the specialized nature of the industry. Health care organizations differ significantly from most employers in that their labor force includes large numbers of knowledgeable workers. These individuals, well educated and technically trained, present unique problems and challenges to human resources professionals when it comes to hiring, retention, and problem solving. The terminology and product are also unique. In addition to health care human resources experience, a college-level degree is suggested. Since psychology, people skills, and management expertise are mandatory for success in human resources, a liberal arts or sociology degree is preferable to a degree in a science such as math or business. (Human resources professionals often train and counsel other managers in staff management techniques.)

It is also important that adequate clerical support be available. The recordkeeping requirements imposed by the various laws are monumental and generate enormous amounts of paperwork. The human resources manager should be relieved as much as possible of clerical duties in order to proceed with setting up systems, counseling, and organizing the department.

The ambulatory care administrator can assist in the creation of the human resources department by establishing organizational policy regarding human resources functions and by notifying all staff about the new department. The human resources manager will need strong administrative support to be successful.

Perhaps the first step the new human resources manager will take is to identify all personnel records and centralize them in confidential personnel files in the human resources office. Personnel records are frequently scattered in managers' offices throughout the organization. Managers may be reluctant to release this information and the authority it represents to the human resources manager. Therefore, it is vital to the success of the new human resources department that the organization establish policies regarding the department's functions and that the policies be publicized to the management staff.

Once the human resources manager has gathered the personnel data from throughout the organization, official personnel files for all employees must be set up. The manager should also review current policies, both written and unwritten, regarding the organization's employees. With this information, departmental policies and procedures can be recommended that are consistent with the organization's policies and practices as well as with applicable laws and regulations. The recommended policies and procedures would pertain to hiring, terminations, wage increases, and so on.

The human resources manager who is establishing a new department can encounter resistance from established departments, which often hesitate to release confidential information about employees. The managers of these departments should be assured that confidentiality is the credo of the human resources manager. The sensitivity of the issue of confidentiality is also the primary reason that the ambulatory care administrator should hire an experienced human resources practitioner to set up a new department. Professional-ism and fairness are the keys to success in human resources. Because of the complexity of personnel issues today, the human resources functions should not be assigned to a secretary or attached as an adjunct to payroll. The special-ized knowledge and experience required to manage human resources in today's ambulatory health care business demand a skilled manager.

Laws, Regulations, and Company Policies

Laws and regulations such as those discussed above in regard to employment are established by regulatory bodies and apply to all employers within that particular jurisdiction. For example, civil rights laws are federal laws and apply throughout the United States. Cities or counties may also have laws or ordi-nances that apply only to local employers (e.g., laws regulating smoking).

Company policies are defined or established by each employer, and they are unique to each employer. Policies may either be written or established through "practice," that is, through the actual implementation of procedures or the ways in which the employer and the management representatives deal with the employees. Policies must conform to the laws and regulations of the jurisdic-tion in which the organization does business. A policy that contradicts the law is imprudent and will cause the organization more problems than having no policy at all.

Ideally, company policies should be written. An organization may establish policies through an "official" manual, employee handbook, memos, letters and similar methods. The method by which an organization communicates with employees is also the method by which it establishes policies. Formal written policies should be clear, concise, and accurate. Once policies are written, they should be dated, numbered, and included in manuals or handbooks. The written policies should be reviewed regularly to ascertain that they continue to conform to actual policies and practices and to laws and regulations.

The human resources department acts as a clearinghouse for policies and practices that may violate various laws and regulations applying to the employer-employee relationship. The human resources manager is knowledgeable about the ever-changing employment laws and strives to provide current, accurate advice and counsel regarding personnel issues to the organization's management staff.

HOW HUMAN RESOURCES HELPS TO CUT COSTS

Besides preventing problems with government agencies and litigious appli-cants and employees, a human resources department can perform other valuable services. It can affect the profitability of an organization by assisting in the management of its most important asset, its employees, and it can accomplish this by playing an active role in the following areas:

- recruitment
- retention
- benefits administration
- worker's compensation and safety
- unemployment claims administration

Recruitment

Today's shortage of skilled health care employees demands creativity in the recruitment function. Newspaper advertising alone is often not sufficient to attract appropriate candidates. Skill is needed to devise innovative recruiting methods, and marketing expertise is required to bring new hires to the organization. A key factor in successful recruiting is timeliness responding to applicants. Experienced, qualified health care applicants often have several job offers from which to choose. A quick response to an application or inquiry gives an organization a clear advantage in a highly competitive job market.

Due to pressing operational needs, many line managers neglect hiring responsibilities until a staffing crisis occurs; then they hire the first person who appears to meet the minimum qualifications for the job. Often this person is a poor or marginal performer, which compounds the manager's staffing problems. Good labor management begins with the recruitment process. The human resources department serves as the recruiting center for the organization. A professional human resources manager can relieve line management by providing qualified candidates for jobs and assisting management in the selection process while ensuring compliance with antidiscrimination laws and company policies.

Retention

More important than recruiting and selecting quality employees is an ambulatory care organization's ability to retain its valuable human assets. Recruitment and selection is an expensive process. Advertisements, telephone calls, management time spent in interviews, and training time are all costly. Therefore, it is more efficient for an organization to allocate resources to retain current employees rather than constantly strive to replace those who leave. Human resources personnel can assist ambulatory care administrators by establishing and maintaining an effective retention program for the organization.

A plan for retention of employees and reduction of turnover will affect many facets of the employer-employee relationship. As a centralized staff department, the human resources department can coordinate the organization's employee retention program, which will result in reduced overall employment costs as well as increased production by allowing line managers more time for operational duties.

Benefits Administration

Employee benefits can add 25 percent to 40 percent or more to an organization's labor costs. They constitute a hidden but very stiff expense for an employer. It is vital that employee benefits be controlled so that the employer receives the greatest value for the benefit dollars expended. In other words, the benefits package must be competitive so that good employees can be recruited and retained, but its costs must be analyzed and controlled as part of the total cost for labor.

Human resources professionals are skilled in benefits administration. They can assist an ambulatory care organization by monitoring its employee benefits so as to control costs and maintain a competitive benefits package for recruiting and retention purposes.

Workers' Compensation and Safety

Employers are required by both federal and state laws to provide employees with worker's compensation benefits for on-the-job injuries. Employers must also provide a safe working environment for employees. Failure to due either can result in significant fines and expensive court settlements.

Human resources professionals are skilled in the administration of worker's compensation and safety programs. They can assist ambulatory care administrators by either lowering worker's compensation insurance rates (if the organization has a worker's compensation insurance carrier) or minimizing required reserves (if the organization is self-insured for worker's compensation). Human resources professionals can also assist in the design, implementation, and administration of an organization's safety program, an important component of an overall program to reduce on-the-job injury and illness costs.

Unemployment Claims Administration

Effective administration of unemployment claims can result in significant cost savings for an ambulatory care organization. Although unemployment compensation laws vary from state to state, human resources professionals practicing in each state are trained in that state's statutes. Careful adherence to the employer's reporting requirements and the legal deadlines can help support the company's position in unemployment claims, resulting in lower unemployment taxes for the organization.

ORGANIZATIONS WITHOUT A HUMAN RESOURCES DEPARTMENT

Despite the advantages of having a human resources department, many health care organizations, either because of size or financial constraints, do not have one. What can an organization without a formal human resources department do to avoid problems with government agencies and control employment costs? Use of sound, comprehensive employee policies is the key. This section presents issues and suggestions for administrators in ambulatory health care who do not yet need to hire a full-time human resources professional.

All organizations are subject to an investigation by the EEOC or state agencies if a discrimination claim is filed by either an applicant or an employee. Preparation for an investigation is extremely time consuming and costly, and there is of course the risk of having to pay penalties and fines. As a means of avoiding problems with antidiscrimination laws and regulations, the ambulatory care administrator must become familiar with the organization's recruitment and selection process, concentrating on such areas as the application form, the interviewing procedure, and preemployment tests.

Application Forms

The application form must meet stringent federal and state requirements regarding its content and the questions it asks of job applicants. Sections that overtly or covertly require information about the applicant's race, religion, sex, national origin, handicap status, medical status, marital status, veteran status, or age must be avoided. As an example, an application should never ask for a photo of the applicant, since photos can be used to determine race, age, and sex. Neither should the application ask for the year of high school graduation, because this date indicates the applicant's age.

Employers are required by laws to maintain affirmative action statistics (e.g., race, sex, age, and veteran status of applicants and employees). But how does one acquire the necessary information without violating antidiscrimination laws? The answer is to devise a method that obtains the data through the employment application but that records and stores the data separately from the application forms (see Exhibit 31-1). Thus, although this sensitive demographic information about applicants and employees must never be used in hiring, promotion, transfer, or termination actions, it can still be recorded and made available to government agencies upon request. The employment application form can also protect an organization from wrongful termination charges and serve as a tool in discharging unsuitable employees. For example, if an employee falsifies responses on an employment application, it may be grounds for immediate dismissal without recourse. Careful wording is essential for ensuring the legality of an employment application. Ambulatory care administrators should submit the organization's employment application to a labor attorney or human resources consultant for review prior to use. This review can prevent expensive fines and save litigation costs for the organization. Appendix 31-A is an example of an employment application used successfully by a large health care organization.

Interviewing

An ambulatory care organization's management staff should be trained in proper interviewing techniques. The ambulatory care administrator should establish an employment interviewing procedure that avoids discriminatory practices and ensures the selection of qualified applicants. The procedure should provide guidelines regarding good interview techniques and questions that should not be asked during an interview. For example, management representatives should never question a female applicant regarding the number of children she has unless the same question is also asked of all male applicants. All questions regarding child-care arrangements, marital status, and transportation to work should also be avoided, since such questions may imply discriminatory practices.

Skillful interviewing techniques can disclose information regarding many of the above concerns without overt questioning of the applicant. Interviewing is a skill; it must be learned. Ambulatory care administrators should ascertain the interviewing skill level of the organization's management staff and work with them toward improvement. The management staff should know the categories of individuals specifically provided protection under the antidiscrimination laws. Once again, ignorance of the laws is no defense against government charges. It is in the best interest of the organization that the management staff be thoroughly trained in the avoidance of discriminatory employment practices.

When selecting an individual for a job, the manager should utilize a straightforward and objective approach. Is this the best candidate? Why? The answers should relate to bona fide requirements for the job, not superficialities (e.g., age) or the interviewer's personal preferences (e.g., a preference for a female

Exhibit 31-1 Applicant Survey

Voluntary Affirmative Action Information *(Completion of information below is voluntary.)*

Applicants are considered for all positions, and employees are treated during employment without regard to race, color, religion, sex, national origin, age, marital or veteran status, medical condition or handicap, or any other legally protected status.

As employers, we comply with government regulations, including affirmative action responsibilities where they apply.

Solely to help us comply with government recordkeeping, reporting, and other legal requirements, we request that you please fill out the Voluntary Affirmative Action Information. We appreciate your cooperation.

This data is for periodic government reporting and will be kept in a *Confidential File* separate from the Application for Employment.

YOUR COOPERATION IS VOLUNTARY. _____

(PLEASE PRINT)   Date_____

Position(s) Applied For _____

Referral Source: ☐ Advertisement   ☐ Friend   ☐ Relative   ☐ Walk-In   ☐ Agency
                          Name of Source *(if applicable)* _____

Name _____ Phone (_____) _____
            LAST   FIRST   MIDDLE   AREA CODE
Address _____
            NUMBER   STREET   CITY   STATE   ZIP CODE

Voluntary Survey

Government agencies at times require periodic reports on the sex, ethnicity, handicapped, veteran, and other protected status of applicants. These data are for analysis and possible affirmative action only. SUBMISSION OF INFORMATION IS VOLUNTARY. Please be advised that your survey is NOT a part of your official application for employment. It is considered confidential information that will not be used in any hiring decision.

Check one: ☐ Male   ☐ Female

Check one of the following:

   Race/Ethnic Group: ☐ White   ☐ Black   ☐ Hispanic
                               ☐ American Indian/Alaskan Native   ☐ Asian/Pacific Islander

Special Employment Notice to Disabled Veterans, Vietnam Era Veterans, and Individuals with Physical or Mental Handicaps.

Employers are subject to 38 USC 2012 of the Vietnam Era Veterans Readjustment Act of 1974 which requires that they take affirmative action to employ and advance in employment qualified disabled veterans and veterans of the Vietnam Era.

Check if any of the following are applicable:

   ☐ Vietnam Era Veteran   ☐ Disabled Veteran   ☐ Other Veteran

Section 503 of the Rehabilitation Act of 1973, as amended, requires employers to take affirmative action to employ and advance in employment qualified handicapped individuals.

Are you handicapped?   ☐ Yes   ☐ No

If yes, please explain _____

_____

medical assistant). If the candidate is selected, can the selection be justified based upon the job criteria? Although it is virtually impossible to remove all prejudices in the selection of job applicants, careful consideration and truthful responses to the above questions should assist the conscientious manager in selecting the best applicant for the job while avoiding discriminatory employment decisions.

Many human resources consultants specialize in management development techniques, including interviewing and selection methods. They can provide ambulatory care organizations with training in these areas if it is needed and relieve the administrator of these specialized and controversial duties.

Employment Tests

Under federal laws, any employment test must be validated as directly job-related and as an indicator of success on the job. For example, a test requiring mathematical skills equivalent to those of a high school graduate for applicants to qualify for a janitorial position is most likely not job-related and is therefore potentially discriminatory. Should a minority applicant who failed to qualify for the janitorial job challenge the organization by filing a complaint with the EEOC, the company would have difficulty justifying the requirement for expertise in mathematics. In this example, the organization could be subject to fines and would incur legal costs in its defense of the inappropriate employment test.

The ambulatory care administrator should monitor the selection procedures of management representatives for questionable techniques involving employment tests. Although the term *employment test* is broadly defined to encompass all of the techniques that are used in the selection process, including but not limited to the application form, the interview, and the employment physical, written employment tests are most often a cause for concern. All written employment tests should be reviewed and validated before being used in the organization's selection process. Human resources consultants can assist the organization in the validation of its selection procedures, including written employment tests.

RETENTION TECHNIQUES

Retention of current employees should be a priority for ambulatory care administrators. Establishing an effective retention program requires a multipronged approach.

First, a review of the current wage and salary structure and benefits package should be conducted. An organization must offer its employees basic security items (e.g., a fair wage and competitive benefits) in order to attract and retain quality people.

Examination of the wage and salary structure should answer these questions: Is the salary structure competitive for the area from which the organization recruits most of its employees? If not, what factors in the structure need change, and what would be the cost of changing them? When establishing or changing a wage and salary structure, an ambulatory care administrator must know the organization's policy and philosophy in regard to wages and salaries. For example, does the company want to be competitive in both wages and benefits? Some organizations may feel that since they offer significant nonfinancial benefits such as location, prestige, or career ladders, they need not compete on salary and benefits. Should a company be high in one and low in another? Does the organization desire to be a leader in compensation issues or just competitive? Answers to these questions, along with information regarding the company's financial status, must be available to the administrator prior to establishing a wage and salary structure.

Once a fair, equitable, and competitive wage and salary structure is established, it is vital that the information regarding the compensation improvements be related to the employees. Retention of good employees depends upon good employer-employee communications. It is motivating to employees if they know that the company is competitive in its compensation package and is striving to remain so.

Retaining employees may also depend upon the advancement opportunities offered by the organization. Good employees are motivated by opportunities for advancement. Ambulatory care administrators should review the organizational structure to find and create career pathways for outstanding promotable employees. If there are areas where these pathways exist, the information should be communicated to the employees. When there are no pathways, the administrator should search for ways to create them.

It is interesting to note that not all employees respond to promotional opportunities. For example, whereas a person eager to advance to a management position would enjoy working for an organization with ample promotional opportunities, this may not be an incentive to an individual seeking stability and predictability in a job. The potential for career movement is not important to some employees. Managers must learn to be adept at recognizing employee personality types. This is an invaluable talent in the recruitment, selection, and retention of employees.

An effective employee retention program should also include a review of the employee benefits package, including group insurance benefits, paid time off, and other perquisites. The review should answer such questions as these: Is the current benefits package competitive for the local area? What enhancements are needed to ensure competitiveness, and what is the cost?

The organization's goals and philosophy should be considered when reviewing the benefits package. For example, certain benefits such as retirement plans and vacation accruement promote employee longevity. Organizations should consider enhancing those plans as a way of increasing retention rates and decreasing recruitment costs.

Currently, there is substantial competition among employers regarding the health insurance benefits they offer. Many organizations are seeking to reduce rapidly increasing group health insurance costs by shifting the higher premium costs to the employees. However, prudent employers must consider all of the costs incurred by a reduction of health insurance benefits and seek alternatives to merely increasing the employees' share of the premiums. Astute job applicants and employees shop for employers who offer not only competitive wages but also good benefits at low cost to employees. A key element in retaining employees is a comprehensive, low-employee-cost benefits package.

Many employees leave an organization because of unresolved employee relations issues such as inequitable enforcement of company policies and perceptions of unfairness or favoritism. Retention of good employees depends upon the establishment of a plan for dealing with employee relations problems and complaints.

Ambulatory care administrators should establish an official problem-solving procedure involving several levels of management, including the top official of the organization. This procedure should be widely publicized throughout the company to all employees, and the administration should ensure that it is equitably followed by all management staff.

Why is an equitable problem-solving procedure so important in the retention of employees? Problems, complaints, and disagreements between staff and management are inevitable. The deciding factor in good employee relations is how difficulties are handled. If dissension is ignored, it will result in further conflict or loss of employees. In either case, the result is a disruption in the effective functioning of a work area. The goal of a problem-solving procedure is to (1) identify problems before they become disruptions; (2) provide employees with an outlet to air dissatisfaction; and (3) identify policy, procedure, and personnel issues within the organization that should be addressed. An effective problem-solving procedure administered evenhandedly serves as a valuable resource for the management staff as well as an excellent means for employees to elicit a response to their complaints.

Exit interviews are a good method to determine why employees are leaving a company's employ. Used correctly, they can be an effective employee relations tool. Ambulatory care administrators interested in good employee relations should establish an official exit interview policy. All resigning employees should be encouraged to provide an exit interview prior to the termination date. An impartial party should be assigned to conduct the interview (never the immediate supervisor). The interview questions should be structured to reveal why the employee is resigning and what the employee thinks about the job, the company, the benefits, and other issues. Interview statistics should be recorded and tabulated, with repetitive problem areas identified for research and investigation.

The goal of an employee retention program is to reduce employee turnover by the most cost-effective means. The methods listed above will aid in identifying problem areas that warrant the attention of the organization's top management.

CONCLUSION

The human resources function is vital to the success of today's ambulatory care organization. Human resources personnel can assist the organization in caring for its most important and costly asset, its employees. Prudent management of the employer-employee relationship is essential for survival, and effective human resources policies will allow the organization to gain the edge needed to thrive in the highly competitive health care market. Even before the establishment of a formal human resources department, there are many steps a smaller health care organization can take to improve its employee relations posture.

SUGGESTED RESOURCES

Reference Book Series
Bureau of National Affairs, 1231 25th Street, N.W., Washington, DC 20037. (800) 452-7773.
Bureau of Business Practice, 24 Rope Ferry Rd., Waterford, CT 06386. (800) 243-0876.

Human Resources Organizations
Society for Human Resource Management, 606 North Washington Street, Alexandria, VA 22314. (703) 548-3440.
Healthcare Human Resource Management Association, 201 N. Figueroa Street, 4th Floor, Los Angeles, CA 90012. (213) 250-5600.
Merchants and Manufacturers' Association (California only), P.O. Box 15013, Los Angeles, CA 90015. (213) 748-0421.
Hospital Council of Southern California, 201 N. Figueroa Street, 4th Floor, Los Angeles, CA 90012. (213) 250-5600.

Appendix 31-A

Employment Application Form

Application For Employment   **Friendly Hills HealthCare Network**

We consider applicants for all positions without regard to race, color, religion, sex, national origin, age, married or veteran status, the presence of non-job-related medical condition, or handicap, or any other legally protected status.

(PLEASE PRINT)   Date of Application_____

Position(s) Applied For _____

Referral Source: ☐ Advertisement ☐ Friend ☐ Relative ☐ Walk-In ☐ Agency

          Name of Source *(if applicable)* _____

Name _____
          LAST   FIRST   MIDDLE

Address _____
          NUMBER   STREET   CITY   STATE   ZIP CODE

Telephone (_____) _____ Social Security Number _____
          AREA CODE

If you are under 18, can you furnish a work permit? ☐ Yes ☐ No

Have you filed an application here before? ☐ Yes ☐ No If yes, give date_____

Have you ever been employed here before? ☐ Yes ☐ No

If yes, under what name _____

Are you employed now? ☐ Yes ☐ No

May we contact your present employer? ☐ Yes ☐ No

Can you, after employment, submit verification of your legal right to work in the U.S.?
☐ Yes ☐ No
(Proof of citizenship or immigration status will be required upon employment.)

Name of friends and relatives employed by Friendly Hills HealthCare Network _____

_____

On what date would you be able to work? _____

Wage/salary you are seeking _____

Are you available to work? ☐ Full Time ☐ Part Time ☐ Weekends ☐ Temporary

Can you work on any shift? ☐ Yes ☐ No

If no, what shifts can you work? _____
                              ☐ Days   ☐ Afternoons   ☐ Nights

Are you on lay-off and subject to recall? ☐ Yes ☐ No

Have you been convicted of a felony within the last (7) years? ☐ No ☐ Yes
(A conviction will not necessarily be a bar to employment, in that factors such as age and time of the offense, seriousness and nature of the violation and rehabilitation will be taken into account.)

If yes, please explain _____

_____

EMPLOYMENT EXPERIENCE

Start with your present or last job. Include military service assignments (but do not list dates of military service and type of discharge) and volunteer activities. Exclude organization names which indicate race, color, religion, gender, national origin, handicap or other protected status.

Employer _____ Telephone (_____) _____
Address _____ City/Zip _____
Job Title _____ Supervisor _____
Reason for leaving _____
Dates Employed: From (Mo./Yr.) _____ To (Mo./Yr.) _____
Hourly Rate/Salary: Starting _____ Final _____
Work Performed _____

Employer _____ Telephone (_____) _____
Address _____ City/Zip _____
Job Title _____ Supervisor _____
Reason for leaving _____
Dates Employed: From (Mo./Yr.) _____ To (Mo./Yr.) _____
Hourly Rate/Salary: Starting _____ Final _____
Work Performed _____

Employer _____ Telephone (_____) _____
Address _____ City/Zip _____
Job Title _____ Supervisor _____
Reason for leaving _____
Dates Employed: From (Mo./Yr.) _____ To (Mo./Yr.) _____
Hourly Rate/Salary: Starting _____ Final _____
Work Performed _____

Employer _____ Telephone (_____) _____
Address _____ City/Zip _____
Job Title _____ Supervisor _____
Reason for leaving _____
Dates Employed: From (Mo./Yr.) _____ To (Mo./Yr.) _____
Hourly Rate/Salary: Starting _____ Final _____
Work Performed _____

If you have worked under another name, please list _____

Special Skills and Qualifications

Summarize special skills and qualifications acquired from employment or other experience. _____
_____
_____

Typing speed, if applicable _____

Other machines which you operate _____

Do you have knowledge of medical terminology? ☐ Yes ☐ No

Do you have previous health care experience? ☐ Yes ☐ No

If so, where? _____

EDUCATION
Elementary
School Name/City/State _____

Years Completed/Degree (Circle)   4   5   6   7   8

High School
School Name/City/State _____

Years Completed/Degree (Circle)   9   10   11   12

Diploma/Degree _____

Describe Course of Study _____

College/University
School Name/City/State _____

Years Completed/Degree (Circle)   1   2   3   4

Diploma/Degree _____

Describe Course of Study _____

Graduate/Professional
School Name/City/State _____

Years Completed/Degree (Circle)   1   2   3   4

Diploma/Degree _____

Describe Course of Study _____

Describe Specialized Training, Apprenticeship, Skills and Extra-Curricular Activities

_____

_____

_____

_____

_____

Honors Received: State any additional information you feel may be helpful to us in considering your application. _____

_____

_____

_____

_____

Professional Licenses and Certifications (Includes Driver's License):

Type _____ State _____ Date Issued _____

Exp. Date _____ Number _____

Type _____ State _____ Date Issued _____

Exp. Date _____ Number _____

Type _____ State _____ Date Issued _____

Exp. Date _____ Number _____

Type _____ State _____ Date Issued _____

Exp. Date _____ Number _____

Type _____ State _____ Date Issued _____

Exp. Date _____ Number _____

Type _____ State _____ Date Issued _____

Exp. Date _____ Number _____

Indicate languages other than English that you speak, read, and/or write.

	FLUENT	GOOD	FAIR
SPEAK			
READ			
WRITE			

Give name, address and telephone number of three references who are not related to you and are not previous employers. _____

_____

_____

_____

_____

Applicant's Statement

I certify that answers given herein are true and complete to the best of my knowledge.

I authorize investigation of all statements contained in this application for employment as may be necessary in arriving at an employment decision.

I understand that neither this document nor any offer of employment from the employer constitutes an employment contract unless a specific document to that effect is executed by the employer and employee in writing. If hired, my employment may be terminated with or without cause, and with or without notice, at any time at the option of either Friendly Hills HealthCare Network or me. I understand that no management representative has any authority to enter into any agreement contrary to the foregoing.

I agree to take a physical examination, which will include a drug and alcohol screening, at any time at the request of the company and at no personal expense to me, and agree that the examining physician may disclose the findings to the company or an authorized agent of the company.

In the event of employment, I understand that false or misleading information given in my application or interview(s) may result in discharge. I understand, also, that I am required to abide by all rules and regulations of the employer.

_____

Signature of Applicant   Date

_____
For Personnel Department Use Only - Do not write below this line

COMMENTS:

_____

Authorization To Hire

Name _____

Requisition No. _____

Department Name & No. _____

Job Title _____

Date of Employment _____

F/T_____P/T_____Hours per pay period _____Rate _____

Supervisor Name _____

Shift _____

Manager/Director _____ Date _____

Remarks _____

_____

32

Effective Ambulatory Patient Scheduling

Michael L. Wiley

THE NEED FOR SCHEDULING

Webster's Dictionary defines scheduling as a timed plan for a procedure or project. For a medical group, the key word is definitely "timed." The primary goal of any appointment scheduling system, either manual or computerized, is to arrange a timetable for patient visits in such a manner that the physicians' and patients' waiting times are kept to a minimum.

In the current environment of rapidly escalating health care costs and increasing competition, medical groups need to evaluate every facet of operations for fiscal responsibility. Ensuring the efficiency of physician schedules, especially in a large, busy group practice, can be extremely cost-effective, not only in actual dollars but also in the patients' perception of service.

Inefficiencies in employee staffing and production equate directly to additional payroll costs and employee FTEs, and scheduling usually is reevaluated whenever profits start shrinking. However, in a prepaid managed care setting a less obvious cost of inefficient scheduling is the expense of hiring additional but "unnecessary" physicians. If a medical group with 100 physicians can realize a 10 percent increase in the number of patients seen through more effective scheduling, the same number of patients could be seen with 10 fewer physicians. This is quite an incentive to evaluate efficiency.

Just as important is the need to maintain a high level of patient satisfaction. The length of time that a patient spends scheduling an appointment over the phone and sitting in the reception area to see the physician can play a large part in the patient's evaluation of service. Continued significant delays in physician accessibility could cause individual patients as well as entire managed care plans to seek other medical groups for service.

APPOINTMENT SCHEDULING PACKAGES

Before starting the search for a computerized appointment scheduling package, it's important to be sure that computerization is actually necessary. If there are no serious operational problems with the current system, even if it is manual, then stop looking. There's no need to fix something that isn't broken! Installing a new scheduling system is a lot of work. It involves a great deal of planning and research, significant hardware and software costs, and a commitment of personnel time for system installation and training.

Different members of the group will have different reasons for wanting a patient scheduling system installed. If all members do not have their needs satisfied, then the risk of failure in project approval and implementation increases dramatically. Consequently, a new system should be viewed from the standpoint of the end user, the data processing department, the administration, and the finance department.

End users generally want more efficiency and better access to information. Time must be taken to study the current scheduling process. Rarely is there anyone who fully understands all aspects of the scheduling process for all departments, so reliance should not be placed on a single individual for all information. It is important to interview all employees and supervisors who are involved with appointment scheduling in order to include all those departments that are affected by aspects of the present system. Remember that implementation of a new system should not only fix existing scheduling problems but minimize new problems. Medical records, nursing, and other departments will undoubtedly have vital input on current deficiencies and on future benefits a new system could provide.

Unfortunately, because appointment scheduling systems use computers, the data processing department is too often inappropriately given the primary responsibility of overseeing all aspects of the project—from requirements planning, system selection, installation, and training through to implementation.

Responsibility of any project should reside primarily with the department that will use it. Data processing staff should concentrate on hardware and software issues as they relate to compliance with MIS goals and strategies. Hardware issues include equipment standardization, maintenance and repair planning, and system connectivity. Software issues include data conversion and input, interfaces with existing company packages, data security, data backup, and downtime contingencies and procedures.

Administrators are generally concerned with long-term business strategies. They must analyze the procedures of the proposed system to verify that the procedures coincide with company goals. In many large groups, appointments are generally not made at the receptionist locations of individual physicians. Instead, there is a "central appointments" area where designated staff schedule most appointments. Hence, part of the justification for a computerized system may be that it will allow the central appointments department to schedule appointments for the home office and for any satellite offices.

Justifying an appointment scheduling system financially involves establishing that there will be an acceptable return on investment. Unfortunately, a clear-cut financial justification is not always possible. One must look instead at the system's potential for improving patient service, increasing employee and medical staff productivity, and providing physician scheduling standardization.

If there are justifiable reasons for changing or implementing a system, it would be appropriate to start compiling a list of the strengths and weaknesses of the current scheduling system. The analysis should pinpoint two types of system features: "must have" features and "nice to have" features. It is a mistake to try to determine right away what type of hardware will be needed. Software is always the most important part of a computerized system. There will probably be at least three packages that fulfill the majority of feature requirements. These packages may be listed on a spreadsheet side by side to see which one comes the closest to satisfying all the requirements. Only after a software package has been chosen should the hardware options be evaluated.

TYPES OF APPOINTMENT SCHEDULING

There are basically three different kinds of scheduling: individual scheduling, block scheduling, and a combination of these. In individual scheduling, a unique-time-of-day appointment is made for each patient. For example, Exhibit 32-1 shows Dave Prime scheduled at 8:30 for 15 minutes, Vince Jackson at 8:45 for 10 minutes, and William Gault at 8:55 for 15 minutes.

Exhibit 32-1 Individual Scheduling

TIME	PATIENT NAME	APPT REASON
8:30 am	Dave Prime	Illness - New Patient
8:35 am	"	"
8:40 am	"	"
8:45 am	Vince Jackson	Recheck
8:50 am	"	"
8:55 am	William Gault	School Physical
9:00 am	"	"
9:05 am	"	"

Note that Vince Jackson is not scheduled until after Dave Prime's appointment is completely finished, and likewise William Gault starts only after Vince Jackson has been seen. Obviously, it is very important, when using this method, to assign an appropriate length of time for each patient's visit. This is done by describing and determining the necessary time for each of the various problems for which a patient might be seen and then setting the length of each appointment based on the applicable description. When the difference between the scheduled appointment time and the time actually needed to see the patient is too great, there is a risk that either the physician will have to wait for the next patient to arrive or the next patient will have to wait past the scheduled time to be seen by the physician.

Further complicating this process is the occasional failure of a patient to be prompt or even to arrive at all. If the patient arrives late or fails to come in, the physician again runs the risk of wasting time waiting for the next patient to arrive. Block scheduling greatly reduces this risk. In this system, multiple patients are scheduled at the same time. For example, Dave Prime, Vince Jackson, and William Gault would all be scheduled at 8:30. However, since the sum of the appropriate lengths in minutes is 40 (15 + 10 + 15), the next available block of appointments would be at 9:10 (see Exhibit 32-2).

This method does a good job of minimizing the physician's waiting time but unfortunately not the patients'. If all three patients arrived at the same time, Vince Jackson would wait 15 minutes while Dave Prime was being seen, and William Gault would wait another 10 minutes while Vince Jackson was with the doctor.

Exhibit 32-2 Block Scheduling

TIME	PATIENT NAME	APPT REASON
8:30 am	Dave Prime Vince Jackson William Gault	Illness - New Patient Recheck School Physical
8:35 am	"	"
8:40 am	"	"
8:45 am	"	"
8:50 am	"	"
8:55 am	"	"
9:00 am	"	"
9:05 am	"	"

A combination of individual and block scheduling can also be used to reduce the risk of physician and patient waiting times. For example, blocking might be used only at the beginning of the day, at the start of each hour or portion of the hour, while the rest of the day is booked using individual scheduling. The doctor will always be slightly behind schedule but not enough to cause long waits. Patients who are late or fail to make appointments will not have as much effect on the waiting times. One variant of individual scheduling involves occasionally overlapping appointment times throughout the day, and another involves reducing appointment lengths to 90 percent of the actual time needed.

BASIC FUNCTIONS

A basic appointment scheduling system must be flexible enough to allow variations in scheduling criteria among different staff members. The fundamental building block of any system is the system definition. This definition, which describes the physician, the weekly schedule by day, and the amount of schedule time by reason for visit, creates the basic pieces needed to build a flexible system.

In the first step, the medical staff for whom appointments can be made are described. Included is information such as staff member names, identifying numbers, specialities, license numbers, supervising physicians (for nonphysician staff members), starting dates, and termination dates. It's very helpful if this information is automatically input into other computer systems so that staff member information remains synchronized between systems at all times. If there are frequent physician staffing changes, starting and termination dates make it simple to restrict appointments to the period between a physician's first and last days.

Next a workday master schedule must be devised. This will identify what times are normally available for appointments for each day of the week. For example, a physician may have open times on Monday and Friday from 8:30 AM to 12:00 PM and again from 2:00 PM to 5:00 PM, on Tuesday and Thursday from 10:00 AM to 12:00 PM and from 2:00 PM to 5:00 PM, whereas Wednesday might be an off day (see Exhibit 32-3).

These schedules require a significant amount of work if the system does not automatically create them. Monthly schedules are also a consideration if routine monthly meetings infringe on the time normally set aside for appointments. Time of day is an element that must allow flexibility. Can appointments be scheduled every 5 minutes (e.g., 10:05 AM) or are they required to be in 10- or 15-minute increments starting on the hour? It may help to reduce patient confusion and increase promptness if appointment times are given to the patients rounded off to the previous quarter hour (e.g., 10:05 AM or 10:10 AM would be rounded off to 10:00 AM).

Exhibit 32-3 Physician Master Schedule

	Mon	Tue	Wed	Thur	Fri	Sat	Sun
12:00– 8:25 am	Off	Off	Off	Off	Off	Off	Off
8:30– 9:55 am		Off	Off	Off		Off	Off
10:00–11:55 am			Off			Off	Off
12:00– 1:55 pm	Lunch	Lunch	Off	Lunch	Lunch	Off	Off
2:00– 4:55 pm			Off			Off	Off
5:00–11:55 pm	Off	Off	Off	Off	Off	Off	Off

The final step is to delineate reasons for appointments and assign each reason a time length. This is the most critical step in defining the system. A thorough study should be made of existing physician-patient encounters, with the focus on visit times. Significant differences among physicians in time spent for the same reason will cause waiting time problems if the reason is a common one. In such a case, try to break the single reason down into several different reasons with varying time lengths. A common set of appointment reasons for the entire practice keeps spellings consistent and meaningful. Abbreviations should always be standardized to avoid confusion. Although physicians in the same specialty may be required to set aside the same amount of time for a reason, not every one in the company can work at the same speed, so it's important that varying times be allowed.

Schedule modification is another crucial step for a basic package. Expected changes like vacations and unexpected changes like obstetrical deliveries will necessitate modification of the normal weekly schedule. Ease of use is greatly desired when modifications occur frequently. Can multiple days be marked for vacation at once or does each day need to be changed individually? What happens to patient appointments when a physician is unexpectedly absent? Can they be rescheduled easily? Are patients' daytime telephone numbers included along with information from the canceled appointments so that they don't have to be rekeyed when the patients are contacted? In some systems, the number of times a particular patient's appointment has been canceled by the doctor is automatically indicated. Patients with appointments canceled more than once may then be given priority for new appointment times or be scheduled as "emergency work-ins" with another physician.

Finally, there is the need to be able to display, cancel, or reschedule an appointment at the patient's request. It is surprising how often patients lose track of appointment dates and times. In large groups, it is also common for patients to arrive on time but forget which doctors they are scheduled to see. The system must allow an inquiry by patient name or medical record number to discover these appointment details. In order to encourage patients to call when they cannot keep an appointment, the cancellation and rescheduling process must be quick and simple. When appointment slots are at a premium, it is advisable to give these calls priority so that open times are reentered into the system as soon as possible.

ADDITIONAL FUNCTIONS

Most companies need more than just the basic functions. Since all medical groups are different, it is hard to create a universal "must have" list, but some additional functions that should be considered are as follows:

- Immediate notification of the medical records department when an appointment is made for today or tomorrow. This provides as much time as possible to locate and deliver the patient's medical record to the physician before the appointment time. This is especially critical when multiple physician offices and multiple medical record file rooms are involved, requiring the transportation of charts between offices.
- Automatic generation of visit slips with charge codes or descriptions tailored to the individual physician. Printing may be delayed until the patient arrives so as to conserve visit slips.
- Automatic search for the next available appointment based on a requested physician, specialty, office location, day of the week, or time of day.
- Twenty-four-hour scheduling for departments with multiple shifts or around-the-clock coverage.
- Multiple appointment coordination when additional physician, room, or equipment dependencies exist.
- On-line help to provide immediate field values and instruction.
- Interfaces with existing patient registration, HMO eligibility, HMO coverage, and other related data bases.

WHAT TO ASK VENDORS

The previous experience and reputation of a prospective software vendor should be investigated carefully. The following questions should guide the inquiry:

- How long has the company been in business? A new company may not have staff with previous health care experience. It is very difficult to design an adequate scheduling software program without knowledge of health care organizations.

- How long has the program been on the market? A new product may not be thoroughly tested. Every new program will have some problems when it is first released. The purchaser cannot afford to spend time helping uncover programming bugs.
- How many times has this program been installed? The more companies that have already "tested" this program, the better. If only a few, problems may arise that no one else has uncovered.
- Where is the company's home office? Local companies are always easier to deal with. They generally have a larger local client base so there are more opportunities to visit some of their customers. Whether it is the time difference or the distance, out-of-state companies often seem to have difficulty answering phone calls when problems occur.
- How often are software upgrades made available? User-oriented companies generally offer software enhancements every 6–12 months. Find out when the last release occurred and whether the company encourages user suggestions and incorporates them in its upgrades. Many large vendors help form user groups that share experiences and problems. In return, the groups allow the vendors to discover what enhancements would be most appreciated.
- Is hardware and software maintenance available? Software maintenance should usually be obtained from the vendor. Normal fees average between 12 and 18 percent of the sales price, but be sure to find out if software upgrades, itemized lists of new release changes, and updated documentation are free with this coverage. Training is generally not included as part of an upgrade package, but it should be available for a fee. Unless your company has the time and employee experience to assist in the maintenance of computer hardware, it will make problem determination less complicated if the vendor handles both hardware and software coverage. However, if the vendor is not local and does not have a contract with a local firm for hardware repair, have backups for critical pieces of equipment or expect a longer downtime.
- What computer hardware is required? Try to standardize equipment whenever possible. This will help users become more familiar with the equipment as they move throughout the company, make it more economical to purchase backup equipment, simplify training, and make future computer interfaces easier. If some computer hardware is already owned and has a good working record, try to buy similar hardware.
- What operating system and programming language is used? Obscure software should be avoided. The vendor will have an easier time supporting upgrades and enhancements that use a common operating system and

programming language, because programmers will be less costly and easier to find.

- Is the source code available? Without access to the source code, changes to or enhancements of the programs cannot be made. You may never need to make any changes, but why take the chance? Most vendors do not include the source code with the system without a significant price increase. This may make the purchase too costly. In this case, have the vendor place the source code into an escrow account. In the event that it goes out of business, ownership of the source code will default to you.

- What training and documentation is included as part of the purchase? Good documentation and user training is vital to a successful implementation, since employees cannot use something they do not understand. If onsite training is available, use it. Also be sure that plenty of assistance is available for system installation, definition, and setup.

- What is the real cost? Do not just include the cost of hardware and software. Be sure to add in hardware and software maintenance, remote communications installation and monthly fees, employee time off and overtime during training, and consultant fees.

STATISTICS

Measurable statistics are very important, both during the implementation and after final conversion. Select critical indicators and compare the new system and the previous system to show project successes and failures. Also, do not implement the new system throughout the entire company immediately. Begin with one of the more problematic areas and use the relevant department as a pilot. This will not only make the rest of the installation easier but will help identify any serious problems before they can affect the whole implementation.

Statistics are also important for assessing employee and physician performance. Many organizations are developing productivity standards to help physicians, employees, and managers evaluate job performance. Patient scheduling statistics are very helpful in establishing staffing standards as well.

Exhibits 32-4 and 32-5 show report samples summarizing scheduled appointments. Exhibit 32-4 summarizes appointments booked by time of day and the offices at which they were scheduled. The column labeled CA lists the numbers of appointments scheduled by the main office's central appointments department, whereas the codes 00 through 50 signify remote office locations. This report not only tracks total daily statistics but also assists in planning staffing requirements for each office.

Individual employee productivity in the central appointments department is listed on a daily and month-to-date basis in the central appointments summary

Exhibit 32-4 Appointments Booked by Scheduling Site

	CA	00	01	02	04	06	07	08	11	12	50	TOTAL
6:00 am	1	8				2	1					12
7:00 am	94	52	19	6	8	18	9		4			209
8:00 am	79	96	31	14	28	29	37	11	15	5	1	346
9:00 am	75	151	28	14	37	52	41	23	4	12	8	445
10:00 am	68	127	29	11	41	51	54	16	3	6	14	420
11:00 am	60	127	23	17	27	36	60	14	3	7	15	389
12:00 pm	47	75	19	22	20	28	44	15	5	5	9	289
1:00 pm	54	80	19	6	7	20	39	9	6	1	19	260
2:00 pm	53	111	17	15	14	12	54	10	4	2	8	300
3:00 pm	44	91	22	22	16	43	51	13	2	8	14	326
4:00 pm	48	110	11	17	16	25	50	12	4	5	16	314
5:00 pm	36	56	9	11	6	8	24	10	1	1	23	185
6:00 pm	15	12		1			8				25	61
7:00 pm											16	16
8:00 pm											12	12
9:00 pm											9	9
10:00 pm											10	10
TOTALS	674	1096	226	156	220	324	472	133	51	52	199	3603

(Exhibit 32-5). By using this summary, staff members may track and monitor their own performance.

Supervisors can use averages to establish and adjust expected workload levels for the department, and they can use the individual statistics as part of the annual employee performance evaluations.

Physician productivity statistics are also valuable. The physician productivity summary (Exhibit 32-6) contains information on patient visits, appointment hours booked, and average patient visits per hour. In addition, ancillary statistics show totals for patients for which tests were ordered, procedures, and charges.

For each physician, statistics are summarized by the various health plans, such as HMO senior plans, HMO commercial plans, and fee-for-service/PPO plans. Percentages are calculated for visits, lab procedures, and x-ray procedures against total visits. This type of operational data helps identify physician adherence to clinical guidelines and utilization criteria, necessary components of a cost-effective medical practice.

Exhibit 32-5 Central Appointments Summary

ASR432	Friendly Hills Medical Group Central Appointments Summary	Date: 10/2/90 Time: 3:21:48
Date: Mon Oct 1 1990		
User Name	*Today*	*Month-to-Date*
Jeri Adams	115	2221
Dolly Donately	101	1952
Cheryl Johnson	9	1495
Patti Powell	102	1845
Lupe Rodriguez	121	2414
Lori Rollins	52	2153
Joanne Williams	95	1629
Katherine Wilson	79	1525
Total	674	15234
Average	84	1904

Visits are broken into rechecks (follow-up visits for established patients), new problems (visits for new problems experienced by established patients), new patients, and manual entries (charges recorded for patients not previously scheduled in the appointment scheduling system). Patient visits per hour is a key physician statistic used to measure physician productivity in a prepaid managed care practice. Ancillary tests are listed by number of patients, number of procedures, and total amount charged for all tests.

THE PROBLEMS AND THE PROMISE

Most currently available computerized systems, while certainly enhancing the scheduling process, are still subject to major difficulties. First, they are often unable to convert patient symptoms and complaints into appropriate time slots. Second, the modification of programs to accommodate new or changed physician scheduling rules is often hard to accomplish. Third, training users to the point where they become experts is an arduous task. And finally, the complexities involved in programming an effective appointment scheduling system have forced companies to use larger and more expensive hardware in order to achieve convenient response times. Resolution of each of these difficulties will make computerized scheduling systems more attractive and will result in an expansion of their use.

Appointment scheduling is a complicated process, but it is critical to appropriate utilization of physicians, staff, and facilities. Establishing the proper system is often difficult and always initially costly, but it is essential to the long-term viability of any group practice.

Exhibit 32-6 Physician Productivity Summary

Category	VISITS							LAB			X-RAY	
	Rechk	New Problem	New Patient	Manual	Total	Hours *Booked	*Vst/ Hour	Patients	Procedures	Amount	Procedures	Amount
DR: 227 SMITH												
HMO Comm.	54	88	4	5	151			105	82	2317	6	629
HMO Senior	129	71	8		208			18	86	2628	18	1985
FFS/PPO	8	8	6		22			6	5	171	1	79
Total	191	167	18	5	381	71	5.3	129	173	5116	25	2693
% To Total	50.1	43.8	4.7	1.3				33.9	45.4		6.6	
DR: 300 JONES												
HMO Comm.	40	332	80	4	456			180	282	7452	46	3081
HMO Senior	22	49	12		83			11	44	1330	15	1041
FFS/PPO	9	35	12		56			26	46	1252	4	432
Total	71	416	104	4	595	122	4.8	217	372	10034	65	4554
% To Total	11.9	69.9	17.5	.7				36.5	62.5		10.9	
DR: 151 BROWN												
HMO Comm.	59	295	44	4	402			180	353	10067	47	3776
HMO Senior	20	39	4		63			24	82	2511	2	1018
FFS/PPO	20	37	6		63			36	74	2230	4	242
Total	99	371	54	4	528	106	4.9	240	509	14808	53	5036
% To Total	18.8	70.3	10.2	.8				45.5	96.4		10.0	
*SPEC. TOTALS												
HMO Comm.	2406	6372	608	1082	10468			4633	7571	215606	1295	126653
HMO Senior	1702	1649	141	109	3601			490	2687	91748	487	44069
FFS/PPO	481	1075	201	83	1840			716	1336	38551	260	23814
Total	4589	9096	950	1274	15909	2867	5.5	5839	11594	345905	2042	194536
% To Total	28.8	57.2	6.0	8.0				36.7	72.9		12.8	

33

Emerging Technologies for Ambulatory Care Information Systems

Todd A. Walike

INTRODUCTION

The past few decades have been witness to a dramatic evolution in information systems. In the past, information system technologies merely played a supporting role in providers' business activities, performing such routine tasks as data entry and statement generation. Today, such technologies are increasingly evident in the development of strategic plans. Successful provider groups of the nineties will be those best able to use information system technologies to remain competitive and take advantage of new business opportunities.

This chapter summarizes the evolution of ambulatory care information systems and explores the market forces driving ambulatory care organizations to implement improved information systems. Following a discussion of the trends influencing today's changing ambulatory information systems, some of the emerging technologies are reviewed. The focus is on how these technologies will be used and the potential benefits to be realized from their implementation. The reason for installing new hardware and software, after all, is to achieve the benefits of enhanced patient service, controlled costs, and other improvements that can contribute to the accomplishment of strategic objectives.

BACKGROUND

History of Ambulatory Care Information Systems

Provider reimbursement of the seventies and early eighties was predominately fee-for-service. As a result, management information systems existed primarily for the purpose of recording transactions and generating patient bills and insurance claims. Needless to say, with the emphasis on billings and collections, information systems were oriented toward automating basic accounting functions. Registration, billing, and accounts receivable were the primary applications used by most providers. Responding to user needs, most vendors provided systems of similar functionality. Few reporting capabilities were provided, since they were not usually required by management or requested by outside agencies.

Within this environment of transaction processing and basic user requirements, service bureaus flourished, because they were cost-effective vehicles for processing charges, adjustments, and payments. These mainframe systems offered few on-line capabilities, since they processed most organizational data in batch mode. In this pre-PC period (the personal computer was introduced in 1981 but few business applications were available for several years), "dumb terminals" were the only devices for inquiry and data entry into the main system.

Current Information Systems Environment

Since the mid-1980s, software and hardware improvements have changed the look of ambulatory care information systems. The software products available today have improved dramatically. Users have demanded more timely processing and vendors have responded by developing on-line systems. Patient, charge, and other information is integrated immediately upon operator entry. No longer do users have to wait for an overnight processing cycle to view their current day's work. In addition to improvements in software, there is a greater availability of automated applications, including appointment scheduling, chart tracking, and managed care.

Significant hardware performance improvements have kept pace with software enhancements. As the cost per unit of processing power continues to decrease, minicomputers and PCs are able to perform processing chores that were possible only by mainframes just a few years ago. This reduction in computing costs has afforded most providers the opportunity to perform their data processing in-house.

As a result, most large practices today use minicomputers to perform basic functions, including registration, billing, and appointment scheduling. The PC is used to support administrative functions such as word processing and electronic mail. It also facilitates analysis of data through the use of data base and spreadsheet software. Furthermore, data from the minicomputer can be downloaded and manipulated on the PC to provide more flexible reporting than that provided by the central system.

Forces of Change

Many factors will influence the use of new technologies in ambulatory care organizations but none to a greater degree than the emphasis on cost reduction.

For over a decade now, health care costs have been scrutinized by the government and private payers in an effort to reduce health care costs or at least slow their rise. For years, Medicare has been cutting back on covered services and reducing reimbursement rates. In 1992, the Resource-Based Relative Value System (RBRVS) takes effect as another means of controlling ambulatory care costs. With falling revenues, providers will look for every opportunity to lower operating costs. Use of new software tools such as executive information systems (EIS) will allow management to better control and monitor overall business activities. Personal computers and PC networks will gain greater popularity, since they will offer low-cost solutions for meeting physicians' systems requirements.

Managed care will continue to have a significant impact on the technologies implemented within ambulatory care organizations. Medical groups and other capitated providers will be less concerned with fee-for-service information systems than with software applications able to receive timely member eligibility information and to control outside referrals and hospital admissions. In addition, sophisticated claims systems will be needed to process discounted fee-for-service, subcapitation, and other various referral reimbursement arrangements.

Quality-of-care requirements also will influence the technologies employed during this decade. In an effort to improve patient care, reduce costs, and retain key business relationships with HMOs and other managed care organizations, providers will perform outcome studies, develop treatment protocols, and monitor established standards through review of physician profiles. These requirements will quickly change the focus of ambulatory information systems from financial operations to clinical care. No longer will effective information systems strictly be "charge-capture" and billing systems. Instead, ambulatory information systems will be complete medical record systems able to track and report on, for example, routine preventive procedures, outliers, physician treatment patterns, and patient outcomes. These systems will provide opportunities for physicians and other health care professionals to improve decision making and patient care.

EMERGING TECHNOLOGIES

Provided below are some of the emerging technologies that, in the future, will be common components of most ambulatory care information systems. The focus has been placed on those areas that have undergone the most recent improvements and have the best chance for implementation or expanded usage in the next few years. This list is by no means comprehensive, emphasizing only those technologies with the most current potential. In fact, right now there are even newer technologies emerging that soon will assist ambulatory care organizations in improving patient care and increasing efficiency and profitability.

Executive Information Systems

An executive information system (EIS) is primarily a reporting tool that summarizes key data. Information is presented in tabular and graphical formats, providing a quick snapshot of critical business indicators and an overview of operations. An EIS for an ambulatory care organization is a software package that stores and processes data that has been downloaded from the central clinical and financial systems. An EIS is useful for performing historical, concurrent, and forecasted analyses. Some of the reporting areas to which an EIS could be applied include patient visits, employee productivity, and prepaid plan profitability. By design, an EIS presents information in summary fashion yet offers the "drill down" capability of supplying the details of a particular summary item upon request. Some EISs are integrated with office automation functions such as word processing and electronic mail. These systems also may be able to tap into data bases such as Dow Jones and Compuserve (see Figure 33-1).

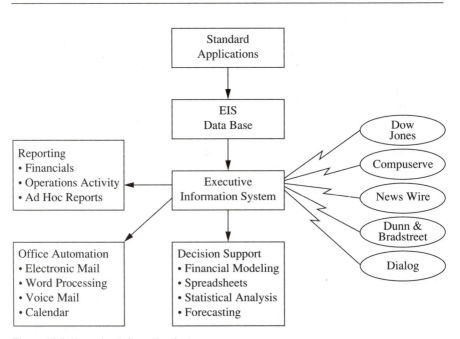

Figure 33-1 Executive Information System

EISs will become prevalent within more ambulatory care organizations in the near future as the products become less expensive and more fully featured. Already an EIS for the PC can be purchased within the $300 to $1,000 range. Many of the newer systems also provide the ability to extract data from existing systems to build a new EIS data base.

As discussed earlier, the increasing power of the PC will change the way providers process data. The EIS is one example of this new approach. Centralized systems still may be the main receptacle for data, but tools such as the EIS will provide CEOs and other executives with the flexibility to view information in ways they desire rather than those designed by the vendor's programmers. The EIS will be management's tool, and, once set up, it will require little intervention by the MIS department. It will allow users to quickly design and modify their own reports instead of waiting weeks and sometimes months for the vendor or MIS department to find time to respond to their requests. In summary, the EIS will provide many benefits including greater user access, more flexible and timely reporting, and more meaningful information, which together will be used to improve management's decision making.

Electronic Data Interchange

Electronic data interchange (EDI) is a technology for standardizing electronic transactions between various organizations' systems (see Figure 33-2). As the health care industry continues to follow the lead set years ago by the banking industry, an increasing array of automated transactions will streamline the operations of ambulatory care organizations. EDI's impact on ambulatory care will be twofold: (1) Submission, receipt, and processing of claims and other third-party transactions will be automated; and (2) data interfaces among the organization's differing systems (e.g., clinic, managed care, laboratory, radiology, etc.) will be simplified.

EDI is viewed by the health care industry as a critical technology for eliminating mountains of paperwork and reducing administrative overhead. The rising cost of processing paper claims has caused the government and many private payers to emphasize electronic submission. In addition, providers are becoming more and more disgruntled with slow claims settlement by payers. Medicare, for example, has extended to 60 days the possible payment cycle for paper claims. Managed care also has introduced many other transactions such as patient encounters, eligibility verifications, referral authorizations, and preadmission certifications. These transactions have significantly increased the volume of information passed between providers and payers. Processing this information manually via a paper record is very costly. The magnitude of transaction volumes has also placed an added burden on the HMOs and other managed care organizations.

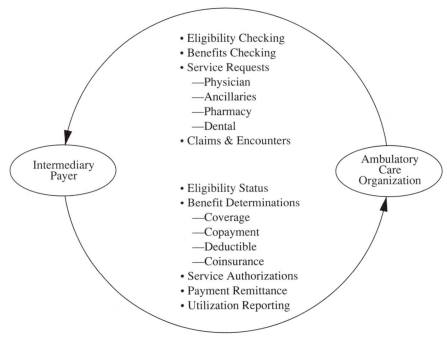

Figure 33-2 Electronic Data Interchange Overview

EDI owes its impetus to the government, private payers and HMOs, but ambulatory care organizations also can benefit. Electronic submission of claims and other transactions through a clearinghouse or a private payer network means faster processing. With little or no intervention by data entry and claims processors, claims adjudication and settlement cycles can be reduced. This results in improved cash flow for the providers, who will no longer have to offer the interest-free financing to payer organizations that results from lengthy reimbursement cycles. Submitting claims electronically through a clearinghouse provides other benefits, including fewer paper claims, less in-house processing, and automated editing of claims. Electronic submission results in a higher percentage of "clean" claims and fewer payer rejections and resubmissions. Using a clearinghouse or other third party also reduces the processing costs required when claims are submitted to multiple payers; instead of submitting claims in various formats to multiple payers, providers submit a single format to the clearinghouse. Rather than having all providers responsible for system changes and sending claims to different payer locations, the clearinghouse becomes the focal point, assuming responsibility for payer system modifications and submissions.

EDI's growing popularity also is due in part to the development of new transactions. One of these is eligibility verification, which is requested by outpatient facilities prior to providing services. Automating this process, which in effect allows on-line access to eligibility information, will greatly reduce costs incurred today by ambulatory care organizations. With on-line eligibility access, the need to maintain and access outdated paper rosters will be eliminated. More importantly, services will only be provided to eligible members. Providers will be notified of ineligible members in time to refuse service or bill the patients when services are rendered.

One of the most significant impacts of EDI will be felt by providers when EDI expands to accommodate claims settlement functions. At that time, the provider, through the use of a patient charge or debit card, will receive payment virtually on the same day the services were provided. Faster claims adjudication and settlement, more timely eligibility checking, and other EDI benefits will result in improved cash flow, fewer concerns regarding outstanding receivables, and a greater physician focus on patient care.

EDI will improve the efficiency of transaction processing within the ambulatory care organization as well. Transaction standards, similar to those identified by HL7 and MEDIX within the inpatient environment, will simplify the interfaces among various ambulatory care systems, including registration, appointment scheduling, managed care, laboratory, radiology, medical records, and others. These standards will streamline the implementation of a multivendor system and reduce interface programming costs. Most importantly, these standards will allow a provider to select systems because they best meet its overall needs and not simply because they can be easily interfaced with existing systems.

PC Networks

PC networks, though not a new technology, soon will play an expanded role in providing management information services. A network generally consists of a server (i.e., a PC on which resides network and application software) and multiple PCs and printers, all connected through a common cabling scheme. The network software allows users to access applications on the server and share resources such as disk drives and printers.

PC networks will become more prevalent within the next several years because they provide a way of addressing unique needs unmet by central systems. A wide variety of inexpensive and easy-to-use software development tools (relative to those for minicomputers) are available for PCs and PC networks. These tools can provide custom programs for applications such as patient relations and marketing, software usually not provided by large system vendors. Some smaller system vendors already have developed some modules such as managed care to supplement providers' basic systems.

PC networks will be more attractive to many provider groups because their price-to-performance ratio is superior to that of minicomputer systems. PC networks can be installed for about one-third the price of comparable minicomputers. In addition, hardware maintenance costs are approximately one-sixth those of minicomputer systems. What currently is holding back a wave of network implementations is the lack of ambulatory care software. But as the hardware performance of these systems continues to improve, vendors anticipating a large potential market will begin developing network software. In the next several years, as the software inventory grows, PC networks will become as common as minicomputers are today.

Imaging

Imaging technology is probably the hottest technology today in ambulatory care organizations. It includes scanners for creating a digital image from paper documents or a direct interface with other systems capable of generating images (see Figure 33-3). Images have relatively large storage requirements, and therefore mass storage devices such as optical disks are usually key system components. Imaging technology will be used more for storing and retrieving digital images. However, the potential exists for integrating image technology with business applications such as claims processing. This merger of image and text applications will reduce costs by eliminating the rekeying and manual processing of document originals such as referral claims.

Imaging in conjunction with the on-line medical record finally will offer the capability of maintaining a consolidated record that is up-to-date and easy to retrieve. The current medical record consists primarily of text data, including visit information, notes, and laboratory reports. Other sources of information, such as patient pathology slides and x-rays, often reside in the departments that performed the relevant procedures. The integration of imaging and the on-line medical record will allow physicians at any location equipped with a PC and high-resolution monitor to view the complete record—from SOAP notes and test results to the original slides, x-rays, and MRIs.

Imaging, as a new technology, still has several "negatives" that will forestall its widespread implementation. First, imaging remains a very expensive technology. The purchase price of scanners, PCs, high-resolution monitors, an optical disk jukebox, and imaging and application interface software for a claims processing application can exceed one million dollars. In addition, the retrieval of images takes more time than the retrieval of text. Image files are larger than text files, and it may take several seconds to a few minutes for an

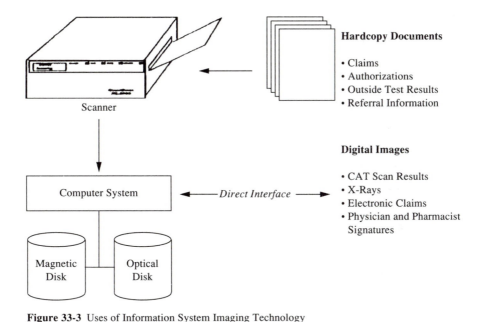

Figure 33-3 Uses of Information System Imaging Technology

image to appear on a display device. Nevertheless, as the performance of these systems continues to improve and the prices continue to fall, imaging applications will be used much more extensively in clinical and administrative departments.

Enhanced Applications

In the next several years, expanded and more fully featured managed care and medical records software is likely to become available. Because of the increased physician demand for more timely data, the expansion in prepaid tracking and reporting requirements, and the continuing emphasis on quality of care, these applications will undergo significant change.

The development of integrated on-line medical records is currently one of the primary goals for many ambulatory care organizations (see Figure 33-4). It is no wonder that this is the case, since physicians at some outpatient facilities have access to patient charts only 60 percent of the time. Access to the paper chart has decreased recently as consolidations of provider groups have occurred. IPAs as well as large medical groups with several satellites and special service locations pose a logistical problem for timely medical record delivery.

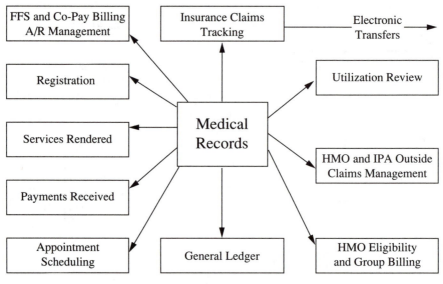

Figure 33-4 On-Line Medical Records

As patients are shuttled among the satellites for various specialty services, it becomes increasingly difficult to ensure that the charts are available where needed. Some organizations have even incurred the administrative expense and coordination nightmare of maintaining duplicate charts at each location.

On-line medical records will virtually eliminate the huge expense associated with requesting, pulling, transporting, and filing patient charts. Some medical groups estimate these costs at several dollars per chart request. On-line medical records will provide access from any location, including the main clinic location, satellites, the hospital, or even the physician's home. In conjunction with an imaging application, on-line medical records will contain all patient demographic and coverage information, problem lists, vital statistics, physician notes and reports, orders, and test results. On-line medical records will also display x-ray, MRI, and other images. Because they are stored on magnetic or optical disks, they will be more easily indexed and organized than paper charts, facilitating access by medical staff.

Although reduction of administrative costs will be one major benefit, improved quality of care also will be achieved. As medical records integrates with other applications such as data entry, order entry, laboratory, and radiology, updates to each record will be immediate. Providing easy access and up-to-date information should greatly improve decision making and overall patient care.

The increasing emphasis on quality and the rise of managed care have created the need for new applications within the ambulatory care organization.

Managed care software has been available for several years. However, the complexities of such software have increased in order to accommodate additional processing and reporting. For example, medical groups today may have dozens of reimbursement arrangements with referral providers that must be monitored and updated. As ambulatory care providers share in more of the risk with HMOs and others, the need increases for sophisticated concurrent review, utilization management, and physician profiling systems.

Advanced Human Interfaces

Other technological innovations will make their way into the ambulatory care environment. These tools, described as advanced human interfaces, will use differing means to achieve the same end. Mobile terminals, bar coding, and voice recognition systems are three innovations that will facilitate data inputting by providing an efficient and more natural computer interface (see Figure 33-5).

Mobile terminals looking much like notebooks or clipboards will be used by physicians to capture patient and visit data at the office, hospital, patient home,

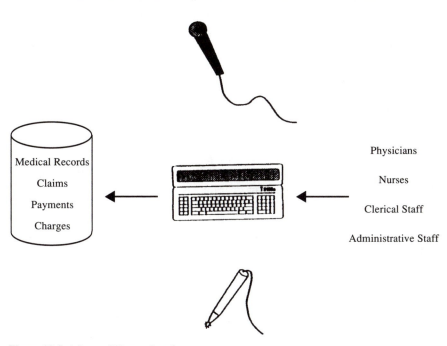

Figure 33-5 Advanced Human Interfaces

or other locations. Information will be gathered at the point of service without the need for a dedicated link to the main computer. A physician will be able to either attach the device to a standard telephone line for on-line processing or key information into the mobile unit and at a later time upload it to the main system for processing and storage in the permanent data base. Since the physician will record information directly into the system (as opposed to the common practice of recording visit information on paper, then keying it into the computer), fewer data entry errors will occur. Use of these devices also will reduce the amount of paperwork, since encounter tickets, batch sheets, and other data entry controls would be eliminated.

Bar coding currently is used in hospitals for inventory control and chart tracking, but similar technology will soon be very evident within the ambulatory setting. Using bar code labels and some type of reader, such as a light pen, provider organizations will more easily and accurately track charts and inventory and enter data. Efficiency will be improved, because bar code readers can recognize and record a patient chart number or a procedure code on an encounter ticket much more quickly than the eye can read and fingers can type. Productivity can be increased five- to eightfold by using bar coding rather than conventional keyed entry. Bar code devices also are extremely accurate, as evidenced by error rates of a fraction of a percent. As more system vendors modify applications such as data entry and chart tracking to accommodate this technology, these devices will gain even greater acceptance.

Voice recognition systems are employed in a few organizations, but wide use of this innovation is still probably years away. These systems are worthy of mention, however, because they use the most natural of all communication tools, the human voice. Voice recognition devices, usually PC-based, receive human voice signals and convert them to binary text and numerical codes for processing and storage. Any type of input could be considered for this technology, but its greatest use will probably be in the recording of medical chart information. The physician can record patient information, progress notes, operative reports, or consults, and the system will immediately update the patient chart, eliminating the transcription cycle. With this technology, the computer performs the transcription at the time of physician dictation.

The three innovations described above will dramatically change the way ambulatory care organizations are structured. Virtually every function, including registration, data entry, and medical records entry, will be decentralized. These systems will afford "one-time" input, eliminating the need to transfer data from paper (e.g., encounter ticket) or tape (e.g., physician notes) to the computer via the keyboard. Administrative costs for word processing, data entry, transcription, and other functions will be dramatically reduced. Perhaps more important, at least for physicians, patient information will be more accurate and up to date.

The big advantage of the technologies mentioned above is that clinical and administrative personnel will be able to more easily, naturally, and productively tap into the power of the computer. Instead of requiring users to change the way they work to accommodate the computer, the computer will be able to accommodate their activities.

CONCLUSION

Ambulatory care organizations are changing dramatically in response to fee-for-service revenue reductions, the increasing influence of managed care, and more stringent operating and reporting requirements of the government, private payers, HMOs, and others. New technologies can assist providers with this change by lowering costs and improving patient care. Realizing these key benefits through the timely implementation of emerging technologies will allow providers to remain competitive in the health care marketplace. As ambulatory care organizations begin to chart their strategies for the twenty-first century, today's emerging technologies must certainly be considered carefully in helping providers achieve their clinical and business goals.

34

Selecting an Ambulatory Care Information System

Brad L. Armstrong

INTRODUCTION

So you want a new computer system? According to Machiavelli, "there is nothing more difficult to take in hand, more perilous to conduct, or more uncertain in its success, than to take the lead in the introduction of a new order of things." Indeed, the quickest way to strike terror into the hearts of physicians and administrators alike is to suggest converting to a new computer system. Their fears are not entirely unjustified. Just about everyone has had experience with installing computer systems that took too long, cost too much, and never quite did what was promised. Nevertheless, since very few medical group practices are willing to return to the old ledger card days, choosing the right computer system is a significant concern. This decision is further complicated by its wide impact on nonphysician personnel and the range of technology that is available today.

If planned and managed properly, however, a system can be selected and implemented that provides substantial benefits to the medical provider while minimizing disruption of its operations. This chapter addresses many of the questions regarding the selection and implementation processes. The focus will be on the needs of larger medical organizations, although many solo practitioners have similar requirements.

CRITICAL ROLE OF COMPUTERS IN AMBULATORY PRACTICE

Today's physicians, whether in solo or group practices, are confronted with an increasingly complex operating environment (see Figure 34-1). Changing government regulations have introduced new administrative requirements such as the use of the Resource-Based Relative Value System (RBRVS). The rise of managed care has put pressure on physicians to assume more risk and to contain costs. Increasing competition from other physicians, hospitals, and

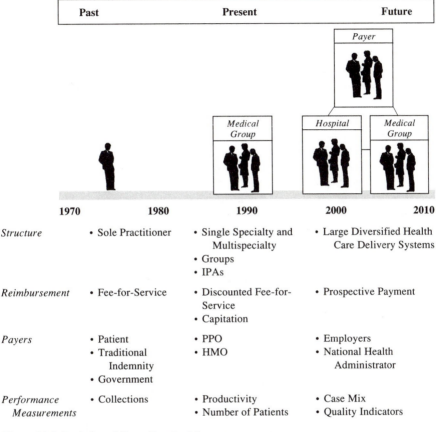

	Past	**Present**	**Future**
	1970 1980	1990	2000 2010
Structure	• Sole Practitioner	• Single Specialty and Multispecialty • Groups • IPAs	• Large Diversified Health Care Delivery Systems
Reimbursement	• Fee-for-Service	• Discounted Fee-for-Service • Capitation	• Prospective Payment
Payers	• Patient • Traditional Indemnity • Government	• PPO • HMO	• Employers • National Health Administrator
Performance Measurements	• Collections	• Productivity • Number of Patients	• Case Mix • Quality Indicators

Figure 34-1 Evolution of Group Practice Management

HMOs has forced them to devote even greater attention to profitability and patient service. In the future, a growing emphasis will be placed on the measurement and improvement of quality using a variety of severity, pattern, and outcome indicators.

In this environment, success can no longer be achieved solely through happy patients and regular rate increases. Instead, it requires streamlining operations, increasing physician productivity, assessing profitability by payer and patient type, and providing distinguished patient care. More and more, groups are relying on their computer systems to give them a competitive advantage in managing these increasingly complex set of variables. Organizations without adequate systems may be limited in their ability to attract and retain new patients.

Assessment of Need

It is safe to assume that many individual physicians and most groups have some type of computer system. The question is whether it is the right one. The answer is not always easy to determine. Of course, there will always be a certain amount of dissatisfaction with any system. So how does one know when it is time to change?

Figure 34-2 indicates symptoms of common computer system problems. One of the most serious indications is slow response time. Usually, this symptom first will be noticed during the scheduling of appointments. The average time it takes to look up a patient on the system should be less than three seconds. Three to five seconds is probably acceptable. Transactions taking longer than five seconds, however, have been found to adversely affect user satisfaction and productivity. The primary cause of poor response time is inadequate hardware, although it also can be caused by inefficient software design or insufficient communications capacity.

Another major reason for considering a new computer system is that the current system lacks adequate functionality to support the group's business needs. This occurs frequently when the software vendor or the in-house programming staff cannot keep up with the group's changing business requirements. For example, many in-house- and vendor-developed systems have diffi-

Symptoms	**Problems**					
	Insufficient Hardware Capacity/ Upgradability	Limited Software Capabilities	Poor Software Design	Lack of Integrated Systems	Poor Vendor Support	Inadequate Data Communications
Poor Response Time	✓		✓			✓
Frequent System Downtime	✓		✓		✓	✓
Manually Intensive Operations	✓	✓		✓		
Management Lacks Critical Information		✓	✓	✓		
MIS Always Fighting "Fires"	✓	✓	✓	✓	✓	✓

Figure 34-2 Information Systems Problem Diagnosis

culty supporting the prepaid eligibility and claims processing functions. Even if the group's software includes certain features and capabilities, they may be difficult to use. For instance, some systems require manual intervention to generate secondary billings, whereas others perform this task automatically. A lack of functionality usually requires a larger administrative staff to process the extra paperwork.

Insufficient management reporting is often a critical systems weakness. The ability to generate not only standard operational but new ad hoc reports is becoming increasingly important to group administrators. It affects the group's ability to evaluate cost-containment initiatives as well as analyze profitability by patient and payor mix. Insufficient reporting could be caused by a lack of standard reports or inefficient reporting tools. In contrast, many systems now have easy-to-use report generators that greatly accelerate customized report development. Another roadblock to effective reporting may be an inability to enter and store important information.

There is no magic formula that will indicate the exact time to upgrade a computer system. If the group is experiencing a number of the symptoms described above, or if the present system has been installed for more than three years, perhaps alternatives should be considered. Because of the rapid rate of hardware and software advancement (see Figure 34-3), the potential rewards from a new system are worth investigating on a periodic basis.

CHOOSING THE RIGHT COMPUTER SYSTEM

Sorting through the seemingly endless systems possibilities can be a daunting task. However, if the right people are involved and a realistic approach (see Figure 34-4) is followed, the organization should be able to achieve its systems objectives.

Who Should Be Involved?

Before any type of system evaluation study is begun, a commitment by senior management as well as the physician leadership is required. One reason is that purchasing and implementing a new system will entail a significant expenditure. In addition, the physicians can be instrumental in gaining the cooperation of staff. During the course of the study, regular reports should be given to senior management by the evaluators or consultants to keep them fully apprised of project progress and any roadblocks encountered. Key physicians, managers, and staff members should bear primary responsibility for identifying system requirements and evaluating alternatives. Since these individuals will

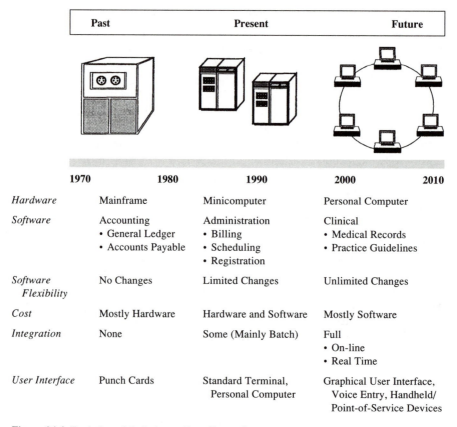

	1970	1980	1990	2000	2010
Hardware		Mainframe	Minicomputer	Personal Computer	
Software		Accounting • General Ledger • Accounts Payable	Administration • Billing • Scheduling • Registration	Clinical • Medical Records • Practice Guidelines	
Software Flexibility		No Changes	Limited Changes	Unlimited Changes	
Cost		Mostly Hardware	Hardware and Software	Mostly Software	
Integration		None	Some (Mainly Batch)	Full • On-line • Real Time	
User Interface		Punch Cards	Standard Terminal, Personal Computer	Graphical User Interface, Voice Entry, Handheld/ Point-of-Service Devices	

Figure 34-3 Evolution of Ambulatory Care Computing

be major users of the system, they should actively participate in choosing it. Additionally, they will play a crucial role in making the system work and achieving the projected benefits. Usually, someone from the MIS Department leads the project, assists in developing plans and requirements, and participates in the system selection decision. However, the primary goal of the MIS department should be to facilitate rather than to dictate the correct decision.

The question frequently arises as to whether outside consultants should be utilized. Consultants can be very valuable in providing insight into various alternatives, identifying approaches employed by similar organizations, and assisting with planning and selection methodologies. Since system conversions occur infrequently, a consultant can temporarily supplement the staff assigned to choose and implement a system, thereby eliminating the need to hire additional personnel. Because of their experience, consultants should be able to

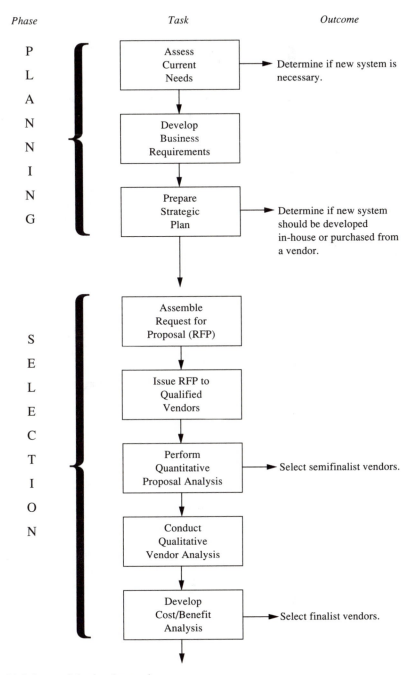

Figure 34-4 System Selection Approach

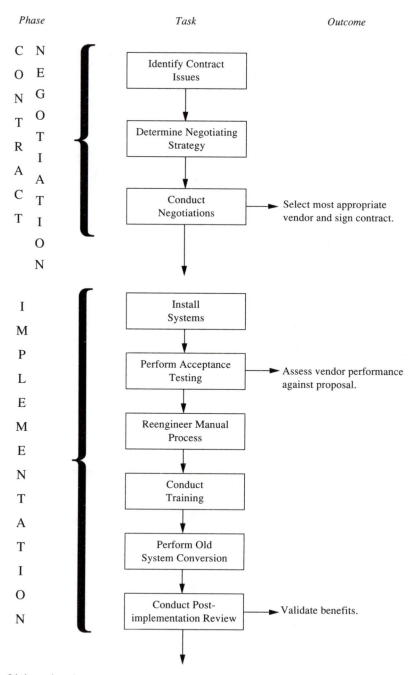

Figure 34-4 continued

accelerate the transition process. However, hiring outside assistance should not be seen as a way to abdicate responsibility. If a consultant is used, the organization itself should fully participate in any work that is performed. Also, the consultant should preferably be independent of any hardware and software vendors and have extensive experience with medical practices.

Developing a Plan

Before making any purchase decisions, a plan should be developed that outlines the group's information systems strategy. An effective plan will map the group's business goals and objectives into specific MIS actions. Potential application areas to be considered include the following:

- registration
- appointment and resource scheduling
- insurance and patient billing
- accounts receivable
- accounts payable
- general ledger
- fixed assets
- budgeting
- payroll
- personnel management
- purchasing
- inventory management
- chart tracking
- order entry and results reporting
- eligibility
- referral authorization
- referral claims management
- utilization and productivity management
- medical records
- radiology
- laboratory
- pharmacy
- case mix and case decision support
- financial and management reporting
- office automation (word processing, electronic mail, etc.)

Make or Buy?

As a plan is being formulated, the decision must be made to either program in-house or buy a packaged program from a vendor. Invariably, those who already have packaged systems would like more of the flexibility and control that in-house development offers. On the other hand, organizations with home-grown systems long to be free from large programming staffs and extensive lists of overdue system change requests. There are advantages and disadvantages with either approach. Table 34-1 lists indicators that can aid in deciding between a make or buy approach.

The optimal approach for most practices is probably somewhere in between—a package but with some modifications. Despite the trend toward increased size, most group practices are still not large enough to justify in-house programming staffs. Most packaged system vendors have a large investment in their systems, an investment that cannot be matched by a single group. Therefore, it almost always makes sense to investigate packaged systems before considering internal alternatives. Software purchased from a vendor usually will have less bugs, better documentation, and additional useful features that were not thought of when specifying system requirements. However, since a packaged system will rarely meet 100 percent of the group's requirements, some customization may be needed. These changes should be kept to a minimum in order to easily install future vendor software releases. In a packaged environment the MIS Department should focus on working with the tools provided by the vendor to accommodate the group's processing and reporting needs.

Table 34-1 Information Systems Make or Buy Indicators

Indicators	Make	Buy
Business Requirements	Very Unique	Standard
Ogranization Size	Large	Small to Medium
Software Availability	Minimal	Many Vendors
Attitude toward Risk	Risk Taker	Risk Averse
Funding	Large Budget or Unlimited	Limited
Ongoing Enhancements	Many	Few
Degree of Integration	High	Minimal
User Disposition	Participative, Demanding	Uninvolved
Business Environment	Dynamic	Stable
Availability of Technical Personnel	Many Available Locally	Few Available

VENDOR SELECTION

Regardless of whether a package or custom approach is chosen, hardware and software vendors will still be needed. This section discusses the steps to be followed in selecting a packaged system vendor. As mentioned previously, a plan will streamline and accelerate the selection process. Although there are many hardware alternatives such as mainframes, minicomputers, and PC networks, hardware should be a secondary consideration. Many organizations have bought leading computer hardware only to discover later that very little software was available for their machines. If possible, hardware and software should be proposed by and purchased from a single (usually software) vendor who is accountable for the performance of both. Otherwise, problems could lead to vendor finger pointing.

Identifying Qualified Vendors

There are literally hundreds of vendors offering systems designed for medical practices. Because of the evaluation time required, it is usually not practical to include more than six vendors when selecting a single system. Therefore, it is imperative that the group only consider established vendors with a proven track record. Low-priced joint development offers from questionable organizations rarely succeed. Listings of hardware and software vendors are published by the Medical Group Management Association and *Computers in Healthcare*. Additional sources include trade shows and other physician groups.

Developing a Request for Proposal

The primary tool used in selecting new systems is the request for proposal (RFP). This document summarizes an organization's current systems environment, its projected business expansion and growth plans, and the application features and reports it desires. Also included are instructions for vendors regarding proposal preparation, evaluation, and required time frames. A thorough RFP is key to reducing misunderstandings and determining the most appropriate hardware and software vendors for the practice. It should provide information about practice needs without specifying how those needs should be met. In this way, responding vendors have the latitude to propose innovative solutions that best fit the organization's goals and objectives. Among the sections to include are the following:

- rules of proposal preparation
- organization background and system overview

- application requirements
- transaction volumes and data retention
- general requirements and system features
- hardware requirements
- vendor questionnaire
  —vendor information
  —hardware and system software
  —application software
  —vendor cost summary
  —references

Recently, questions have been raised by groups and vendors alike about the necessity of the formal RFP process. Alternatives have been sought such as the "try before you buy" approach where prospective purchasers actually operate a test version of a system over a period of one or more weeks. This type of evaluation methodology can provide significant insight into the appropriateness of a particular system for the group, but it is impractical for evaluating several vendors at a time in a competitive bidding situation. Another drawback of this approach is that, without a detailed proposal, system performance guarantees will be difficult to obtain, thereby exposing the group to unnecessary risk.

Vendor Evaluation Techniques

Once the RFP has been issued and the responses have been received (typically in about three to four weeks), great care should be exercised in evaluating each proposal. Vendors are anxious to make a favorable impression and will often begin contacting group personnel even before the RFP is issued. They have polished presentations and marketing materials that are designed to highlight the strengths of their systems. Unless a methodical and comprehensive evaluation approach is used, the final decision may be unduly swayed by sales techniques rather than solid vendor credentials. At all times, the medical organization and not the vendors should control the process. If possible, a single contact person should be appointed to work with the vendors to schedule meetings, ask follow-up questions, and provide feedback. Throughout the selection study, each evaluator should not rely on memory but should write down objective observations regarding system strengths and weaknesses.

The first step in the evaluation process, defining evaluation criteria, should have been completed before the RFP is issued. These criteria would include the following:

- software
  - —competitive cost
  - —extensive standard features and reports
  - —comprehensive capture of required data
  - —ease of implementation and use
  - —availability of inquiry and referencing tools
  - —flexible software configuration options
  - —good system and user documentation
  - —high system integrity and auditability
  - —excellent stability and reliability
  - —ease of modification
  - —comprehensive maintenance and updates
- hardware
  - —high price:performance ratio (for proposed applications)
  - —availability and ease of implementation of future upgrades
  - —ease of installation and operation
  - —comprehensive system utilities
  - —minimal environment requirements
  - —availability of software applications and tools
  - —extensive networking and communications
- vendors
  - —broad product and industry knowledge
  - —experience with similar organizations
  - —long-term commitment to medical practice market
  - —strong financial performance
  - —contract flexibility
  - —high level of service and support
  - —continuous product improvement
  - —ability to meet required implementation schedules
  - —active user groups
  - —outstanding references

The next step is to assign a numerical rating to each vendor proposal. One way to do this is to assign points to each possible vendor response as defined in the RFP. For example, if the vendor indicates that a requested feature is already a standard part of its system, it would receive the maximum score of six points for that feature. If this feature could be provided only through a major software modification, a score of one point would be assigned. A percentage grade would then be calculated for each RFP section based on the total points received and the maximum possible. An overall grade would be assigned to each proposal based on a weighted total of all the sections. The section weightings would be determined by the group in advance based on perceived importance.

At this point, it may become obvious that one or two vendors should be eliminated from further consideration because their proposals do not adequately meet the organization's needs. The remaining vendors should be invited to demonstrate their systems to the evaluation committee. At the same time, reference calls should be made to known vendor clients (not necessarily limited to those that have been listed in the proposals). These reference calls should attempt to identify specific features that clients like or dislike about the systems rather than deal with generalities. Most references are happy to talk at length about their systems, but an interview guide or questionnaire prepared ahead of time can facilitate the gathering of information. Important information to obtain includes

- system configurations and volumes (for comparison)
- system response time and downtime statistics
- strengths and weaknesses of various applications
- custom software developed
- performance and responsiveness of vendor
  —training
  —implementation
  —maintenance and support
- any surprises encountered
- reasons why this vendor was chosen (would the vendor be chosen again?)
- other clients to contact
- important contract provisions
- additional considerations

The results of demonstrations and reference calls should help narrow the field to two or three finalists, and actual visits to the clients of these vendors should be made. The goals of the site visits are similar to the goals of making the reference calls, but the visits provide an opportunity to speak with more people and to validate system performance in a real workplace.

System Costs

Although each vendor should have included a detailed cost schedule in its proposal, some "hidden costs" may have been omitted such as sales tax, conversion costs, custom programming, cabling, site preparation, and shipping fees. Sometimes the proposed hardware configuration may be inadequate for future growth and the price of upgrades should be added to the proposed costs. A schedule should be prepared for each finalist vendor so that one-time and ongoing maintenance costs can be compared.

Potential Benefits

One of the most critical tasks in selecting a new system is identifying the potential benefits to be derived. Throughout the selection process, personnel will have increasingly greater expectations about the advantages of a new system. It is important, however, to document the benefits and establish accountability for achieving them.

A first step in assessing the future impact of a new system is to determine how current business operations will be changed. A new computer system should provide substantial improvements in cost, service, and revenue. However, the organization will not achieve the full potential of the new system if appropriate changes in the way it conducts and tracks its business are not made. Existing procedures have evolved around the current systems. "Reengineering" is necessary to take advantage of new features and capabilities and to eliminate unnecessary activities. This process involves looking at every critical function that is currently performed and asking if and how it could be done better using the new system. Improvements resulting from reengineering should then be combined with other tangible and intangible benefits to justify the increased costs of the new system.

Since the success of the new system depends on the cooperation of the MIS department, the users, and the vendor, it is imperative that they all be involved in projecting measurable system benefits. They can then be responsible for achieving the benefits once the system is implemented. This procedure also ensures that estimates are reasonable and conservative.

The potential benefits of a system suitable for a group practice include the following:

* financial benefits
  —accelerated collection of outstanding receivables
  —reduced write-off of bad debt
  —increased collection of patient copayments
  —improved cash management
  —better tracking of insurance billings
  —reduced supply and postage costs

- —lower staff costs
- —reduced space requirements
- administrative benefits
  - —improved staff and physician productivity
  - —reduced errors
  - —enhanced employee morale
  - —reduced staff turnover
- patient care benefits
  - —increased availability of patient chart information
  - —reduced waiting times
  - —greater scheduling flexibility and coordination
  - —increased availability of physician reference information
  - —better quality measurement and control information
  - —streamlined patient flow
  - —reduced exposure to professional liability lawsuits
- management reporting benefits
  - —expanded collection of patient and service information
  - —increased availability of practice analysis data
  - —enhanced ad hoc reporting tools
- public relations benefits
  - —improved public perception
  - —stronger contracting position
  - —better patient communications

To calculate projected benefits, first determine a unit of measurement (e.g., patient visits or prepaid enrollment might be used to measure physician productivity). Next, determine the current baseline standard. Then make assumptions for improvements based on user and vendor estimates, observations from other groups, and live simulations. Applying the estimated improvement factors to the current baseline should indicate the actual benefit expected. Benefit dollar estimates may then be calculated using estimated unit costs such as cost per visit. As indicated in Figure 34-5, timing of benefits should also be considered, since there is approximately a one-year time lag between new system expenditures and realized benefits.

Making the Final Decision

Upon completion of the analysis, the last step of the evaluation is to select the preferred vendor. After the summary comparison of the finalist vendors is

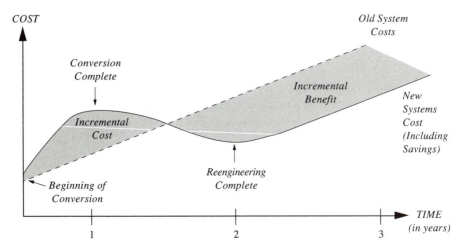

Figure 34-5 Realization of Benefits

---

reviewed, a selection team meeting should be held to agree on the most appropriate vendor. If a disagreement occurs, the cause is usually a difference of opinion regarding the organization's needs or a vendor's qualifications. To resolve disagreements, tangible examples should be presented during the decision meeting. If a consensus still cannot be achieved, then one of the following actions should be taken: additional research should be conducted, it should be agreed that the majority opinion will prevail, or it should be agreed that senior management will cast the deciding vote. Whatever the decision, however, all must be committed to its successful implementation.

NEGOTIATING A PURCHASE CONTRACT

There are many approaches and strategies that can be used to achieve favorable contracts. Since there are many books published on the art of negotiation, this section focuses on the terms and conditions of the contract itself. The organization should keep in mind that for large system purchases all terms are negotiable and most vendor contracts are written to protect the vendor. At the same time, signing a purchase agreement is the first step in forming a partnership that could have a great impact on the purchaser's ability to compete in the health care marketplace. Since the contract is so critical, it is wise to begin negotiations before a final vendor is selected. In this way, items such as price discounts and performance guarantees can be considered in choosing a preferred vendor.

The following are some of the terms and conditions that could be negotiated as part of the contract:

- price discounts
- system response time guarantees
- acceptance testing provisions before and after installation
- payment terms tied to major deliverables and completion of testing
- RFP response guarantees
- specified maintenance, support, and training levels
- specified problem resolution procedure
- lock-in of future hardware, software, and service discounts
- guaranteed compatibility with existing systems
- custom software and interface development
- royalties for major development projects
- limited price increases for maintenance and other items
- expanded license to include potential business ventures
- provision of source code

In conducting negotiations, the first step is to review the vendor's standard contract thoroughly and identify all of the issues to be discussed. Then the buyer's position and priority rating (high, medium, or low) should be determined for each issue. These priorities should then serve to guide the negotiating team.

MAKING IT WORK

Choosing the right system is a significant accomplishment. However, how that system is implemented can greatly affect its success or failure. Management should take primary responsibility for the success of the project while working in conjunction with staff and the vendor. As with the previous phases of the selection project, a comprehensive implementation plan, with a project organization structure that involves management, the MIS department, and users, should be developed. The areas to be addressed include

- project administration
- site preparation and cabling
- hardware installation
- software installation

- application support file development
- acceptance testing
- system conversion
- custom software development
- organization reengineering and procedure revision
- training
- post-implementation review

As previously mentioned, one of the primary goals of the implementation is realization of projected benefits. That is why a significant amount of attention should be paid to reengineering and redesigning the current organizational structure and procedures to take full advantage of new system features and capabilities. During subsequent post-implementation reviews, actual benefits should be compared to those projected, and any variances should be explained and corrected if necessary.

CONCLUSION

In the current health care environment, medical group administrators are finding that risk, when appropriately managed, can yield significant returns. Similarly, purchasing a computer system has many risks that, if managed, can also yield substantial benefits to the group. Therefore, the first goal in choosing a system is to minimize the risks by obtaining management, physician, and user participation and commitment; determining expectations in advance; employing a thorough selection approach; and negotiating a solid purchase contract. The second goal is to maximize the benefits of the system by determining specific, reasonable, and measurable improvement targets; establishing user and vendor accountability; and following an implementation approach that takes advantage of the new system capabilities. The achievement of these goals should help the ambulatory medical organization to meet the challenges it faces today and will face in the future.

35

Facilities Design

Robert Hanna and Susan Andrea Ritchie

INTRODUCTION

Outpatient medical facilities were historically located and designed more for the convenience of physicians than for the convenience of their patients. A physician would find a town or city where he or she wished to reside or where medical services were in demand and there established an office practice. Most often the practice location was a part of, or at least in close proximity to, the physician's home. Hospitals were not a consideration in locating the office. House calls were invoked for patients too sick or injured to travel to the physician's office. In many parts of the United States, the office is still located in the physician's home, even though house calls are rarely made. Before dismissing the home office as completely anachronistic, note that it does have the one major advantage of giving patients much greater access to a personal physician both night and day, a degree of access lacking in the large medical office complex or hospital emergency room of today.

Individual physicians as well as smaller group practices are now more likely to be found in specially designed medical office buildings. These medical office buildings are usually independent, but increasingly they are part of a hospital–medical office complex. Since this book is primarily concerned with the large outpatient group practice, this chapter discusses the suitability of locations and facilities from the provider viewpoint as well as from the patient viewpoint.

LOCATION

The location of a group practice should be determined by four different considerations:

1. accessibility
2. visibility

3. image

4. expandability

Accessibility

Parking

In many parts of the country today, particularly in large cities and their suburbs, parking is perhaps the major determinant of medical office location. Ideally, parking should be easily available, provide convenient access to the physician's office, and be free of charge. Close-to-the-entrance handicapped parking is a necessary patient convenience. Because of patient turnover, delays in seeing patients, and the labor-intensive nature of medical practice, an outpatient facility requires more parking than, for example, an accounting or architectural office. In many municipalities, this increased need for parking is built into the local ordinances, which might mandate five or even six spaces for each thousand square feet of medical office space leased or owned. Since these onerous requirements exist, many otherwise suitable locations become unacceptable such as modern industrial parks, independent nonmedical office buildings, and many shopping centers.

Because of parking constraints, many medical groups opt for renting space in a new building built for their purposes and to their specifications. Another solution is to rent in an office or light-industry complex during its early formation. At that time the vacancy factor might still be high, and the landlord might therefore be more willing to provide adequate parking for a medical tenant at the expense of future tenants whose parking needs may not be as great. Parking structures, paid parking, and street parking are generally considered burdensome to customers and are best avoided whenever possible.

Having employees park offsite is still another strategy for escaping onsite parking restrictions. However, this is not usually in the best interests of employee relations and often incurs increased potential liability for the safety of employees and their vehicles. Employees should of course park away from the more convenient parking areas, saving these for patients. The same is true, in most cases, for physicians. Given the dominance of outpatient medical care, it is no longer the case that every physician needs an automobile immediately available for hospital trips or house calls. It is probably not good patient relations to make an elderly patient on crutches walk 50 yards and then cross through a designated physician parking area. Many group practices simply assign a few close slots and label them "Call Physician," "Emergency Physician," or "Courier." Finally, a patient-sensitive parking layout should include easy automobile access to the office entrance, with convenient patient dropoff and pickup points in addition to adequate, well-located handicapped parking.

Demographics

Assuming that the patient parking issue can be satisfactorily resolved and there are still choices available, the demographics of the group's patient population may be used to help determine which office site is preferable. A survey of addresses of existing patients will quickly uncover the location that is most convenient for this group. However, if the practice is intent on developing a prepaid managed care practice, demographic information obtained from HMOs active in the area could be very useful, since it might reveal a preponderance of potential patients in an alternative area. Similarly, if the practice's marketing strategy is to market to areas where there is above-average population growth, demographic information can be used to find these areas. The demographic analysis of populations has become very sophisticated, is readily available (usually at low cost), and should be utilized whenever possible in finding suitable locations for facilities.

Convenience

In addition to handy parking, other convenience factors include proximity to the patients' homes or places of work and proximity to the physicians' primary hospitals. Marketing studies have demonstrated that in most communities patients offer no resistance to traveling five miles to see a physician and little resistance to traveling up to ten miles. Families, of course, would generally prefer the office to be located near home, whereas single younger patients might prefer a location near work. People are more willing to travel a greater distance for tertiary or subspecialist care than for primary care, which is needed far more frequently. Thus, the makeup of the particular practice is still another consideration to take into account.

All of these factors need to be carefully noted and prioritized when considering alternative practice locations. Again, since outpatient care is becoming increasingly dominant and outpatient surgicenters, imaging centers, and the like are becoming increasingly prevalent, the nearness of the medical office to hospitals is now less important in determining location. Many groups involved in prepaid medicine contract with several different hospitals or change hospital affiliations for financial or quality reasons. But proximity to hospitals still may warrant consideration if the practice encompasses strong hospital-department specialties such as obstetrics or cardiovascular surgery.

Visibility

In a competitive situation, visibility of the facility may be an important factor. The location listed in a brochure from an HMO or other managed care organization becomes more meaningful if the patients can relate to the address mentioned. Similarly, when new clients are on their way to the facility for the first time, perhaps with an ill family member in the vehicle, they will be grateful if they can immediately locate the proper approach and entrance. A main thoroughfare is preferable to an obscure side street. Well-located traffic signals expedite entrance and egress. A stand-alone facility is simpler to identify than an office buried in a large building, sequestered deep in an office complex, or hidden in a long strip of shopping center storefronts.

Signage is an important element of office design as well as a tool for increasing visibility. Adequate signage should never be taken for granted but should be researched prior to the signing of leases or purchase agreements. Again, municipalities differ greatly with regard to sign ordinances, as do building developers, so it is absolutely essential to have signage fully described in all medical office leases, including the size and placement of signs. And of course signage within the office complex is equally important for patient access and convenience. Interior signs should be simple to follow, be coordinated, and have lettering that makes it easy for the elderly to read them.

Many physicians assume that medical practices have considerable leverage in obtaining variances from local governments in areas such as signage, parking, building height, and so on. They reason that, since the provision of medical care is such a vital function for any community, politicians will bend to their wishes and developers will be desirous of having them as tenants. In most cases this is an erroneous assumption. The fact is that medical practices do not generate sales tax revenues, they overutilize parking, and they add to downtown congestion. Most municipalities would much rather see the inauguration of a new automobile dealership or sporting goods store than a large medical office. To overcome this negative bias, it is necessary for medical practices to carefully develop good relationships with local politicians, exercise humility in seeking their input, and actively involve them in the planning process.

Image

The image projected to patients is another important consideration in office location. Since quality of care is an important patient concern, the office and its setting must try to convey the appropriate message. Clean lines, lack of clutter, and simple, crisp signage are generally associated with quality in the eyes of patients. Again, a stand-alone facility at some distance from the nearest fast-food or dry-cleaning establishment and with pleasantly landscaped parking is probably ideal. But a positive image is not inconsistent with a location in a new and modern general office complex or industrial park, especially if there is proper signage. Shopping centers can also be suitable if the landscaping is attractive and there are complementary quality shops and restaurants and an illusion of space.

Expandability

One common denominator of progressive group practices, especially those developing expertise in managed care, is growth. For this reason, when seeking location, room for expansion is a vital consideration. If leasing is being considered, there should be provisions put in the lease that give the practice right of first refusal of adjacent space as it becomes available. In some cases, expansion of the building and addition of a parking building are also possibilities. Somehow, in every lease, the issue of the availability of more space should be addressed. It is obviously far better to explore this issue at the beginning of the lease relationship than at the end of the lease period. Again, to allow more maneuverability for expansion, leases should generally be kept to five years or less, with subsequent options, unless the organization is assured that future expansion can be accommodated.

It should be apparent after examining all the factors to be considered in selecting an appropriate office location that the ideal site is seldom found. Office location is therefore usually a compromise. Each practice must develop a strategic plan, organize its priorities, and evaluate its politics prior to the important decision of where to locate.

FUNCTIONAL PLANNING

For the purpose of functional planning, a group practice must define the population it intends to serve. This will dictate which services should be provided and what sort of internal layout will be necessary for the office. A practice with a large percentage of older patients, for example, might require more space for internal medicine, orthopedics, and ophthalmology. Younger populations are heavy users of family practice, obstetric, and pediatric departments, and hence space would be needed for mothers to park strollers and for a children's play area. A prepaid or managed care practice may require extra areas for radiology and laboratory services so as to keep these in-house rather than referring patients to outside fee-for-service providers.

Patient traffic through the office is a prime consideration, since an inefficient flow will severely hamper the ability to complete patient visits quickly. If the practice is located in a multistoried building, the elevator might be the nucleus of the office and might determine how it functions. Corridors must be wide enough to allow free access and mobility of patients in wheelchairs; handicapped persons do not want to be viewed as burdens or obstructions. Although there may be wheelchairs in the corridors, there also must be sufficient space for patients and staff to move freely. The width and length of hallways are usually addressed in local building and fire codes, which vary from city to city. Therefore, space planners and architects need to be familiar with local regulations. Functional planning is a very complex and intricate process, and even experienced administrators would do well to consult professional office planning experts.

BUILDING DESIGN

Each outpatient practice facility includes three basic types of space: public space, medical space, and administrative space. The relationship of these spaces varies considerably depending on the practice style. Many fee-for-service groups do little more than share being on call. They may have no centralized services other than possibly laboratory or radiology services. Each individual practitioner would have his or her own reception area, exam rooms, and patient medical records. As physicians in a group interact more with each other, the degree of centralization and sharing of administrative services increases. In the more sophisticated, larger group practices, even physician offices might be shared, with specific exam rooms designated to individuals on a daily basis. This section deals with the requirements of group practices with some degree of centralization.

Public Space

Public space comprises reception areas and corridors as well as entrances and exits. Ideally there should be two entrances: one for patients and one for physicians and staff. This enables physicians to enter and leave without meeting patients in the waiting room and allows staff to take their required breaks. Similarly, physicians and staff generally prefer not to share toilet facilities with patients, so public space can be subdivided into patient space and staff space.

A nationwide mandatory code requires medical facilities to be designed to accommodate the handicapped, thereby making it necessary to create entrances and passages that are easily identifiable and free of barriers. If the facility is on an upper floor, at least one elevator must be roomy enough for a gurney. Codes may also require staff areas and patient facilities to be suitable for the handicapped.

The reception room is where patients get their first impression of the practice. This room should be comfortable and cheerful, with appealing colors, soft lighting adequate for reading, and attractive furnishings. Its size can be determined by the patient population and the physicians' work habits. The greater the volume of patients seen daily, the larger this area will need to be. The dimensions of the room should ideally accommodate the number of patients scheduled in an hour, with space for one accompanying friend or relative. Again, sufficient space must be allocated for handicapped patients.

In designing the reception room, it is important to ensure easy access to the reception desk. The patient should be able to enter the room and proceed to the reception desk without difficulty. The reception desk should be arranged so as to allow staff members to cover for each other during breaks and absences. A centralized and efficient layout will reduce the number of staff required and considerably lower overhead costs. Since the reception staff usually maintain the appointment bookings, they must be able to see each patient upon arrival and before leaving. They need to have a good view of the reception room so that they can keep patients informed about waiting time. Many studies indicate that waiting is a major frustration for patients. It is very important that, if a doctor is behind schedule, the receptionist staff be able to regularly inform patients how long they might have to wait. Finally, patients in the reception area should of course have ready access to restrooms and drinking water.

Medical Space

Laboratory

Both the laboratory and the radiology unit (assuming laboratory and radiology services are provided in-house) may be made more efficient if they contain their own small reception and waiting areas. Specific counter and equipment requirements for the working laboratory are dependent on the type and number of procedures to be performed. In other words, the design of the laboratory must take into account the needs of the patient population.

One common laboratory shortcoming is a shortage of electrical outlets. This shortcoming can be even more damaging if the time comes for expansion.

The laboratory must provide space for two functions: specimen collection and laboratory analysis. A draw chair and table, work counters 30 to 36 inches in height, knee space for seated technicians, and a refrigerator for storage and possible freezing of specimens should generally be provided for when designing the laboratory.

Radiology

In planning the radiology area, consideration must be given to the weight and size of the equipment. For example, the upper stories of a multistory facility may not structurally accommodate heavy equipment. A 10-by-12-foot room is usually adequate for most x-ray machines, although enhancements such as mammography or ultrasound equipment may require additional space. Usually the ceiling needs to be at least 9 feet high. The area should also contain a place for patients to dress (ideally a 3-by-4-foot alcove with doors for privacy), a control area for the technician, and a room for film-processing equipment. Although radiology equipment can be broken down into components, it is advisable to provide at least a 3-foot-wide door in this room for ease in moving the equipment. The patient dressing area should contain a safe place to store or lock up patient valuables, and there should be carpeting so that patients do not have to walk barefoot on a cold floor to the radiology room.

The radiology room itself generally does not need a sink or prep area, although a nearby restroom would be beneficial for certain fluoroscopy procedures. Two or more walls of the x-ray room, depending on the location, must be shielded to protect passers-by from radiation scatter. Data from the radiation physicist's report will inform the designer about which walls must be shielded, the thickness of the shielding, and the height of the shielding panels. Commonly the door to the room must also be shielded. Such doors often become very heavy and must have a heavy-duty closer. The control partition, if located within the room, must also be shielded. It is possible to install prefabricated control partitions with glass viewing panels, which are available from various suppliers. If the control area is located outside the x-ray room, there must be a protected glass window to enable the operator to observe the patient at all times. This control area normally occupies a space 3 feet by 3 feet.

There are considerable variations in the size of radiology equipment, power requirements, and other specifications. Therefore, it is essential to obtain and coordinate all equipment data before proceeding with the work. A shielded cassette pass box used for transferring exposed and unexposed film back and forth between rooms should be placed in the wall between the darkroom and the radiology room. A centralized film storage area with heavy-duty shelving will be needed as well.

The manufacturers' literature will specify utility requirements and critical distances between equipment. Sometimes additional structural supports are needed in the ceiling to support the weight of the x-ray tube stand. In the case of a new installation, the equipment distributor will assist the consultant in designing the room and locating the equipment in the room. Decisions regarding the room configuration and the equipment to purchase will depend upon the expected type and size of the patient population and the expected growth.

General Medical Space

Good traffic flow is essential to the efficiency of a medical office. Nurses are usually responsible for controlling patient traffic to and from the exam rooms, so the nurses station and exam rooms might best relate to each other as parts of a module. Such a module should also include a physician's office.

The primary functional consideration regarding exam rooms is size. An exam room of 8-by-10 feet is probably large enough to comfortably allow a full-size exam table, a built-in sink cabinet with optimal storage above, a stool on casters for the physician, a guest chair for the patient, a treatment stand, and perhaps a small piece of portable medical equipment. If space permits, a dressing area for patients is a nice touch. This area, partitioned by a curtain, needs to be no larger than 3-by-3 feet, which is enough space to contain a chair, clothes hooks, hangers, a mirror, and perhaps a shelf for hand-carried items.

A second functional consideration is the position of the examining table. The standard table is 27 inches wide by 54 inches long, with stirrups at the foot if it is to be used for pelvic or urologic examinations. The table also has a pullout footboard that extends the length of the table to about 6 feet. The foot or stirrup end of the table should be angled away from the door as well as away from the wall so that the doctor has access to all sides of the patient and so that the patient is out of view of passers-by in the corridor if the door happens to be opened during the exam. If the handicapped code allows, the exam room door should be hinged so that it opens away from the wall. Although this might seem awkward, it is helpful in an exam room because it shields the patient from the corridor if the door is opened during an examination and it gives the patient added privacy while dressing.

Whatever the final design of the exam rooms, the key to creating a productive and efficient medical office area is the relationship between the exam rooms, the nurses station, and the support areas. Time spent by staff traveling between telephones, the nurses station, and the exam rooms can be greatly decreased if this relationship is a good one. The nurses station is where the staff perform a variety of tasks such as weighing patients, taking temperature, communicating via the telephone, and handling paperwork. The size of the station depends on the number of aides who will use it, the type of medical practice, and the functions to be performed by the aides. The number of aides can be estimated on the basis of each physician's practice requirements. A patient restroom adjacent to the exam rooms and nurses station facilitates examinations and the handling of urine specimens.

A family practice suite might function best with a large nurses station. Since a wide variety of medical procedures are performed, from minor surgery to casting fractures, it would be impractical to store adequate supplies and equipment in each exam room. Therefore, the nurse must prepare the exam room with any special supplies, injections, dressings, and instruments that are anticipated for a particular visit. Many of these items can be stored at the central nurses station, where there might even be an autoclave for sterilization of instruments as well as equipment for performing certain laboratory procedures.

For a pediatric suite, it might be desirable to have both a well-child waiting room and a sick-child waiting room. If space is limited, sick children could be handled by having an entrance to the suite near an exam room. The entrance might have a buzzer or bell for summoning a nurse to let in a sick child, who could then be ushered into the adjacent exam room immediately.

A special procedure or multipurpose room is often benefical to have. It should be larger than an exam room (13-by-13 or 18-by-13 feet, depending upon need), with enough space for storage of surgical supplies, dressings, and special equipment. An electrical floor outlet should be located at the exam table for minor surgery equipment and endoscopy. This room could also serve as a casting room if a plaster trap is provided for the sink. Extensive counter space and a sink are essential, and an autoclave may be desirable. The lighting must be considered early in the planning stage, including whether it should be portable or installed overhead. The number of procedure rooms required again depends upon the specific needs of the particular medical practice.

Administrative Space

Administrative space comprises the accommodations for the business office manager, medical records staff, and other centralized administrative staff. It should be versatile and flexible, whether modular in design or with a specially devised area for each activity. Either way, the plans should include the possibility of future growth.

The business office is the financial heart of the outpatient facility and is responsible for such critical functions as patient billing, credit and collections, accounting, and insurance. Today, virtually all medical offices are computerized and have sophisticated software applications that handle appointment scheduling, patient billing, insurance billing, accounting, collection letters, statements, insurance claim tracking, and operational data. If an integrated software system is to be employed, it is critical that it be properly planned, with appropriate allowance for space for both equipment and operators. In a prepaid practice, administrative space should be augmented to provide room for activities such as checking eligibility, processing claims, and coordinating benefits. A modern and progressive group practice requires administrative space for human resource functions, staff training, utilization review, and quality assurance as well as at least one meeting room.

The convenient storage of medical records is also highly important. In order to provide continuity of care for patients, accurate records must be maintained where they are easy to retrieve. It is important in the planning stage to project the future needs for medical chart storage. The design must include provision for the number of new patients expected to be added to the practice each month.

That number should be projected forward for five years (the length of most leases) and added to the existing number of charts. Medical records should be located where they can be accessed easily by the receptionists, nurses, and business office staff.

To ensure confidentiality, many management staff members need private offices. These offices should be accessible to physicians as well as patients. Also located in the central administration space should be an area for the PBX operator. Most advantageous would be a small, quiet room designed for comfort and located away from public view.

Storage

In a modern medical office, efficiency depends on the existence of adequate storage space. Storage areas should be at least 6 feet square, with two or more walls having adjustable shelving for office supplies, medical supplies, and housekeeping items such as cartons of toilet paper, paper towels, and tissue. Ideally, one storage area should be provided for each medical office or module. Larger practices generally require offsite storage and warehouse facilities as well.

Heating, Ventilation, and Air Conditioning

The heating, ventilation, and air conditioning (HVAC) requirements of medical offices are specialized, in that they involve the physical comfort of patients and staff. For example, patients, sometimes clad in only a gown, usually spend more time in exam rooms than staff or physicians, so warmth is a priority. The central reception room, on the other hand, is made to accommodate many people, which adds to the air conditioning load. A nurses station or office, where fully clothed staff move about, has still different temperature requirements.

Various factors must be considered in designing a functional HVAC system, including

- lighting load
- room occupancy
- equipment load
- comfort level based on room functions
- outside heat load from windows, roof, etc.

It is recommended that a competent HVAC consultant and contractor be utilized to ensure the system is adequately designed and installed.

Plumbing

A medical office building demands a greater amount of plumbing than a standard office building. Each exam room and each procedure room should be equipped with a sink for handwashing, and each nurses station needs facilities for handwashing and equipment cleaning. There should be restrooms for patients and staff, with facilities for the handicapped. If the office has a lab and radiology unit, a restroom must be provided in this area. Radiology will also need pipes going to the film processor and a floor sink for draining the processor. The darkroom should have a sink large enough to wash the rollers when the processor is being serviced. Given these heavy requirements, plumbing represents a major portion of the building cost. It also may impair a landlord's ability to rent the building to other tenants after the expiration of the lease.

Electrical

In blueprinting any office, the electrical specifications must also be well thought out. This is especially true for the medical office. Adequate outlets must be provided in exam and procedure rooms. In addition to standard outlets, service must be furnished for autoclaves, exam lights, and other specialty items.

The laboratory and radiology departments have specific electrical needs. Equipment suppliers should furnish the conditions and wire schematics for each device. It is advisable to employ a competent electrical engineer so that proper circuits and proper panels are supplied. The engineer may specify isolated circuits for monitoring equipment and dedicated circuits for radiology. If a computer is used, an uninterrupted power supply is helpful so that programs are not lost in the event of a power failure. It is convenient to provide ample wiring for telephone and computer lines during the installation of electrical conduit. This wiring must be separate from the electrical conduit, but it can be positioned adjacent to it to conserve cost.

Other Concerns

One need that is commonly overlooked is space for refuse. To avoid the possibility of objectionable odors that could enter the building, the waste area should be situated away from but adjacent to the building. Infectious waste must be handled in accordance with regulations, which vary from locality to locality. Unless the local code specifies otherwise, infectious waste should be kept in a locked container in a secure area until properly disposed of. A significant liability is involved in the storage and handling of infectious waste, making it imperative that it is disposed of properly.

Besides the foregoing functional considerations, various permits and licenses must be obtained before the occupancy of a new office can occur. The following is a partial list:

- business license
- elevator license
- fire department inspection
- utilities hook up
- refuse collection

Checklist

The following is a partial checklist of major items that the builder must include in the final plan. An astute administrator is well advised to double-check these items, since many contractors have limited experience with outpatient medical facilities.

Code Review

- Occupancy load
- Number of required exits; separation of exits
- Illuminated exit signs
- Radiation shielding
- Fire separations
- Handicapped bathrooms and other accessibility requirements
- Elevator

Partitions

- Sound control
- Extension of partitions above suspended ceiling
- Fiberglass batting (sound)
- Texture of finished wall (specify)
- Durable and cleanable finish for walls (specify)
- Special ceiling heights, if required

Doors

- Hollow versus solid core
- Pocket doors (not recommended due to higher cost and lower acoustic value)
- Door closers (heavy-duty)
- Hardware, keying of locks, key schedule
- Door finish (painted or stained, plastic laminate)
- Type of door frame (welded hollow metal or wood)
- Width and height of doors (specify)
- Carpet height—plus pad, if any (specify)

Plumbing

- Wrist or foot pedal control faucets
- Acid resistant waste pipes, as necessary for special conditions
- Sizes of sinks (specify)
- Vacuum breakers (darkrooms), as required by code
- Separate shut-offs for each fixture
- Floor drains in darkrooms, hot-water heater room, janitorial closets
- Toilet fixtures and accessories
- Handicapped toilet facilities

Communication Systems

- Telephones
- Intercom
- Signal lights for exam rooms, nurses stations, and physician offices
- Annunciator panel
- Music system (speakers)
- Location of telephone terminal panel (requires electrical outlet)
- Interior signage

Mechanical Systems

- Location of hot-water heater (if electric, requires outlet) and floor drain
- Exhaust fans (bathrooms, darkrooms, labs, cast rooms) for maximum quietness of operation

- Interior zone sizing and thermostat location
- Return air system design
- Acoustic criteria and sound insulation for exam room privacy
- Equipment location and accessibility for service
- Replacement filters

Casework

- Style of construction and types of drawer glides, hardware, and hinges (specify)
- Support blocking in walls (or ceiling) to carry x-ray view boxes, cassette pass boxes, x-ray equipment, special light fixtures, casework, and certain pieces of medical equipment (specify)

Lighting

- Lighting for special areas
- Exit and emergency lighting system
- Switching diagram
- Lamp wattages (specify)
- Color of grid (spine) for suspended acoustic ceiling (specify)
- Acoustic tile (specify)

Electrical

- Special outlets, 220-volt lines, and floor receptacles (specify)
- Height of outlets (specify)
- Outlets over countertops (should run horizontally and if near sink outlets must be G.F.I.)
- Location of main and remote circuit breaker panels
- Location of phones
- Layout for main telephone room and incoming service
- Electrical data for equipment and other systems to be installed (specify)

Building and Other Codes

Fire Protection Requirements

- Nonflammability of material
- Exiting requirements

- Emergency illumination
- Storage of gases
- Firefighting equipment
- Electrical systems
- Fire and smoke detection systems and alarms

Handicap Requirements

Federal and state codes mandate the handicap requirements regarding the following:

- Location of ramps, curb cuts, parking stalls
- Placement of exits
- Interior design configurations
- Dimensions of elevators and restrooms
- Door widths
- Placement of restroom fixtures and accessories

Construction Requirements

- Minimum sizes of rooms and various departments
- Location and number of windows
- Minimum ceiling heights
- Relationship of various rooms to one another
- Planning and programming decisions with regard to function
- Accommodation of equipment (spaces for gurneys, drinking fountains, public telephones)

Energy Conservation and Environmental Impact

State and local codes mandate energy conservation and regard for the ecological impact a proposed building will have on the environment. The code classifications may fall under the jurisdiction of city, county, state, or federal codes.

Codes Relating to Medical Facilities

Code requirements for medical offices are numerous and often confusing. The local building code will determine the type of construction for a particular medical facility.

Although state building codes vary, the following items are generally subject to regulations:

- Width of corridors
- Number of exits
- Handicapped bathrooms
- Separation of exits
- Length of dead-end corridors
- Ceiling heights
- Emergency and exit illumination
- Construction of partitions
- Fire separations
- Radiation shielding
- Fire detection devices or sprinkler system

Care should be taken during the planning and design stages to ensure compliance with all code requirements. A preliminary review with the local building department "plan checker" would be appropriate.

Required Exits

The number of exits is based on the proposed occupancy load or the number of people using the space. Approved exits must lead directly out, and doors may have to open in the direction of egress. Exits may not be through kitchens, storage rooms, or spaces used for similar purposes. All exits must be clearly marked and accessible in case of fire.

Separation of Exits

When more than one exit is required, each must be separated by a specified distance proportional to the size of the space in order to provide sufficient access to the outside if there is a fire.

Stairs and Doors

Stairwells with fire-resistive enclosures and self-closing fire doors are intended to function as smoke-free evacuation towers in case of fire. The stairs must be sufficiently wide to enable people on stretchers to be evacuated if necessary.

Fire Alarms and Extinguishing Devices

Sprinkler systems may be required in many facilities, particularly in laboratories, large storage areas, or hazardous areas that are often unoccupied. Smoke or heat detectors and alarms are advisable where sprinklers are not feasible or required.

Floor and Wall Coverings

After all is said and done, a clean-looking, attractive, color-coordinated facility has great appeal to patients. Certain color schemes are restful, others may be discomforting. Unless a staff member has demonstrated some degree of talent for interior decorating, hiring an expert consultant is to be recommended.

Index